HANDS HEAL:

Communication, Documentation, and Insurance Billing for Manual Therapists

SECOND EDITION

Hands Heal

Communication, Documentation, and Insurance Billing for Manual Therapists

SECOND EDITION

Diana L. Thompson, LMP

Licensed Massage Practitioner
Seattle, WA

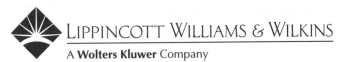
LIPPINCOTT WILLIAMS & WILKINS
A **Wolters Kluwer** Company
Philadelphia • Baltimore • New York • London
Buenos Aires • Hong Kong • Sydney • Tokyo

Editor: Peter Darcy
Managing Editor: Eric Branger
Marketing Manager: Christen DeMarco
Production Editor: Jennifer Ajello
Compositor: Maryland Composition
Printer: Data Reproductions Corp.

351 West Camden Street
Baltimore, Maryland 21201-2436 USA

227 East Washington Square
Philadelphia, PA 19106

Printed in the United States of America

Second Edition, 2001

Library of Congress Cataloging-in-Publication Data

The Library of Congress Cataloging-in-Publication data has been applied for.

The publishers have made every effort to trace the copyright holders for borrowed material. If they have inadvertently over-looked any, they will be pleased to make the necessary arrangements at the first opportunity.

To purchase additional copies of this book, call our customer service department at **(800) 638-3030** or fax orders to **(301) 824-7390**. International customers should call **(301) 714-2324**.

Visit Lippincott Williams & Wilkins on the Internet: http://www.LWW.com. Lippincott Williams & Wilkins customer service representatives are available from 8:30 am to 6:00 pm, EST.

05
4 5 6 7 8 9 10

Reviewers

Richard H. Adler, JD
Attorney at Law, Adler◆Giersch PS
Seattle, Washington

Lori L. Bielinski, LMP
Tacoma, Washington

Barbara Frye, LMP, GCFP
Author of *Body Mechanics for Manual Therapists: A Functional Approach to Self-Care and Injury Prevention*
Seattle, Washington

Terry Graham, PT
Private Practice, Physical Therapy
Seattle, Washington

Elliot Greene, MA, NCTMB
Silver Spring, Maryland

Elisabeth Sliney, LMT
Practitioner and Lecturer
Based in Akron, New York

Mary Sharon Long
Nationally & Maryland State Certified Massage Therapist
Private Practice, Massage Therapy
Catonsville, Maryland
SeniorTouch LLC, Owner
Massage Programs for the Elderly
Baltimore, Maryland

Foreword

The licensed massage practitioner has so much to offer the individual consumer and the health care community. More and more massage practitioners are realizing the importance of their work and creating greater awareness and momentum about the benefits of massage therapy.

Despite the gains that are being made with individual consumers, non-massage health care practitioners and insurers remain reluctant to embrace massage therapy as an integral part of modern health care. This reluctance stems from a list of issues, including lack of practice guidelines and standards of care, perceptions of professionalism, effective chart note documentation, and responsiveness to the communication needs of other healthcare professionals.

Seen in this light, Diana Thompson's book is a very timely and much-needed bridge to overcome these real and perceived obstacles surrounding practice guidelines, professionalism, treatment protocol, and documentation. Diana Thompson brings forth unending experiences in understanding patient needs, figuring out what is important to the referring doctor, and satisfying insurance companies in the paperwork process. She brings practical information to life by blending years of experience, stories, and humor that will undoubtedly make this book required reading for all massage students, as well as those practitioners wanting to work more closely with medical doctors, osteopaths, chiropractors, and physical therapists. It will also help practitioners have an easier time in dealing with insurance companies.

The value of this book is multi-dimensional for the massage practitioners and the massage profession. The practitioner will find practical, simple, and easy-to-use information and forms that comprehensively capture relevant information. Paperwork will become more efficient and effective. The profession benefits immensely because it raises the bar on expectations within and outside the massage profession concerning communication, documentation, and professionalism.

This book facilitates the mission of each licensed massage practitioner and massage therapy association seeking greater access for the consumer to obtain massage treatment and care, relief for illness, injury, and disease, as well as those wishing to obtain maximum health. Diana Thompson has made a very valuable contribution. It is now up to each licensed massage practitioner, massage therapy organization, and massage school to join her in advancing a most worthy cause.

Richard H. Adler
Attorney at Law, Editor

Preface

Background of Hands Heal *and Manual Therapy*

Hands Heal was conceived in the early 1990s. At that time, complementary and alternative medicine was receiving a lot of press and catching the attention of mainstream health care systems. Massage therapists, bodyworkers, movement therapists, and energy workers were receiving patient referrals from physicians, many for the first time. Increasingly, manual therapy services were being covered by insurance plans.

Not everyone in allopathic medicine greeted the complementary providers with open arms. Skepticism was widespread. Many questioned the validity of manual therapies. Insurance carriers demanded statistics and scientific studies proving that treatment was curative and not palliative. Few were found. Independent medical examinations were implemented early in personal injury cases, and health insurance utilization review boards audited practitioners, both in an attempt to deny or to limit the use of manual therapies.

In this atmosphere of litigation and peer reviews, charting focused on proving the legitimacy of the practitioners and their modalities. I wrote the first edition of *Hands Heal* to prepare massage therapists for the charting requirements of those skeptical times. My information was based on years of experience in the early stages of the integration of massage therapy into health care. My teachers were chiropractors, attorneys, and insurance adjusters. I was videotaped for depositions, gave testimony in court, submitted narratives to lawyers, and saw my charts reviewed by utilization management panels. On the up side, when my claims were denied, the decisions were reversed after I submitted convincing progress reports; I filed liens with county court houses and requested letters of guarantee from attorneys, and as a result, I received payment in full when everyone else was asked to cut bills in half. I wanted to share what I had learned.

Much has changed in a short time. Manual therapies are now considered a viable treatment option for many people and are a covered benefit in an increasing number of insurance plans across the US. As a result of this widespread integration of manual therapies into private health care benefit packages, charting requirements have also changed. The focus of documentation is shifting from legitimizing the practitioners and validating manual modalities to proving that the treatments improve patient outcomes and cost less than traditional treatments. The shift demands progress-oriented functional outcomes reporting, a style of charting recently adopted by physical therapists and other health care providers. Progress is apparent when the patient's quality of life improves. Quality of life is measured through functional outcomes—the patient's increased ability to participate in activities of daily life.

Current research supports the emphasis on functional outcomes. A randomized trial studying the effects of various alternative therapies in treating persistent low back pain was conducted at the Center for Health Studies in Washington State. Dan Cherkin, PhD, Senior Scientific Investigator, concluded that therapeutic massage is an effective treatment for persistent low back pain because massage significantly improved the patient's ability to function (for example, ability to walk up stairs and put on socks). There was not a statistically significant reduction in symptoms, though there was a correlation between massage and the reduction of medication (Cherkin D, Eisenberg D, Street J, et al. Randomized trial comparing traditional Chinese medical acupuncture, therapeutic massage, and self-care education for chronic low back pain. Arch Intern Med 2001;161).

As manual therapists, if we persist in trying to demonstrate patient progress through a reduction in symptoms, we are less able to provide our patients with encouraging results or prove the curative nature of our modalities. Rather, if we demonstrate patient progress through improved function, we will successfully validate manual modalities.

This shift in charting is exciting. Practitioners and patients alike enjoy the focus on improving function. Setting functional goals and charting functional outcomes engages patients in their healing, inviting them to participate in all levels of healing. Functional outcomes reporting fits into a SOAP format with few adjustments, and the second edition of *Hands Heal* makes the transition to functional outcomes reporting easy.

Changes in This Edition

In addition to the inclusion of functional outcomes, there are several significant changes to *Hands Heal*. First, I replaced *Massage Therapy* with *Manual Therapy* in the title. My intent is to include all hands-on healing arts. The term *manual therapy* embraces all forms of soft tissue, spinal, and bioenergetic manipulation, as well as postural re-education. Soft tissue manipulation is the primary technique of massage therapy, physical therapy, and the extensive array of bodywork specialties. Chiropractors and osteopaths practice spinal manipulation. Bioenergetic manipulation focuses on the energetic fields of the body (Reiki, therapeutic touch, Polarity, etc). Postural re-education specialists include Feldenkrais, Aston Patterning, and Alexander Technique, to name a few.

The second change evident in the title is the inclusion of communication and insurance billing with documentation. These topics are natural and necessary additions. Communication and the therapeutic relationship are integral to documentation; we have nothing to write if we are not engaged with our patients. Patients are involved in every level of healing, from providing information to choosing and implementing their care. Their involvement hinges on our relationship with them; if we are honest, respectful, and encouraging, they may trust us and open themselves to change. My intent throughout the second edition is to emphasize building productive relationships with those ultimately responsible for healing—the patient—and shift the focus away from our need to prove that we are legitimate health care providers. Skillful communication enables us to accomplish and document patient outcomes, the only proof we need.

Insurance billing is included at the persistent urging of my colleagues. At first it was overwhelming. Once I committed to the project, however, it became clear what was needed. Many texts on insurance billing specialize in the regulations of a particular state and provide information that is quickly outdated. This book provides tools that are universally applicable to the verification and reimbursement needs of personal injury, workers' compensation, and private health insurance billing across the US. It does not provide information detailing which insurance plans cover what modalities, nor does it instruct you on which CPT codes to use. State regulations vary, and plans differ in their inclusion of manual therapies. Rather, you learn from this book how to communicate with the individual carriers, verify each patient's benefits, accurately complete the billing forms, record payments, and resolve or appeal unpaid claims. This information is not time-sensitive because you learn the skills necessary to adapt to changing codes and procedures.

In addition, there are changes to the SOAP format. In the second edition, the SOAP format is no longer modified for massage therapists. Traditionally, the Assessment section records the practitioner's diagnosis of the patient's condition. Massage therapists do not have diagnostic scope. Therefore, I previously advocated using the Assessment section of the SOAP chart to record the changes in the patient data as a result of the massage. With the inclusion of functional outcomes reporting, the Assessment section is allocated to recording functional goals. As a result, massage therapists no longer need to modify the SOAP format to make use of all categories. Continue to omit the diagnosis from the Assessment section unless your scope of practice permits it. Record the results of your treatment in the Objective section of the SOAP chart, consistent with other professions. Use the Assessment section to record functional goals.

Also new to the second edition is an entire chapter devoted to charting wellness sessions. Manual therapy enhances wellness in addition to treating health conditions. Regardless of its intent, manual therapy is a health care service and therefore must be documented. However, extensive documentation using the SOAP format is not necessary in wellness care. In the second edition, I offer a new format called the HxTxC chart, appropriate for wellness care, sports venues, and spa environments.

Pedagogical and Text Features

A vast array of stories, exercises, and quotes are included to enhance learning. In keeping with the native southwestern designs used in the first edition, I have assigned the following symbols to identify the three categories listed above:

- Storyteller (stories): the storyteller, weaving tales of the ancient ones, invites you to learn from those who came before us.
- Bone Game (exercises): the dice, carved from the bones of animals, invite you to learn through play.
- Wise One Speaks (quotes): the wise, old owl, invites you to learn through the wisdom of others.

Throughout the book, there are words in bold type and phrases italicized. The bold-faced words make up the glossary. The italicized phrases represent what can be written on the SOAP charts.

As always, it is not my intent to offend anyone with my choice of words. Therefore, I wish to explain my terminology. My goal is to be inclusive and representative of the diversity within complementary health care professions. However, the words I choose may not be the terms you use in your practice. Please insert words appropriate to your profession and beliefs where you find it necessary to do so. For example, I refer to manual therapists as *practitioners* or *health care providers*; you may call yourselves *educators* or *therapists*. I use the term *patients*; you may prefer *clients* or *students*. I say *referring health care*

xii

HANDS HEAL:
COMMUNICATION,
DOCUMENTATION,
AND INSURANCE BILLING
FOR MANUAL THERAPISTS

provider instead of *primary care provider*, so as not to imply that physicians are the only acceptable primary care.

Finally, only three of the original paragraphs from the first edition of *Hands Heal* remain unchanged in this edition. You will find *Hands Heal: Communication, Documentation, and Insurance Billing for Manual Therapists* to be current, comprehensive, and critical to the integration of manual therapy into mainstream health care systems. It is my belief and intention that integration will positively influence the current health care environment.

Acknowledgments

To all of you who generously shared your stories, appreciation, and feedback at conventions and workshops, thank you for providing much of the material for the second edition.

Thank you Kerry Ann Plunkett, Eileen Stretch, ND, and Alternáre Health Network for the opportunity to embrace the needs of managed care documentation. You planted the seed for the second edition.

A special thanks to Lori Bielinski and Deborah Senn, the Washington State Insurance Commissioner, for your dedication to complementary medicine and for setting national precedence in complementary and alternative health care integration; and the law firm of Adler◆Giersch, PS, for your commitment and service to manual therapists. Without your work there would be little need for this book.

I offer my warmest respect and heartfelt thanks to the people who made this book possible: my guardian angels Richard Adler and Lisanne Yuricich who taught me what I know and gave me the opportunity to share it; my behind-the-scenes editor Alice Bloch, who makes words sing; the staff at LWW who raised the ante on professionalism and quality; and my reviewers whose brilliant insights shaped the final product. To Duane Hobbs, the designer of the new forms, Lori and Janelle Otterholt for assistance with the glossary, Coleen Rene for the energy charting consult, Barb for surfin' the net, and Terry for going over Chapter 6 just one more time. Thank you Sari Spieler and Clint Chandler for carrying a heavier portion of our workshop responsibilities while I was experiencing tunnel vision with this project. Annie Thoe, LMP, GCFP, and Anne Wardell, LAc, LMP, thanks for keeping my body healthy. I especially loved those sessions to unleash my mind and boost my creativity!

I am especially grateful to Richard—I cannot thank you enough for sharing your wisdom, Duane for clearing my plate so I could be still and have creative thoughts, and Jackie Espejo Phillips for removing fear from my vocabulary. Without your support emotionally and financially, this would not have been possible.

I dedicate this edition to my beautiful wife, Jackie, who patiently loves me during this personal growth experience called writing. You *espejo* my soul.

Contents

SECTION *A*

Communication

CHAPTER 1

Communication and the Therapeutic Relationship

*T*he Creator gathered all of creation and said, "I want to hide something from the humans until they are ready for it. It is the realization that they create their own reality."

The eagle said, "Give it to me, I will take it to the moon."

The Creator said, "No. One day they will go there and find it."

The salmon said, "I will hide it on the bottom of the ocean."

"No. They will go there, too."

The buffalo said, "I will bury it on the plains."

The Creator said, "They will cut into the skin of the earth and find it even there."

Then Grandmother Mole, who lives in the breast of Mother Earth, and has no physical eyes but sees with spiritual eyes, said, "Put it inside them."

And the Creator said, "It is done."

(A story from a Sioux friend told to Gary Zukav, author of *The Dancing Wu Li Masters* and *Seat of the Soul*, reprinted with permission, "In Search of the Soul," *Life Magazine*, 12-97.)

Let's change one word in this poignant story and pretend the Creator said, "It is the realization that they create their own *health*." The change does little to affect the message, yet this new twist proposes a powerful and significant concept for health care providers and patients to consider: individuals possess the ability to heal themselves. In reality, we exercise that ability every day, when we make simple choices about what to eat, or seek care when we need it, or survive against overwhelming odds. All of us possess a life force that is tenacious and enduring, undiminished until the moment of our death. That life force drives us toward health.[1]

Therefore, the patient may be the best person to involve in the healing process. The patient has all the data, takes all the risks, and implements much of the solution. When actively involved in their own healing, patients develop their self-confidence and sense of responsibility, as well as becoming less dependent on their caregivers.[2] Our role as health care practitioners must expand to include providing our patients with opportunities for self-discovery—illuminating and expanding their unique strengths and tapping into their internal wisdom—and empowering them to heal themselves.

Introduction

In the past, the interview was used only to gather information about a patient's symptoms and health history. The medical model demanded that the expert—the physician—collect data that would lead to an accurate assessment of the patient's condition. Once a diagnosis was assigned, the standard of care for the patient's disease was administered.[3]

Today, allopathic and alternative health experts alike recognize the flaws inherent in the traditional approach. First, human beings are individuals and respond uniquely to identical treatments. Second, a growing body of evidence indicates that emotions are responsible, at least in part, for disease. Some researchers believe that 90–95% of all patients who visit physicians have physical symptoms that are directly caused by emotions.[4]

Consequently, the central focus of the interview process has shifted from collecting data to building relationships. Health care providers from all disciplines embrace the patient-practitioner relationship as their primary asset. One purports that the relationship *is* the therapy.[5] Some claim that trust is imperative to patient satisfaction and compliance,[3, 6] others, that trust or lack of it affects the results of any care provided.[4] Cardiologist Herbert

Benson writes, "Belief or faith—whether it's deep in the mind or heart or focused on some outside object, like a physician—can play a key role in generating a response in the body."[4]

Trust is the key component to building meaningful relationships. Once the bond of trust is formed, patients will confide in us, provide insight into their conditions, and lead us to solutions that fit their lifestyles.[6] Trust is established when patients feel understood. Unless patients believe the practitioner really understands what they are trying to say, they are unlikely to believe the practitioner has their best interests at heart or can be of any use to them.[3] Dean Ornish, MD, in the book *Kitchen Table Wisdom*, puts it like this: *"Providing people with information—facts—is important but usually not sufficient to motivate them to make lasting changes in diet and lifestyle. If it were, no one would smoke. We need to work on a deeper level . . . to create a place safe enough for people to talk about what's really going on in their lives, to tell their stories, without fear of being judged, abandoned or criticized. Then, when people are really heard, are they likely to make lifestyle changes."* (Reprinted with permission, Remen, *Kitchen Table Wisdom: Stories that Heal*, Riverhead Books, New York, 1996.)

This chapter first presents the communication skills we need for building relationships with our patients and includes exercises for developing those skills. It then describes the goals of interviewing patients and recommends approaches for reaching those goals. These are two tremendously huge topics. Entire books have been written on both subjects: interpersonal communication skills and interviewing skills. The chapter introduces the subjects, but more importantly, I encourage you to explore these complex subjects further. Good communication skills are essential to the therapeutic relationship and good recordkeeping. Some of these skills sound simple but are much harder to effectively incorporate them than they appear. Practice by role playing with peers, perform the exercises in this book, attend workshops that will advance your communication skills, and read books devoted to the subject. Invest as much time and energy in mastering communication as you devote to advancing your manual techniques. A suggested reading list is provided. (See Figure 1-1)

1. *Kitchen Table Wisdom: Stories that Heal*, by Rachel Naomi Remen (Riverhead Books, New York, New York, 1996).
2. *Interviewing for Solutions*, by Peter DeJong and Insoo Kim Berg (Brooks/Cole, Pacific Grove, California, 1998).
3. *Messages: The Communications Skills Book, Second Edition*, by Patrick Fanning, Matthew McKay, and Martha Davis (New Harbinger Publications, Oakland, California, 1995).
4. *You and Me: The Skills of Communicating and Relating*, by Gerard Egan (Brooks/Cole, Monterey, California, 1977).
5. *ABC's of Effective Feedback: A Guide for Caring Professionals*, by Irwin Rubin and Thomas Cambell (Jossey-Bass Publishers, San Francisco, California, 1997).
6. *People Skills: How to Assert Yourself, Listen to Others, and Resolve Conflict*, by Robert Bolton (Simon & Schuster, New York, New York, 1979).

Figure 1-1. Resources for Communication Skills

Interpersonal Communication Skills

A successful relationship with patients requires a variety of communication skills, both verbal and nonverbal. When you develop and use these skills, you lead patients to discover and accomplish their goals for health. You can enhance patient cooperation and motivation not by overcoming patient resistance, but by offering practical feedback that invites patients to focus on their strengths instead of their pain. The interviewing skills introduced in this chapter will not only assist you in gathering information for your treatment plan, but will also help your patients to change their attitudes and summon the strength and wisdom to heal on a deeper level.

The following sections present detailed examples of various communication techniques that promote successful relationships with your patients.

BE PRESENT

No person can fully comprehend another, but with practice, guidance, and self-awareness you can learn to talk with a patient.[6] Talking can seem so simple, but it takes a great deal of skill to be present with someone, especially a person in need. Illness often makes a person feel vulnerable or weak, and thus anxious about taking risks and sharing personal information. It has been estimated that without realizing it, people inject communication barriers—such as becoming argumentative, beating around the bush, or withdrawing—into their conversations over 90% of the time when one or both parties have a problem to be dealt with or a need to be fulfilled.[2] A commitment to be present and available for your patients is the first step in manifesting trust and respect, the cornerstones for a productive relationship.

Being fully present for each patient is nearly impossible. We are easily distracted—by the last patient who has suffered an unjust tragedy, the afternoon lecture we are rehearsing nervously in our minds, or the menu for tonight's dinner. We habitually jump to conclusions by coming up with the quick fix for the minor solutions while the deeper concerns have yet to be uncovered, making value judgments based on a patient's appearance, or hearing a familiar situation in the patient's words and filtering the information through our own experience. Or we show up with a personal agenda—the drive to succeed, a desire to contribute, an eagerness to practice new techniques or try out new theories—and forget to honor our patients' role in their own health. We are human. These distractions are normal. What is important is your commitment to being present. Notice when you are distracted and bring your attention back to the person in front of you.

We need to do more than feign interest in our patients' stories. If we offer anything less than our authentic self, our patients will see right through us. Robert Bolton, PhD, in his classic book *People Skills*, rates genuineness as the number-one quality of communication, and defines it as being open and honest, present and authentic. The keys to being genuine, as defined by Bolton, are self-awareness, self-acceptance, and self-expression. By cultivating these personal attributes, we will develop the skills necessary for being present and authentic with our patients.[2] Below are some concrete tools and practical exercises for developing our personal presence.

Self-Awareness

In today's fast-paced world, there is little time to sit still. We keep ourselves so busy that we often seek out experts to tell us who we are and what our purpose is in life. Self-help seminars and how-to books are numerous. We don't have time to explore our own ideas or to wait until the answer to our question presents itself. The quick-fix attitude is everywhere.

On the other hand, self-awareness is not just something found on a mountain top or after years of meditation practice. It really can be found inside you—with a little practice. A simple way to develop your self-awareness is by listening to your inner voice.[2] If we are to trust in our patients' internal wisdom, we must learn to recognize our own. We must first acknowledge that we have a sense of inner direction, or intuition, and that we can trust it.[7] Trust in our intuition is strengthened with practice. Make the time to listen to yourself. We regularly tune out our internal voices, or ignore them when they do surface, by overworking, watching TV, or engaging in our habits: eating, drinking, exercise, and so on.[2] Instead, get to know yourself by spending a small amount of time each day being silent. With practice, you will begin to hear the voices inside you and distinguish where they come from. Some may be the voice of your mother, others of past experience, but the voice that softens your belly when it speaks is the voice of your intuition. Your "gut instinct" is literally just that. In Chinese medicine, it is believed that the stomach is the original brain.

Practice using your intuition by placing your hand on your belly during your silent time and asking yourself yes or no questions. If your belly tightens, the answer is no; if it softens, the answer is yes.

▼

BONE GAME 1-1

Separate Self from Patients

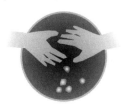

Take five minutes between patient sessions to breathe, stay silent, and be with yourself. It may be helpful to sit in a quiet, dark room with no distractions. During this time, mentally separate from your last patient. You may need to run through the events of the last session and experience the feelings you may have chosen not to express in front of the patient. A medical intuitive told me that to separate from the previous patient, she says, either silently or aloud, "I separate myself entirely—mentally, physically, spiritually, and emotionally—from Darnel. I call back all my energy, and I send him back all his energy."

When you have completed a session, check how you feel. Often the lines blur between our patients' thoughts and feelings and our own. Be clear about who you are, separate from those you interact with throughout the day. Verify your feelings about the day, your work, and your health. Take a few deep breaths and feel the air move into your body. Notice how your body moves to accommodate the air as you breathe in and out. Imagine that the air moving through you is a life force, a warm light pushing life into every nook and cranny of your body. Experience your physical self and your emotional self.

Finally, prepare for the next patient by inviting your internal wisdom to surface during the session. The Upledger Institute, in the CranioSacral Therapy seminars, refers to internal wisdom or inner voices as your "inner physician." You may have other ways of referring to your intuition, in accordance with your belief system. If there is something you need help with, ask for specific guidance. Maybe you want the strength to refrain from judging Sara when she doesn't do her homework exercises, or the confidence to listen to your intuition when you see Clint tense up when he reports he is fine. Affirm your self-awareness skills by saying, "I am whole and separate from

Sara. I practice with skill and provide care that honors Sara as a whole and separate human being. It is my heartfelt intent to be present with Sara, to offer her my understanding and compassion, and to facilitate her healing by tapping into her strength and internal wisdom."

Self-Acceptance

Self-acceptance is about recognizing all aspects of your character, embracing your humanness, and trusting that you are enough. Self-acceptance is not synonymous with self-approval. It is not about ego. It does not mean we have to feel good about our behavior when we are hurtful. Self-acceptance begins by simply recognizing that we all contain parts we may consider negative or frightening. When we do not accept the full range of our feelings and thoughts, we often ignore our inner voice.[2] Fear and denial prevent us from understanding and relating to our intuition. It is impossible to separate the good from bad, to love one and hate the other. Rachel Naomi Remen, MD, attended a seminar of Carl Rogers and reported him saying, "I realize there's something I do before I start a session. I let myself know that I am enough. Not perfect. Perfect wouldn't be enough. But that I am human, and that is enough."[7] When we begin to accept ourselves as being enough, we are able to be present for others.

An essential part of the individual healing process has to do with going within, into the shadow aspects—the aspects that, out of fear, we have denied, disowned, or suppressed. Shakti Gawain, in the book *Healers on Healing*, writes that the reason thoughts or feelings take a negative turn is because we do not accept them or allow them their natural expression. Suppressed anger, for example, may manifest later as violence toward others or toward ourselves in the form of illness.[7] If we can accept the good and the bad in ourselves, we are better able to accept the positive and negative aspects of our patients. Start with yourself; kindness to others begins with kindness to yourself.[8]

▼

BONE GAME 1-2

Practice Acceptance

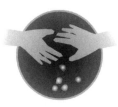

Exercise your ability to recognize a variety of human behaviors or characteristics in yourself.

Pick a day, preferably one with a full patient load. You may have a few patients who push your buttons. If so, pick a day when they have appointments scheduled. If you are in school, use conversations with your classmates for this exercise. The task is to observe the conversations with your patients and notice when your "judgment flag" waves: when the patient does or says something that you form a negative opinion about. Throughout the day, reserve part of your brain for these observations. It is possible to do this exercise and still be present for your patients. Make a mental note of the experience, or jot down a reminder word on a sticky note.

Later that day, take a moment to review the situations that raised the judgment flag, or pull out all the sticky notes and lay them out before you. Give yourself permission to be honest and compassionate with yourself. Hold up the proverbial mirror and see if you have any of the traits you found fault with in your patients. Remember, a mirror should reflect a clear image, not a sermon.[2]

> Repeat this exercise on another day, replacing the judgment flag with the times when you felt admiration for the person before you. Again, make mental or physical notes reminding yourself of the situations, and review them later in the day. See if you can find yourself in their stories.
>
> Practice this several times to strengthen your ability to accept all aspects of yourself. You will then experience deeper compassion for others as well.

Self-Expression

The self-expressive person is aware of his innermost thoughts and feelings, accepts them, and, when appropriate, shares them responsibly.[2] In a patient-practitioner relationship, it is rarely appropriate for the manual therapist to divulge personal thoughts or feelings. A rule of thumb is to share only the information that contributes to the healing relationship. Self-expression is not self-disclosure. It takes a practitioner with a developed sense of self-awareness and self-acceptance to know how to express the true self without revealing personal information.

Talking about yourself can distract the patient. Even though we may intend to create a true healing relationship, in which both heal and both are healed,[7] clear roles must be maintained. The therapeutic relationship requires that the practitioner focus on the needs of the patient. It is possible to express your true self—be whole and complete with your patients—without relating your opinions or life events.

Self-expression can be relayed through your genuine interest in the patient. One of the basic premises in Dale Carnegie's *How to Win Friends and Influence People* is that friends are made by becoming interested in them, not by trying to get them interested in you. He even goes as far to say, "It is the individual who is not interested in his fellow men who has the greatest difficulties in life and provides the greatest injury to others."[9] Avoid imposing on your patients by making them feel they have to take care of you. For example, resist telling your patients that your day got off to a rough start. That information may lead them to filter their own needs so as not to make your bad day worse. Allow them their own process, and keep yours to yourself.

You can demonstrate your interest in your patients by listening to them with your whole body, and by watching their whole bodies and not just listening to their words. Many researchers claim that only a small portion of the understanding one gains from face-to-face interactions comes from words. The results of these studies vary slightly: the importance of verbal information ranges from 7 to 35%, with the rest belonging to non-verbal communication.[2] Be conscious of your facial expressions. Surprise, alarm, worry, distaste, or annoyance easily steal across one's face but should be avoided.[6] Give credence to the expressions that steal across the patient's face.

The therapeutic relationship is not the place for talking about yourself, but that does not mean you should suppress your thoughts and feelings altogether. During the 5 minutes of quiet time between patients, feel those feelings, have those thoughts, and make those faces. Or designate a person with whom you can express your feelings at the end of the day or week. During the session, focus on the patient's feelings. Be so clear in your own thoughts and feelings that you can reflect the patient's words and expressions without distortion. One of the most productive interview skills is that of mirroring for patients, reflecting their innermost thoughts and feelings so that they may realize their inner wisdom. Avoid mirroring their negative thoughts and focus on reflecting their strengths. It is important to show understanding and compassion for their negative thoughts, but concentrate on reinforcing the positive ones.

Consider the potential obstacles to listening during the interview. Earlier, we discussed how easily we practitioners can be distracted. Remember, it is very hard to hear when you are talking.[10] Instead of talking about yourself, ask open-ended questions that elicit information about the patient's situation, how she feels about it, and how it affects her life.

▼

BONE GAME 1-3

Morning Pages

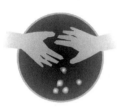

> The best way I have found to get to know myself is to write three pages of whatever comes to mind, every morning, no excuses. This writing is called morning pages, a term I much prefer to "journaling," which feels so formidable and permanent. I learned of morning pages in Julia Cameron's *The Artist's Way*.[11] I scribble thoughts, feelings, and opinions; anger, grief, and desire; gossip, reactions to TV shows, and movie critiques onto those pages, thus sparing my friends, loved ones, and patients. Writing morning pages has helped me sort out emotions and situations, and has allowed me to express myself in ways I can be proud of. I have fewer regrets since practicing a daily writing routine. That alone is worth every minute of "I don't know what to write this morning...." Try it. You will be amazed at what you discover about yourself.

PRACTICE UNDERSTANDING AND COMPASSION
Develop Good Listening Skills

To foster good listening skills during the interview, limit the distractions in the room. For example, turn off the phone ringer. Don't wear clothes that call attention to yourself. Arrange the room so that nothing is between you and your patients: avoid sitting behind a desk or crossing your arms or legs. Be on the same level with your patients; don't sit on the table. Face them and make solid eye contact. Sit on the edge of your seat. Be relaxed, yet alert and involved. Respect their personal space; three feet is considered a safe distance in American culture. Gesture during their stories: nod your head, smile, show concern. Use touch, with permission, to express your compassion.

Listen to the Words and Hear the Feelings

Understanding patients involves grasping both the content and the process of patient communication. The content refers to what the patients say; the process refers to how they say it: their tone, body language, and facial expressions.[3] As mentioned earlier, most information is communicated nonverbally. If we focus on the symptoms alone, we miss the patients' personal reactions to their condition, in essence, we miss the uniqueness of each individual. Information is all around us. Feelings are the energizing force that help us sort our data and use it effectively to shape and implement relevant action steps.[2] Remember, if the patients do not feel understood—both the facts and the emotions—they do not trust the practitioner and the therapeutic relationship is at risk.[3] To strengthen the relationship, explore the patient's feelings while you gather data.

Although you should be attentive to your patients' feelings, do not analyze those feelings or attempt to cross over into a psychotherapeutic relationship unless you are trained and licensed to do so. The goal is to understand how our patients feel about their condition, because their feelings can help or hinder the healing process. Research has discovered that when a person is aggressive and anxious, for example, excessive amounts of norepinephrine and epinephrine are secreted, even at rest. The arteries thicken, and the excess hormones cause blood vessels to constrict. The gradual rise in blood pressure can cause hypertension, stroke, or heart failure.[7] Unless the patient's feelings are considered—verbally or nonverbally expressed by the patient, and understood and reflected by the practitioner—recovery from disease can be an uphill battle.

Patients do not always express their feelings freely. As a culture, we are private with our feelings. Experience may have trained your patients to hide their feelings at first. Until patients feel safe enough to express their feelings, look for alternative ways of gathering emotional information.

Body language is the best way to tap into the patient's feelings. Research shows that words are best at communicating facts, but body language is the primary system for expressing emotions. The behavior of a person—her facial expressions, postures, gestures, and other actions—is an uninterrupted stream of information and a constant source of clues to the feelings she is experiencing.[2]

Reflecting or **active listening** is a tool that can be used to acknowledge emotions you see in a patient's behavior, whether or not they are expressed verbally. Reflecting means repeating, paraphrasing, or summarizing the feelings the patient has expressed either verbally or nonverbally. Use your intuition and read body language if the patient does not name her emotion. Watch for facial expressions, postures, and gestures; listen to voice tone, pitch, and volume. If you are not sure what the expression means to the patient, consider what it might mean to you, and reflect your interpretation for confirmation.

Until you feel comfortable reflecting, adopt the formula "You feel (name emotion) because (name event or condition)."[2] Practice this formula with your peers until it becomes natural. Use the formula to summarize the information the patient (peer) shares with you. For example, "You feel sad because pain prevents you from lifting your baby." Another example: "You feel frustrated because you cannot concentrate on your homework with the headaches." Or, "You feel happy because you were able to garden for an hour without back pain."

Sometimes patients' body language reflects something different from their words. Check by saying, "You say you are happy that you were able to garden for an hour without pain, but you look as though you are sad that the back pain is still a problem and is preventing you from gardening for longer." Another example: "Clint, I heard you tell me that you feel fine today, but I can't help noticing that you are wearing your shoulders like a pair of earrings. Is it possible that you are carrying some tension in your shoulders today?" A little humor, if used with discretion, can also help loosen a person up. Speak with compassion, not with prodding.

Exploring or reflecting feelings can be a useful tool for the following:

◆ Making the patient feel understood
◆ Helping the patient become more aware of her feelings
◆ Encouraging the patient to speak more about her feelings[3]

As a patient expresses her feelings, use **silence** to further explore the patient's emotions. Silence can uncover deep feelings. Don't jump to complete the patient's sentences or to fill up pauses with more questions. If given time to think, patients will often sink a little more deeply into their thoughts and will express the feelings or problems that lie beneath the surface. Too often we make the mistake of focusing on the first thing that comes up in the interview, when the source of the problem is deeper. Your use of silence will add to patients' satisfaction with the therapeutic relationship and to their feeling of being deeply understood.

In the interview, explore the patient's entire relationship with her condition: when and why she experiences it, how the condition affects her daily activities and emotions, and what she is doing to cope with it. **Following skills** are a form of listening skills we can use to discover how patients view their situation. **Door openers**—an invitation to talk—can start things off. These can be as simple as, "You are here because of shoulder pain while working on the computer. Tell me how you feel about this." Open-ended questions can further the search; for example, "What do you notice when your shoulder starts to hurt and you have a deadline to meet?" Reinforce the tools that work for patients by **complimenting** them on being active in their health care; for example, "What a good idea, to stretch while sitting at your desk! It decreases the pain and helps you feel more energized." Lead them to explore additional ways of handling their stress and promoting physical healing; for example, "What could you do to remind yourself to stretch regularly even before the pain begins?"

See Through the Other's Eyes

Compassion is another key component to the relationship. We want the patient to feel understood but not judged. Compassion denotes respect for the patient's point of view. It is important when developing relationships to see through the eyes of the other person—through his historical, cultural, and emotional filters. To do this we must set aside our own belief systems, judgments, and expectations about the outcome of the relationship. Respect the patient's personal values and personal space, and allow the patient to be her own person.[2] You will still experience your biases and filters, but you will also demonstrate a commitment to understanding and compassion, and return your focus to what is important to the person in front of you.

▼

BONE GAME 1-4

Gain Perspective

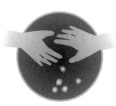

Flip back to Bone Game 1-2: Practice Acceptance. After you have raised the proverbial mirror and looked at the possibility of possessing some of the same qualities as your patient, add the following piece to the exercise:

Evaluate each situation separately. Put yourself in the shoes of each patient—view the situation from the patient's perspective, with the patient's history and values—and see whether you can understand why he acted the way he did.

To be compassionate is to be fair, patient, kind, and consistent.[2] It is unconditional love—concern for the well-being of another—regardless of your opinions of the other person. From a Buddhist perspective, compassion is equal to emptiness. Pema Chödrön describes compassion as being soft and gentle, clear and sharp, open and warm.[8] A person with a well-developed sense of self-acceptance, who has practiced kindness on herself, will have an easier time feeling and expressing compassion for her patients.

HAVE FAITH IN THE PATIENT'S STRENGTH AND HEALING ABILITIES

Later in this book, in the opening story of Chapter 4, there is a patient, Sandee, who is having difficulty believing that her health was improving. Eventually, her manual therapist is able to illustrate Sandee's progress, convincing Sandee of her improvements. Providing substantial proof of her progress was like flipping a switch inside Sandee's head. Suddenly, she had confidence in herself and in her therapy, and was willing to work harder to achieve greater results. Patients' perceptions, meanings, and definitions shift over time and in interactions with others.[3] As practitioners, we must consider that how we think, feel, and act greatly influences how our patients view their health.

According to research, people's perceptions of their own health can actually determine how good their health is. People who feel hopeless about their situation or helpless to do anything about it generally have higher disease rates, are less able to fight infection and disease, and succumb to disease at a much higher rate.[4] Studies show that people who feel helpless have the same physiological response as people who *are* helpless: their heart rate slows, blood pressure drops, the heart becomes prone to arrhythmia, the stomach pumps out less gastric secretion, and there is a decrease in urinary water and sodium. The body secretes the stress hormone cortisol, nervous system activity is slowed, muscle tone decreases, and immunity is suppressed. The body behaves as though it is giving up.[4]

Not giving up—believing that change is possible, even when the patient feels hopeless—is perhaps the most important thing we can do as manual therapists to help our patients be successful in their efforts to heal.[3] We must have faith in our patients, and in their ability to contribute to their own health.

The World Health Organization defines health as "a state of complete well-being in all the aspects of one's life: physical, mental, social, and spiritual—not just the absence of disease."[4] The book *Body Mind Health* provides a comprehensive list, shown here in Wise One Speaks 1-1: Qualities of Wellness. Use this list to develop ways to exhibit faith in your patients' strength and healing abilities and to influence the attitudes and emotions of your patients to promote improved health. If our attitudes influence our patients' perceptions of their health, thereby affecting the outcome, we should make it a point to influence their health in a positive way. When the mental, emotional, and spiritual aspects of wellness are manifested, the physical aspects follow naturally.[4]

▼

WISE ONE SPEAKS 1-1

Qualities of Wellness

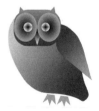

(Reprinted with permission from Hafen, Karren, Frandsen, Smith. Mind/Body Health: The Effects of Attitudes, Emotions, and Relationships. Boston: Allyn & Bacon, 1996.)
- **Sense of empowerment and personal control:**
  –control over one's responses, not necessarily one's environment
  –integrity, the ability to live by one's deepest values
  –feeling heard and respected
- **Sense of connectedness and acceptance:**
  –to one's deepest self
  –to other people
  –to earth and the cosmos
  –to all regarded as good, and to the sources of one's spiritual strength

- Sense of meaning and purpose:
  - giving of self for a purpose of value; a caring sense of mission
  - finding meaning and wisdom in here-and-now difficulties
  - enjoying the process of growth
  - having a vision of one's potential
- Hope:
  - positive expectation
  - ability to envision what one wants before it happens

Sense of Empowerment and Personal Control

Ensuring that patients feel heard and valued—an important component of the sense of empowerment and personal control—is a skill we have already worked on in this chapter. For patients to feel heard, we need to demonstrate that we understand what they say and how they feel. We have discussed a variety of listening and communicating skills that help us do that well. We can create a non-distracting environment, use body language to show we are listening, ask patients about their feelings, and reflect what we hear and see to express our understanding. By accepting what patients say without judging or criticizing, we show that we value what they are telling us.

We can assist patients to live according to their values by listening for what is really meaningful to them and then integrating their values into the treatment plan. If Darnel is deeply committed to playing with his granddaughter and showing her affection but his low back pain prevents the types of activities he is used to, we can help him discover those play activities that will not increase his discomfort and possibly strengthen his low back.

Once patients are doing homework that satisfies needs integral to their core values, reinforce the benefits of the work they are contributing. Compliment them on their ability to affect their health, and they will feel they have some control over their situation. Provide treatment options, and educate patients on the various benefits of each, allowing them to choose their treatment and homework. A sense of control regarding the outcome of the treatment contributes to the speed and quality of recovery, and allows people to take responsibility and act effectively on their own behalf.[4]

Lack of control may have an even stronger negative influence on health than does a high level of stress. Hypertension, anxiety, and pain levels increase, and the immune system is compromised. People who don't believe they can control or change their situation, or who don't believe they are capable of contributing to their healing, slacken their efforts or give up altogether, whereas those who have a strong sense of control and ability exert great effort to master the challenge.[4] It takes little effort on our behalf to compliment people on their efforts and to point out their successes.

Sense of Connectedness and Acceptance

Reflecting patients' words and feelings often helps them more clearly understand their situation, what it means to them, and how it fits into their life, even though all you have done is summarize what they said. The information may seem new to the patient because she is hearing it put together for the very first time.[2] This sense of understanding and being understood can give someone a feeling of connection to the world.

Accept your patients for who they are, to support their own self-acceptance. Your respect for their values gives them space to be who they are when they are with you.

Be an example for your patients. Demonstrate consistency by showing your respect for others as well as for them. Be tolerant and flexible; celebrate diversity. If you are critical of others in front of your patients, they may assume that you are critical of them behind their backs. Have a positive attitude about yourself, your connection to others, your work, your profession, and the things that are meaningful to you.

Sense of Meaning and Purpose

There is no one more valuable to the patient than herself, and nothing more valuable to her than her health. One of my patients has made millions from the stock market as a result of employee stock options. This patient fully acknowledges that all the money in the world is not a substitute for health. Each patient has one and only one body. Give your patients a sense of purpose by involving them in their healing process in a way that is satisfying and fulfilling.

Ask your patients whether there is anything positive in their situation. If they believe there is something to be learned or accomplished from the pain, they can muster up the courage to face it head-on.

Compliment your patients on their strength and wisdom, and help them realize their unlimited potential to grow. Help your patients appreciate the process of growing and learning. They will have much to contribute to others after accomplishing the task at hand.

Hope

A positive expectation is the product of knowing what is possible and visualizing a positive outcome. If we can help our patients understand how their condition is affecting them physiologically, and how the body works to heal itself, they can visualize successful healing and support the results. Rachel Naomi Remen uses visualization to combat terminal diseases. For example, in her book *Kitchen Table Wisdom,* Dr. Remen tells the story of a patient who used an image of catfish to enhance the function of his immune system and battle cancer. The patient visualized " . . . millions of catfish that never slept, moving through his body, vigilant, untiring, dedicated, and discriminating, patiently examining every cell, passing by the ones that were healthy, eating the ones that were cancerous, motivated by a pet's unconditional love and devotion." Dr. Remen compared bottom-feeders eating what does not support the life of an aquarium to white blood cells attacking and destroying cancer cells to help her patient understand that his body was on his side. In the end, he was confident that the daily meditation contributed to his full recovery. (Reprinted with permission from Remen. Kitchen Table Wisdom: Stories That Heal, New York:Riverhead Books, 1996.)

Hope is more than a positive expectation; it is the ability to fight against overwhelming odds and to laugh in the face of adversity. A fighting spirit has been shown to stimulate production of neuropeptides, chemical messengers that stimulate and mobilize the immune system. Humor dissipates stress and accentuates the positive. Laughter increases breath rate, circulation, and oxygen levels; relaxes muscle tension; and breaks the pain-spasm-pain cycle—thus acting as a painkiller.[4]

In summary, physical health is only one aspect of wellness. Wellness includes mental acuity, a zest for living, a tolerance for different ideas. Wellness brings with it empathy, compassion, and a sense of cohesiveness with the rest of humanity. Wellness encompasses a fighting spirit, an optimistic outlook, an attitude of hope.[4] Take care of your patients' physical health, of course, but never omit the wholeness that is human. Whenever you can, maintain perspective, provide encouragement, boost patients' self-esteem, educate and provide options, prove that behavior can lead to positive outcomes, dispel doubts, encourage independence, and be flexible, consistent, positive, and responsive to your patients' needs. Do all this, and they will rise to the occasion and do much more for themselves.

Interviewing Skills: Team Therapy Model

In this book, I propose a new paradigm for approaching interviews called the **Team Therapy Model**. As holistic practitioners, we cannot entirely embrace the medical model, which implies that the expert's perceptions about the patient's condition are more important than the patient's perceptions. As manual therapists, we provide treatment and therefore cannot wholly adopt the intervention-free model of solution-building.[3] Some manual therapists use touch as an additional form of communication rather than for corrective purposes, as in the Rosen Method. Most manual therapy professionals, however, apply manual techniques with curative intent. Therefore, a combination of the two models will serve us best.

The primary goals for the Team Therapy Model approach to interviewing are:

1. Create a relationship
2. Share information
3. Develop goals for health
4. Choose and implement solutions
5. Evaluate progress and provide feedback

The rest of this chapter describes each goal and recommends methods for reaching it.

CREATE A RELATIONSHIP

A deep and meaningful relationship, productive for both patient and practitioner, is the primary goal of the interview process. This goal requires the practitioner to be mindful of the relationship from beginning to end. Creating and preserving a meaningful relationship calls for our constant attention, understanding, compassion, and faith in the patient's personal strength and abilities. To foster a relationship between you and your patients, practice the interpersonal communication skills described earlier in this chapter.

We have countless opportunities to build productive relationships with our patients. The interview process is ongoing. It often begins (through our brochures and phone conversations) before we meet the patient, and it extends beyond the time we spend together. For example, the greeting on our answering machine can encourage or discourage the next step in initiating a relationship, depending upon the impression we make. Asking patients for permission to touch them and informing them of our intentions before massaging the chest may eliminate fear and open up potential for change, rather than promoting resistance. Patients have told me that during times of pain or trauma, they heard my voice in their heads, instructing them to breathe, look, and listen for clues telling them how to take care of themselves. We develop relationships before, during, and after every session, whether we are communicating actively or processing information indirectly. Make the most of these opportunities.

SHARE INFORMATION

Interviewing is an information-gathering process. Your patient possesses all the information you need; you must simply create a trusting relationship in which information flows freely. Ask questions that lead to pertinent information and listen carefully to the replies. Every bit of information from the patient—verbal and nonverbal, symptoms and perceptions—leads to a deeper understanding of the patient, his condition, and the potential solution. Grasping the relationship among the patient, the condition, and the solution is the key to success.

There are two primary obstacles to gathering information: thinking you already know the answer, and being afraid to ask the question.[8] Proctoring countless practical examinations has shown me that it is human nature (or the product of watching television game shows) to leap to conclusions. We are so eager to solve the problem and to be the first to get the right answer that we don't take the time to thoroughly explore the possibilities or look beyond the obvious. We fall into what is most familiar to us. I remember a story I read years ago in a professional magazine. An examiner for a doctoral program in neurology explained that over half the candidates failed the oral examinations, largely, he thought, because they didn't listen to everything the patient said and therefore didn't obtain adequate information. They were too apt to focus on a key phrase or word that pointed to a familiar dysfunction. Instead, they should pursue lines of questioning suggested by the patient's comments and gather additional information on which to base their conclusions.

▼

I received a phone call from a chiropractor who was hosting a student apprenticeship program at her office. I was the faculty liaison. She called to complain that the student practitioner was treating all the patients as though they had rotator cuff injuries. Some patients did indeed have rotator cuff injuries, but others had thoracic outlet syndrome, carpal tunnel syndrome, or whiplash injuries. The student had recently studied rotator cuff injuries in a pathology and clinical treatment class. As a result, she was listening for familiar information and didn't bother to register other important information. Instead of exploring all possibilities, she jumped to the explanation that she had the most immediate information about: if the patient had shoulder pain, it must be caused by a rotator cuff injury.

STORY TELLER 1-1

Explore Possibilities

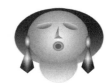

Solving minor problems while ignoring deeper concerns is one of the biggest sources of inefficiency in industry, government, schools, and health care.[2] We leap to conclusions because we are eager to help or be right, we are in a hurry, or any number of reasons. We are desperate to explain our experience, so we force-fit a few pieces of information into familiar scenarios and call it good, rather than searching for more details without the pressure of categorizing the data. Sometimes the process of asking questions and gathering information can be far more important than identifying a cause or pinpointing a dysfunction, because it can lead patients to a better understanding of themselves, their relationship with their bodies, and their role in their own health.

Be more curious than afraid. Often we avoid asking questions when we cannot control or anticipate the response. We are afraid of information we might not understand or feelings that could get out of hand. Someone's story might be more than we can handle, or we won't know what to do with the information once we know it. We fear the patient will think we are asking silly questions or being nosy. If the question arises in your mind, and a part of you believes the answer could contribute to the patient's health, trust your instinct and ask.

▼

STORY TELLER 1-2

Be Curious

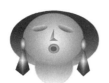

> Do not let fear limit your ability to serve. I remember the first time a patient cried during a session. I handed her a tissue and considered stopping the work I was doing on her legs because it seemed too emotionally difficult for her. I was afraid to break the silence and ask her about it. Eventually, I summoned the courage to say, "I see that you are crying. Shall I stop what I am doing, or would you like me to continue?" She said, "Oh no, please continue. I am crying because I have never been touched in such a respectful and caring manner before." I almost missed out on the most moving comment anyone has ever made about my work.

Explore the data thoroughly; include the patient's thoughts, feelings, behaviors, and experiences. Reflect the content and the context of the patient's story. Affirm the patient's perceptions and your interpretations. Exploring and reflecting patient perceptions is the most important aspect of interviewing skills.[3] When explored and understood, these perceptions help both ourselves and our patients make sense of their health issues and can lead us to understand the relationship among the patient, the patient's condition, and the successful treatment.

What questions are important to ask? It is difficult to determine whether information is helpful before you know what the information is and get a sense of how the patient feels about the information. Leading questions will follow a predetermined path—yours. Open-ended questions allow for individual expression and interpretation from the patient's point of view. Engage in conversation instead of asking an endless stream of questions.[2] The conversation can begin with something as simple as, "Tell me about your health concerns," or, "What are your goals for today's session?" Choose the significant details from the patient's story and listen for clues that provide a direction for further open-ended questions.

Prevent people from rambling. Create purposeful dialogue by interrupting with brief reflections of helpful information.[2] A long-winded story may have had one vital piece of information that can be paraphrased back to the patient, break his chatter, and focus attention on providing deeper insight into the relevant detail.

Some patients have difficulty talking about their concerns or asking for what they want. Take your cues from the intake forms. The patient may find discussing his problems uncomfortable, but have no trouble putting the information on paper. The difficulty may lie in your choice of language or your focus on a particular condition. To let the patient lead you, ask, "What should I know today so we can meet your goals for health?" Compliment patients on what they have done for their own health—even showing up for the appointment. Compliments may help them open up.

Acquiring information from patients is an art. You will need to cultivate a flexible style to accommodate your patients' differences in background and in knowledge about manual therapy and other health matters. It is important to use language that your patient understands, yet still use consistent terminology. As you ask your questions, define any specialized terms that you use. Avoid both speaking down to patients and speaking over their heads.

The Pre-Interview

The patient initiates the relationship by gathering information about you and determining whether you are the right manual therapist for her. Make sure your external image—ads, brochures, office space—attracts the type of patient you are seeking. Identify your target clientele and speak directly to them in your marketing efforts and in the way you project yourself.

Once the patient decides to take the next step and contacts you directly, gather enough information to determine whether you want to pursue the relationship before scheduling the appointment. Find out why the patient is seeking care, and get a few details about her health history to help you decide whether you can and want to be of service or whether a referral is in order. Ascertain in advance whether you need a doctor's prescription or consultation before you can begin treating the patient so that the first session will not be a waste of time for you or the patient.

In advance of the first appointment, share any information you feel is important to prepare patients emotionally and physically for the session: what they can expect during the session, fees, and what to wear, for example. Invite prospective patients to ask questions about your experience, modalities, education, affiliations, and references to assure them that they have made the right choice and to put them at ease. Be prepared to mail information before the first session: your credentials, office policies, intake forms, directions, and so on. Avoid confusion and limit the chances of unmet expectations.

The Interview

Gather information that helps the patient relax, enhances the relationship, and opens dialogue. Begin by asking how the patient likes to be called—Ms. Freeman? Karen?—and tell her how you prefer to be called. Chat a little bit to make her comfortable and to get to know her a little bit. For example: "It's a beautiful day today. Do you have plans to enjoy the weather?" Avoid personal information about yourself; focus on getting to know the patient.

Review how you work and what the patient can expect during the session. For example: "To begin with, I need to understand as much about your goals for health and your expectations of me as possible. In addition, it is helpful to explore how your past may be influencing today's concerns, so I may be asking you a lot of questions. All this can take a while, but I promise that you will get at least a half-hour of hands-on therapy today. In the future we will probably just need 5 or 10 minutes to get me up to speed before we begin the therapy." Even if you explained things over the phone, the information is received differently face-to-face. Watch the patient's reactions to your information, and respond to her needs.

Initial interviews can be extensive and time-consuming. It is advisable to schedule time for the interview in addition to the treatment session. **Insurance companies** may or may not pay for extended initial visits, depending on the **insurance plan** and the type of provider. You should know this in advance of scheduling the appointment. You may have to shorten the first hands-on session, to allow for the extensive interview and stay within the standard treatment time. The information obtained in the interview is critical to safe and effective treatment, and increases efficiency in the long run. It's best to do a complete interview in the first session or two, rather than having information trickle in over time.

Patients may have conditions that make it difficult to sit for extended periods of time. Others may get antsy. Be attentive and respond to their spoken and unspoken needs. Intersperse movement assessment tests with the question-and-answer format. Patients may want to begin the hands-on part of the session immediately. Be flexible and gather information with your patient in sitting, standing, or lying positions. Make sure that you have adequate information before you begin treatment. I suggest that you juggle verbal questioning with hands-on information gathering or relaxation techniques to keep the patient comfortable. Avoid beginning therapy before you have enough information to provide safe treatment.

▼

BONE GAME 1-5

Share Information During a Relaxing Foot Bath!

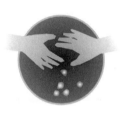

Initial interviews may run upwards of a half-hour for adequate information gathering. A foot bath is a creative way to keep your patients relaxed and the information flowing. If they think they are missing out on precious treatment time answering questions, they might tighten up the lips. A foot bath is a way to ensure that the patient is comfortable and feels that therapy has already begun.

To provide a foot bath for the initial interview, prepare two plastic dish tubs: one with hot water and one with cold water. Before inviting the patient to select a tub, find out whether he has any conditions that would preclude benefit from either bath temperature. If no contraindications are present, invite the patient to choose one or the other, or to alternate them, and adjust the temperature of either by scooping water from one into the other until the preferred temperature is obtained. Tailor the foot bath by providing marbles to roll around underfoot or essential oils to add. Have towels available within reach so the patient may pull his feet out at any time.

Review the intake form and reflect the patient's general goals for health and priorities for treatment. Find out what the patient's goals and expectations are for the visit. Ask, "How can I help you?" or, "Why are you here?" Hearing the patient speak adds to the written information on the form. It also apprises you of any inaccurate presumptions or unreasonable expectations and gives you an opportunity to change these instead of disappointing the patient. Setting reasonable goals is essential to a productive relationship; this subject will be discussed at length in the next section and in the following chapter. Begin the discussion by listening and comprehending the patient's goals for health and for sessions with you. Later, move to shaping and developing the patient's goals with the purpose of tracking outcomes and promoting patient participation.

Explore what treatments the patient has tried and what modalities he is considering trying. "What worked or didn't work?" "Do you have a sense of why the previous treatments did not work?" These questions will make your sessions more efficient, because you can use treatments the patient likes and believes to be effective, rather than spinning your wheels with treatments that have already been proven ineffective.

Use the intake forms to begin a direct line of questioning regarding history and current conditions. Take note of the patient's priorities, and focus on those. You may be interested in the patient's respiratory history, while he is intent on getting attention for a recent knee injury. Make the patient feel that his needs are being met before focusing on less urgent details.

▼

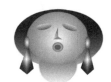

STORY TELLER 1-3
Memories Affect Healing

Explore relationships between current symptoms and previous history. Stimulate the patient's memory in an attempt to connect previous events—traumas, illnesses, repetitive movements—that may have initiated the current condition. Little things may trigger important memories. For example, a patient was watching a large family board an airplane. She noticed and identified with the eldest child's difficulty carrying a younger sibling. There were too many kids for the parents to take care of, so the older kids were helping with some of the younger ones. My patient, too, was the eldest in a large family. Her mother had died when she was young, and she shouldered a great deal of responsibility in caring for her younger siblings. That memory, combined with the interview question, "What kinds of things did you do as a child that might have been stressful to your neck?" pulled it all together for her. She not only had a great deal of physical stress with her younger brothers and sisters clasping their hands around her neck to help her lift them, but she also had the weight of the responsibility of trying to replace her mother. By recognizing the origin of the physical stress and acknowledging an emotional component, she has dramatically reduced the occurrence of her neck spasms.

Gather as much detail about symptoms as possible. Prompt patients with consistent adjectives like *mild*, *moderate*, and *severe* when you explore the details of their symptoms. Using consistent terminology to describe, for example, the intensity of pain, will show progress more clearly over time. It is easier to compare *moderate pain* with *mild pain* than to distinguish between *hurts pretty bad* and *kinda sore*. The ability to prove progress is an important component of documenting information. It will also assist in encouraging patients to participate in their treatment. Once they feel successful, they will work harder to further that good feeling.

Information regarding the patient's medications can be enlightening and helpful in creating a safe treatment plan. The list of medications on the intake form can be daunting at times. Have a **Physician's Desk Reference (PDR)** handy to look up medications and their side effects. Better yet, ask the patient for information. Find out why he is taking the medication, and you may uncover a condition not listed on the intake form. Ask about side effects; manual therapy has the physiological effect of increasing circulation and may increase the metabolic breakdown of the medication.[12] Be alert to an onset or increase in those side effects.

Hands-On Interview

The interview—asking questions, listening, and observing—segues into the hands-on interview—questioning the whole body, listening, observing, palpating, and testing. Make it a point to acknowledge that you are moving from hands-off information gathering to hands-on information gathering. The initial touch affects how the patient will respond to the ensuing physical contact: relaxing into your touch or pulling away, being open to treatment or resisting it. Ask patients for permission to touch them prior to your first hands-on contact. This demonstrates respect and instills trust. It makes the difference between feeling poked and prodded, and being handled with compassion and caring. Tell patients where you are going to touch them and why you are going to touch them there, and ask for their consent before you follow through with the contact. You may need to do this for only a session or two. Once trust is solidified, you can obtain their permission to discontinue the consent questions.

Educate your patients throughout the hands-on interview. Prepare them to stand up, sit down, and walk this way before you put them through the paces. Let them know why you are palpating their neck when it is their back that hurts. Tell them your goals for each modality and invite them to visualize the results you intend. Inform them of your options and allow them to choose which techniques you use.

The interview and the hands-on interview both involve verbal and nonverbal communication. The two may present you with conflicting information. You may hear the patient say one thing, yet you may witness the opposite response in facial expressions or tension patterns. Reflect both findings when this happens, and invite the patient to make sense of the possible conflict. The patient may be unaware of the contradiction. Presenting your findings in a neutral or curious way invites her to work with you to resolve it. This promotes partnership and gives the patient a deeper understanding of herself rather than putting her on the defensive.

▼

STORY TELLER 1-4

Listen With Your Hands

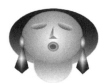

Aisha came in for her monthly session after the holidays and was bubbling with stories of her festivities. After chatting for a moment I asked her, "What do I need to know to be of service to you today?" She replied that she was fine and couldn't think of anything to tell me. I struggled for a moment to release her respiratory diaphragm and then asked her again, and again she replied that she couldn't think of anything. As she said that, her abdominal muscles tightened even more. I informed her that her belly was tighter than usual, but with her holiday glow, it sounded as though there was no stress in her family or social life. I asked her if anything unusual was going on at work. "The mayor is coming!" It was as though she was just remembering. She was in charge of a community service program and had spent the entire week preparing for the mayor's visit on Monday. Her stress level was over the top, and she put the site visit out of her mind to cope. Her body hadn't forgotten. She acknowledged that it was Friday, there was nothing else to do, and she felt prepared for the event. As she spoke about her week at work, her abdominal muscles softened and her diaphragm released. She admitted she could now relax, and she did.

Hands-on information gathering can take many forms depending on the modalities you use. You will use various techniques—palpation assessing system integrity, postural analysis, motion testing, etc.—according to your individual specialty or training as a manual therapist. As you ask questions, the body responds as well as the voice. For example, in

Upledger's CranioSacral training, practitioners are taught to listen for the truth in the body by asking questions, then feeling for changes in the craniosacral rhythm as the patient verbalizes answers. If the movement of the cerebral spinal fluid stops, the answer to the question is significant to the healing process. Develop your individual skills and gather adequate information for determining safe and effective treatment.

The hands-on interview is a mixture of information gathering, treatment, and evaluation. As new information presents itself, treatment shifts to comply. The effectiveness of the treatment application is immediately assessed, providing new data. The interview cycles continuously throughout the hands-on session. Be aware of this and don't reserve the information gathering for before and after only. If necessary, stop periodically throughout the hands-on session to record the information obtained. My Feldenkrais practitioner incorporates breaks into her sessions. Her invitation to rest for a few minutes gives her a chance to take notes without my feeling I'm being ignored.

As you share the information you are gathering with your patient, try not to reflect only negative findings. "This is really tight" or "that feels very congested" over and over again can be discouraging. Instead of judging the patient's joint mobility, ask him to describe what he feels; for example, "How does your shoulder feel when I move it like this?" Asking the same question after you have applied treatment can help integrate the solution, making a mental connection to the physical change. "Now how does your shoulder feel when I move it?" Compliment the patient on his progress. Reinforce the work he contributes between sessions. "Your tissue feels great here. You must be very successful with your stretching routine."

Post-Interview

In the final stage of the interview process, summarize the information gathered throughout the session, and confirm your findings with the patient. Ask the patient which treatment modalities and application locations felt productive and which ones were not so effective. Present your assessment of the patient's progress and response to the treatment. Compliment the patient on her participation during the session, and thank her for contributing to the outcome. Summarizing the information and drawing conclusions about the effectiveness of the treatment increase the patient's awareness of the value of the session, make her conscious of the benefits, and acknowledge her ability to contribute to the outcome.

DEVELOP GOALS FOR HEALTH

So far, we have been intent on building productive relationships with our patients and uncovering information that aids us in providing safe and effective treatments. To be truly effective in producing results, however, we must understand our patients' needs and identify goals that direct the treatment plan and illustrate progress. The goals should be specific, measurable outcomes that both the patient and the practitioner strive to attain.

Health goals are hinted at early in the therapeutic relationship. During the initial consultation, the patient describes the physical complaints and the desired results. Intake forms record health concerns and goals for health. Throughout the interviews, we listen to the patient's needs, explore her symptoms, research her history, and try to understand the impact of the condition on her life. This information leads us to formulate goals that ensure the patient's needs are met.

Develop goals by defining the following:

◆ Function—the goal is based in an activity of daily living.

◆ Relevance—the goal is pertinent to the patient's lifestyle.

◆ Measurability—the results of the goal are quantifiable and qualifiable.

◆ Attainability—the goal can be achieved in a reasonable time frame, given the specific constraints of the goal and the patient's condition.

As you develop goals with the patient, explore the following questions: How does the patient define wellness? What are the patient's expectations of you and of herself? How can you contribute to the patient's vision of health?

Define Patient Needs

First, we must focus on the needs of the patient. Often we have agendas based on what we think is best for our patients. We may see things that need fixing and be eager to impress our patients with our ability to treat their conditions. We may pressure people into fixing problems they are not emotionally or physically prepared to address. Behavioral scientists have noted that the less a person is under pressure from others to change, the more likely change will occur.[2] Therefore, we should fully understand our patients' needs and support them to accomplish *their* goals for health—when and how they choose. We do not have the final say on what is best for our patients.[3]

Help your patients articulate their needs. They may have well-formulated complaints but limited experience transforming symptoms into goals. When needs become palpable, patients can identify significant, tangible goals. For example, Darnel complains of low back pain. He hopes the manual therapist will get rid of his pain. The goal—eliminate pain—can be intimidating and its pursuit frustrating to both the practitioner and the patient. It is difficult to measure changes in pain, in and of itself. It is nearly impossible for the patient to experience progress—a decrease in pain—when he continues to endure pain daily. Do not focus on pain when exploring the needs of the patient. Instead, focus on function: how pain limits the patient's ability to participate in daily activities. We are better able to comprehend the needs of our patients when we understand how their symptoms affect their quality of life.

Function and Relevance

Goals are based on interactions with people, with projects and hobbies, with tasks and responsibilities. Before the patient chooses a goal for the treatment plan, explore what the patient's day would look like if there were no limitations caused by a health condition. Ask the patient to specify activities she can no longer do because of her condition, activities she struggles with, or activities that aggravate her condition. Discuss how the absence of that activity affects the patient's well-being. For example, Darnel can no longer pick up his granddaughter because of back pain, and their relationship is suffering. Headaches cause Arturo to be short with his students, resulting in frustration and a decrease in classroom productivity. Carrie can't go dancing since the whiplash injury and has stopped dressing up and wearing makeup. Lydia, the president of the quilting society, hasn't attended the weekly quilting bee for months because of her arthritis. These situations express a clear image of the effect of the patient's symptoms on his/her life. In these cases, the patient becomes less concerned about being pain-free if she can comfortably resume her treasured activities.

After hearing about the many activities affected by the patient's condition, ask her to choose one activity that she is yearning to get back to. Ensure that the goal you and the patient use for the treatment plan is significant to the patient's life and is something the patient is motivated to achieve. For example, Darnel's low back pain may keep him from vacuuming, mowing the lawn, and washing the car, but he may not be eager to resume those activities. During the interview, we discovered that Darnel's low back pain prevents him from picking up his granddaughter Madi and giving her hugs. Both Darnel and Madi are negatively affected by the loss of intimacy. Rather than select a goal based on a symptom (eliminate low back pain), which is difficult to measure and problematic to experience accurately, develop a goal based on a function (lift Madi and hug her) that is of great importance to Darnel and to his granddaughter. Take the activity Darnel has selected and develop it into a well-defined goal that both you and he can strive to accomplish.

Measurability and Attainability

Once the patient has selected an activity that is basic to everyday life and instrumental in her quality of life, develop a goal that is:

◆ Measurable, so you can identify when the goal has been accomplished.
◆ Attainable, so it can easily be accomplished in the designated time.

Customize the goal to fit the patient's lifestyle, healing abilities, and definition of wellness.

Ascertain the patient's healing ability: how fast she heals and how well she responds to treatment and self-care. The patient has selected the basis for the goal that best fits her lifestyle. It is up to us to develop a goal that she can attain. Explore the patient's typical healing response by researching her health history. How did she heal from other similar conditions? What treatments did she seek out? What was effective? Does she have a history of maintaining self-care routines? Are there any distractions or complications that might affect her healing time? Is she under a lot of stress or stricken with grief? It may be difficult for the patient to focus on healing when her best friend is in a coma because of the same car accident.

Consider typical scenarios similar to the patient's scenarios. Based on your knowledge, how long does it normally take for someone of the patient's age and lifestyle to recover from this type of condition and to resume normal activity? Experience may tell you that frozen shoulder usually takes 6 months to 1 year to resolve. Combine this information with your theory of the patient's healing abilities to develop a reasonable goal for the patient. If Paola is eager to get back to work and has a strong constitution and a history of fast recovery, set goals that involve Paola using her injured shoulder early in treatment.

Understand how the patient defines wellness. It is important for the patient to resume normal activity, but we must grasp what was normal for the patient prior to the onset of the condition. What was the patient capable of? What was her activity level? Her flexibility and endurance? How well did she sleep? What was her appetite like? Was she willing to take risks? Answers to these questions will help you determine the patient's expectations of treatment results. A 20-year-old ballet dancer may have a different expectation of flexibility from a 40-year-old computer programmer.

Gather enough information to determine a reasonable goal for the individual. For example, Darnel wants to lift and hug his granddaughter. Find out what Darnel is capable of doing now and what it would entail for him to be able to lift and hug Madi. How much does Madi weigh? How much weight can Darnel lift without pain in his low back? How much weight can Darnel lift from an elevated surface like a chair or a tabletop? How severe is Darnel's condition? What is his prognosis? Would Darnel be satisfied with finding alternative ways to hug Madi without lifting her?

Set the patient up to succeed. The patient has told you what he wants. Now figure out how close to that goal he can get by next week. Set your sights on a goal he can easily reach. It is important to keep the patient's confidence up so he can focus on the task at hand energetically. Lead him to select a goal he will feel good about accomplishing in the short term. An easy process for whittling a goal down to tangible size is to reflect the desired outcome to the patient and ask what he would consider a reasonable halfway goal. Then ask what would be half of that, then half of that. Ask for baby steps toward the goal. For example, Madi weighs 40 pounds. Darnel cannot pick her up off the floor. A midway goal for Darnel might be to pick her up off a stool. Half of that goal might be to pick up something half her weight off a tabletop. A baby step might be for Madi to climb into Darnel's lap while he is sitting down and sharing hugs. If they are struggling with the process, provide a few examples. Use unrelated goals as examples so the patient doesn't feel he should follow suit. Use the examples to stimulate brainstorming.

Be creative in your suggestions. If Darnel is willing to find alternative ways of getting his hugs from Madi, he might be willing to perform other exercises to get him closer to lifting Madi up on his own. For example, explore with Darnel what objects he could practice picking up when he is playing with Madi. Is there a toy of substantial weight that he could pick up from the table and hand to her? Is there a toy light enough that he could pick it up off the floor and hand to her? Can they make a game out of picking up toys: she picks up a toy from the floor to hand to him, he puts it on the table, then starts the game again by lifting the toy off the table to hand to her?

Once the patient has selected a goal he can achieve by next week, specify the parameters for success. How much does the toy weigh? How high is the table? How many times does Darnel have to lift the toy? How many times a day does Darnel need to repeat this exercise?

Qualify the goal as well as quantifying it. How will Darnel feel when he has successfully achieved the goal? If lifting the toy off the table causes Darnel to increase his pain medication or stay in bed for two days recuperating, it is not a quality achievement. A well-defined, 1-week goal for Darnel would be to lift a 10-pound doll house up from the kitchen table, place it on the coffee table, and lift it back to the kitchen table five times, three times a day, with only a mild increase in pain.

Darnel may have been so focused on the fact that he could not lift his granddaughter that he did not even explore what he could do. Part of setting and developing goals with patients is to help them participate in life, look for alternative ways of living a quality life, and regain their ability to do the things they want to do. This is easily accomplished by setting short-term goals you know they can achieve and motivating them to stretch a little further each week, getting closer and closer to their goals.

CHOOSE AND IMPLEMENT SOLUTIONS

Solutions encompass all of the following:

◆ The patient's self-care routine and homework exercises.
◆ The treatment provided by the manual therapist and other health care providers on the team.
◆ Any belief, act, or intention that brings the patient closer to the health goals already set.

I use the term "solutions" to encourage patient-centered treatment planning. Patients, their family members and friends, the spiritual figures they consult, and the health care team all contribute to the patient's expression of health. The important piece in choosing and implementing solutions is to consult your patients and encouraging their participation in all aspects of treatment.

Discover the patient's strengths. Find out what she is already doing to take care of herself. Use questions about comfort, not pain, to discover the patient's abilities to heal. Focus on the positive whenever possible. Too often we dwell on pain. We ask patients to chart their pain on intake forms; we question patients about their pain during the interview; we ask, "Does this hurt?" when we touch them. Instead of asking how frequently they experienced pain today, ask about when they felt good. Use this discussion to explore their strengths. Find out what was going on around them when they felt good. Did they do something that triggered that good feeling? Help them see how they contributed to the good feeling. Compliment them on knowing what to do to feel better, reinforce that activity as a solution to their condition, and encourage its use. If we are to involve our patients in their healing process, we must tap into the resources already available to them.

▼

> **Consider this quote:**
> "When I focus on what's good today, I have a good day, and when I focus on what is bad today, I have a bad day. If I focus on the problem, the problem increases; if I focus on the answer, the answer increases." Bill W. *Alcoholics Anonymous.*[3]

WISE ONE SPEAKS 1-2

Focus on the Positive

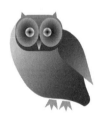

Explore additional ways that patients contribute to their own healing. Brainstorm solutions without clarifying, judging, or dismissing them. Be creative in the search and be open to different ideas. Share in the brainstorming by building on ideas the patient has presented. The goal is to create homework and self-care activities that the patient can successfully apply to improve his health. These discussions may take time in the beginning, but they will save time over the long run. The discussions promote self-awareness and reinforce that the patient is capable of affecting his well-being. The patient will learn from this experience and explore other solutions between sessions. He will be forthright in offering ideas throughout the therapeutic relationship, thus saving you from the process of trial and error. Failed attempts at homework assignments will be reduced because the homework will be the patient's idea. Treatment applications will be welcomed because they were discussed and agreed upon in advance. Show respect for your patients and consider their input in all decision-making.

Educate your patients on the effectiveness of various solutions. They may have several ideas that they are willing to implement but lack particular knowledge about when it is best to use one option over another and how each option works. If patients understand when to try a particular exercise and how that exercise helps them attain their goals, they may be motivated to try it more often. Solutions fall to the wayside when the value is not realized. Teach patients how the body's healing mechanism works, and demonstrate how their solutions affect their health. Invite them to imagine the body healing as they do their homework.

Narrow the list of possible solutions, and discuss the pros and cons of those remaining. A long list of solutions can overwhelm the patient. Select one or two to implement between now and the next session. Plan what, how, when, and where to do it. Remind the patient how it works. Demonstrate proper applications of solutions and correlate them with other activities. For example, teach Darnel proper lifting techniques to prevent reinjury and promote recovery. Invite him to practice his new-found lifting techniques with his granddaughter and apply the same techniques to lifting groceries and laundry.

Be vigilant in pursuing patient-centered solutions. Practitioner-imposed solutions are often unsuccessful. Too often we classify patients as resistant or uncooperative when they do not follow through on assigned homework or self-care activities. Noncompliance is generally attributed to the patient's personal flaws or to some deep-seated pathology. In the medical model, the professional is rarely, if ever, held responsible for the mismanagement of the therapeutic relationship. If the patient shows progress, the practitioner can take the credit and feel competent, but the notion of patient resistance lays most of the blame for lack of progress on the patient and distances the practitioner from responsibility.[3] Steve de Shazer has proposed that what practitioners take to be signs of resistance are, instead, the unique ways in which patients chose to cooperate.[13] Keep in mind that it is your patients' choice to participate in their healing. Do not judge them if they are not successful in their efforts. Take responsibility. It is possible that you selected homework that doesn't fit their lifestyle instead of focusing on their own healing abilities.

Don't give homework to patients who are not committed to change. Giving them tasks to do would only show that you are not listening to them. Instead, ask them to pay attention to what is happening in their lives that tells them the condition can improve, or to pay attention to the days that are better and notice what is different.[3] Wait until patients are able to trust that their health can improve.

Encourage self-awareness before exploring solutions. Provide information and self-care education that heightens patients' awareness of their relationship with the condition. Help them listen and respond to the messages their bodies give them throughout the time between sessions. When patients are ready, teach them to pay attention to internal warning signs—like tension in the shoulders—and to respond before their symptoms get out of hand.

Treatment Options

Treatment is a collaboration. When only one person in the therapeutic relationship is seen as the healer, fixing the problem may be possible, but healing is not. Although the patient may benefit in some ways, she is stuck in a dependent relationship, with little opportunity to experience strength and growth. Each of us has a technique—perhaps several—that we use to treat our patients. It is important to remember that the technique does not heal; the relationship does.[7] The treatment you provide simply facilitates the patient's own self-healing capabilities. Use the technique as another opportunity to listen to the patient, understand her, and help her find her way toward better health.

Typically, patients defer to the expert practitioner regarding treatment choices. They do not know the language of manual modalities or the full expanse of what is available, they do not have experience in the variety of techniques, and they do not understand the pros and cons of the choices before them. None of these facts justifies leaving patients out of the decision-making process. Whatever your treatment techniques, educate your patients on the advantages and disadvantages of each. Discuss the various places on their bodies that the techniques can be applied. Ask if they have any preferences to the style of treatment, the places you touch, or the order of application. Find out whether any technique does not sound appealing and should be avoided. Demonstrate the techniques if necessary. Be flexible. If the patient feels something isn't working at any time in the session, do something else.

Some patients want to respect your expertise and not get between you and your knowledge. When a patient says, "Just work your magic!" you may take this as a compliment, but don't stop there. Your "magic" does not promote shared responsibility. Give the patient a choice, no matter how simple. For example, "Shall we begin the session with you lying face up on the table or face down?" or, "Do you prefer that work on your low back be done while you are prone or supine?" or, "Should I work on your neck to release the pain you feel in your hand?" Most patients are not accustomed to being asked for their input. It may just take a little encouragement for them to discover that they really do have opinions and preferences. Always give patients the option to choose how, when, and where their treatment should be applied. Make sure you give them plenty of information to base their decisions on.

Involve your patients during the treatment itself as well as during treatment selection. As you are working, invite them to notice how they feel before and after a treatment technique. For example, as you move a patient's shoulder, you might notice limitations in the available movement and that the quality of the movement is compromised. Rather than point out the limitations, ask what the patient notices. "How does this shoulder feel to you as I move it? Now move it yourself. How does that feel?" Apply the predetermined treatment and move the shoulder again. "Now how does your shoulder feel?" Show the patient how to perform the same or similar treatment techniques at home to get the same result. Don't make the treatments mysterious or magical. Share your expertise and knowledge, and empower your patients to heal themselves.

EVALUATE PROGRESS AND PROVIDE FEEDBACK

Communicate through all stages of the interview by evaluating the patient's progress and sharing feedback that can strengthen, modify, or correct the results. Progress hinges on all aspects of the therapeutic relationship: communication; trust; faith in the patient's strength and healing abilities; quality of touch; understanding the patient's needs; developing meaningful goals; providing education; and listening to the body, mind, and soul of the patient. If you intend to give quality service, you must evaluate each step of the healing process and elicit feedback from the patient continually.

Evaluate progress by summarizing your observations: what you hear, what you feel, what you see, what you interpret. You can present your summary to the patient immediately after your observation, during the post-interview, or at scheduled reevaluation periods, depending on how pertinent the information is. For example, the patient's response to a treatment technique may be critical if it is the first time the technique has been used or the response was significant. Otherwise, wait until the end of the session to summarize the results. At the end of a series of sessions, evaluate the treatment plan together. Were the goals accomplished? Was the treatment style effective? Which techniques will you continue to use? Receive the feedback with an open mind and heart. Modify your treatment plan to accommodate the patient's preferences.

Use evaluation to reinforce the results of the session. Help the patient experience the changes in his body on many levels: physically, mentally, and emotionally. Often patients leave the session with little awareness of their progress. They may feel better but have no context to understand their experience or words to explain the sensations. Verbalize your findings, demonstrate the increased movement, have them observe the postural changes in the mirror, celebrate the progress. Compliment them on their ability to respond to the treatment and integrate changes. Help them recognize their contribution to the results, and reinforce the effects their homework will have on maintaining and furthering their progress.

Regularly set reevaluation dates. Some patients are shy about giving feedback during the session. They may feel vulnerable on the table, or they may enter a deep state of relaxation that makes it inappropriate to push for feedback. Setting aside time periodically for evaluation can provide a safety net for patients and let them know you are committed to hearing their concerns and responding to their needs.

SUMMARY

Developing the therapeutic relationship is central to the interview process and is even more important than gathering information or accurately assessing the patient's condition. Trust, compassion, and understanding are the cornerstones for creating a productive relationship. Your ability to be fully present for your patients and to exhibit faith in their strength and healing abilities lay these cornerstones in place. Without a strong bond, patients are reluctant to share their concerns, and treatment planning becomes a guessing game.

Concentrate on building the therapeutic relationship while striving to achieve the goals of the interview. Your tasks include:

1. Create a relationship.
2. Share information.
3. Develop goals for health.
4. Select and implement solutions.
5. Evaluate progress and provide feedback.

Communication is critical to achieving the goals of the interview. Employ the following verbal and nonverbal skills:

- Door-openers, open-ended questions
- Active listening: reflecting, paraphrasing, summarizing
- Complimenting
- Body language: eye contact, posture, gestures
- Silence
- Touch

Maintain an open line of communication throughout the pre-interview, interview, hands-on interview, and post-interview. Ensure optimal results for the patient by eliciting feedback with intent to strengthen, modify, and correct the treatment plan.

REFERENCES

1. Remen RN. Kitchen Table Wisdom: Stories That Heal. New York: Riverhead Books, 1996.
2. Bolton R. People Skills: How to Assert Yourself, Listen to Others, and Resolve Conflict. New York: Simon & Schuster Inc, 1979.
3. DeJong P, Berg IK. Interviewing for Solutions. Pacific Grove, CA: Brooks/Cole, 1998.
4. Hafen BQ, Karren KJ, Frandsen KJ, Smith NL. Mind/Body Health: The Effects of Attitudes, Emotions, and Relationships. Boston, MA: Allyn & Bacon, 1996.
5. Taylor K. The Ethics of Caring: Honoring the Web of Life in Our Professional Healing Relationships. 2nd ed. Santa Cruz, CA: Handford Mead, 1995.
6. Bates B. A Guide to Physical Examination. 2nd ed. Philadelphia, PA: Lippincott, 1979
7. Carlson R, Shield B. Healers on Healing. Los Angeles, CA: Tarcher Inc., 1989.
8. Chödrön P. Start Where You Are: A Guide to Compassionate Living. Boston, MA: Shambhala, 1994.
9. Carnegie D. How to Win Friends and Influence People. New York: Pocket Books, 1936.
10. Pye J, Jago W. Effective Communication in Practice: A Handbook for Bodywork Therapists. Edinburgh: Churchill Livingstone, 1998.
11. Cameron J. The Artist's Way: A Spiritual Path to Higher Creativity. New York: Tarcher/Putnam, 1992.
12. Werner R. Pathology for Massage Therapists. Baltimore, MD: Lippincott Williams & Wilkins, 1998.
13. DeShazer S. The death of resistance. Family Process. 1984; 23.

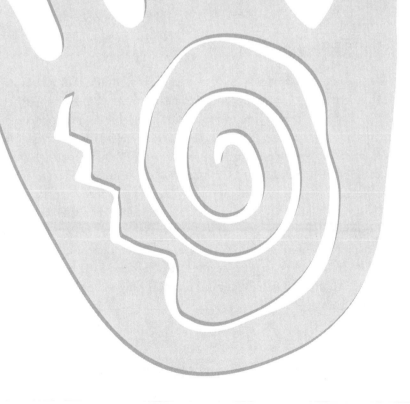

CHAPTER 2

Communication With the Health Care Team

*F*requently, I am invited to speak with doctors and their staff on the benefits of manual therapy. During these discussions, doctors often complain, "I tried referring patients to massage therapists. I never heard back from them. Why should I refer to a therapist who does not apprise me of the patient's status?"

As manual therapists are increasingly included on health care teams, it is important to remember that communication helps to establish rapport, trust, and create productive relationships.

Introduction

Team health care consists of a group of practitioners who have a common goal: to provide complete and complementary care for the shared patient. Groups are defined by the patient, usually with the guidance of a doctor. Members of the group are selected according to the patient's needs and each practitioner's ability to meet those needs. The group members form a team by consulting with each other, sharing information, and providing individualized care. Together, the patient and the practitioners complement and strengthen each other's efforts. The team approach is beneficial to the patient, the practitioners, and the patient's insurance company in many ways, including:

- ◆ Increased safety
- ◆ Increased productivity
- ◆ Increased efficiency
- ◆ Reduced duplication in treatment

Manual therapists are among the **complementary and alternative medicine** (CAM) practitioners commonly added to health care teams today. In the past, manual therapists had little motivation to seek medical referrals and participate in team health care. Consumer demand is changing that. Manual therapists are actively being solicited by consumers, **referring health care providers** (HCP), and medical specialists to participate on health care teams. Consumers visit CAM practitioners nearly twice as often as primary care physicians, and they are willing to pay out-of-pocket to do so. A study in 1999 showed that 27% of Americans had received care in the past 5 years from massage therapists alone. That number was up from 22% in 1998 and 17% in 1997. In addition, 54% of primary care physicians and family practitioners said they would encourage their patients to pursue massage therapy as a complement to medical treatment.[1] All manual therapists need to know how to be productive members of the health care team.

Guidelines for Communication

Communication is expected in health care practices, with or without a team approach to healing. Insurance companies demand a paper trail demonstrating **medical necessity**, functional outcomes, and cost efficiency. Referring HCPs feel the third-party pressure of justifying referrals and the responsibility for results. Reassure referring caregivers by providing them with the necessary paperwork without prompting, and demonstrate competency in documentation and report writing.

Keep correspondence simple and direct. Many doctors do not have time to decipher handwritten chart notes, analyze test results, or discuss issues over the phone. Correspond directly to the referring HCPs through brief letters that summarize important details and report patient progress. Send copies of **SOAP (Subjective, Objective, Assessment, Plan) charts** and test results with the reports if the referring HCP requests them.

Send copies of the reports to all members of the patient's health care team. Do not write additional reports specifically to the adjunctive therapists; simply send them copies of the original letter to the referring HCP. Do not be discouraged if you do not receive the same courtesy. Team health care is not universal. Specialists are expected to report back to the referring HCP, but the reverse is not standard. Set a good example of team communication and send reports to the entire team.

Follow these guidelines when communicating with the health care team:

◆ Correspondence should be word processed on professional letterhead.
◆ Write in a narrative format in letter style.
◆ Use the patient's last name with Mr. or Ms.
◆ Avoid handwritten fill-in-the-blank forms. (Save these for daily note-taking.)
◆ Avoid abbreviations and symbols. (Ditto.)
◆ Provide information clearly and promptly.
◆ Be brief. Summarize details and state progress.
◆ Enclose copies of SOAP charts in addition to reports, if requested.
◆ Send duplicates or photocopies. File the originals.

Document verbal conversations and phone messages. Person-to-person meetings are rare but greatly enhance treatment planning. Voice mail allows information to be shared without calling back or interrupting the patient sessions. Take notes. Record date, time, names of participants, and content in the patient's chart. Follow the rule, "If it isn't written down, it didn't happen."

File all patient-related correspondence with the health care team (letters, reports, e-mails, faxes, phone calls, and meeting minutes) in the patient's chart. If patient files are electronic, attach related correspondence files to the patient's e-file.

Standard Methods of Communication

Use familiar pathways and common language to establish communication and enhance relationships with referring HCPs. Standard methods of communication include:

◆ Introductory letters
◆ Prescriptions
◆ Initial reports
◆ SOAP charts
◆ Progress reports

Communication with the health care team should establish rapport and accessibility, convey professionalism, request information and provide data. Initial correspondence educates others on the benefits of your treatments and how to use your services most effectively. Once contact is established, a prescription will identify treatment preferences and provide billing information. If necessary, call the referring HCP to clarify contraindications and cautions for treatment. After the patient's first visit, an **initial report** will state your plans for treatment. Write **progress reports** every 30 days to update the team on the patient's progress and suggest changes in the treatment plan. Make sure reports are based on and substantiated by information recorded in the SOAP notes.

INTRODUCTORY LETTERS

Introduce yourself to other health care providers in your area. Many referrals are casual and don't name a specific practitioner or style of manual therapy. Physicians, naturopaths, chiropractors, etc., who are well-educated on the various types of massage, bodywork, and movement therapies are better able to serve their patients by providing individualized referrals. Encourage direct referrals by establishing a relationship with HCPs in advance. Send a letter introducing yourself. (See Figure 2-1) Enclose brochures that explain your services, and copies of references, credentials, or professional affiliations. Include articles that demonstrate the benefits of your techniques. Offer to meet at their office or talk on the phone.

Begin by writing to your patient's HCPs. Mention that you share a patient (with your patient's permission, of course.) A built-in recommendation often puts a doctor at ease. Contact providers in your community or neighborhood. Target caregivers whose clientele is like yours. For example, if you specialize in chronic pain, contact the chronic pain clinic in your area. If you are fluent in sign language, write to providers who have patients in need of that service.

An introductory letter states the following:

◆ Credentials and certifications
◆ Experience with similar referrals
◆ Commitment to support their treatment plan and communicate regularly
◆ Specialties
◆ Request for referrals based on your specialties
◆ Education and advanced training
◆ Professional affiliations and references

The first paragraph of the letter should introduce yourself, state your credentials and your intent. *Hello. I am a certified Polarity Therapist. You and I share a patient—Kate Nelson. I wish to take this opportunity to introduce myself and tell you about my work. I enjoy working with other health care providers and I am committed to providing quality care. I hope we will work together.*

The second paragraph states your experience working with similar HCPs. The intent is to demonstrate interest in them, create trust and convey confidence. *I understand that you are fluent in sign language and have many patients with hearing disabilities. I, too, am fluent in sign language and have deaf and hard-of-hearing patients. I am experienced in participating in team health care, communicating regularly, and supporting referring caregivers' treatment plans. Enclosed are samples of my documentation and report writing style. I am looking for doctors to refer to and receive referrals from.*

Next, describe your specialties, modalities, and treatment philosophy. Ask for referrals specific to your area of expertise. *As a Polarity Therapist, I palpate points and patterns in the patient's energy anatomy to assist in the flow of healing energy in the patient's body. I teach a series of self-help exercise techniques to promote self-awareness and create relaxation and balance.[2] I specialize in facilitating healing in patients preparing for and recovering from*

Naomi Wachtel
567 Sunnydale Dr.
Flat Irons, CO   80302
TEL   303 555 8866   •   FAX   303 555 8867   •   EMAIL   wachtel@email.com

Dr. Shawn Hall
1234 Main Street
Flat Irons, CO 80302

Dear Dr. Hall:

Hello! I am new in your area and would like to introduce myself. I am a licensed massage therapist certified in lymphatic drainage. I recently opened an office down the street from you and am looking for a doctor specializing in chronic pain whom I can refer to and possibly receive referrals from.

I am experienced in working with chronic pain referrals. I am accustomed to the needs of chronic pain patients and the level of documentation and communication required to participate on the health care team. Enclosed are copies of SOAP charts and progress reports of a recent chronic pain case, and a letter of reference from the referring physician.

I understand the complications of chronic pain syndrome and am trained to work with the passive congestion of phase two inflammation—a typical component of the condition which hinders healing. I have received advanced training in lymphatic drainage which has been proven effective in resolving the inflammatory issues of chronic pain syndrome. Manual lymphatic drainage has been safe and effective in cases in which long-term use of NSAIDS has failed or is contraindicated. Enclosed are a few articles that detail specific findings.

Enclosed are brochures designed to inform patients about the benefits of manual lymphatic drainage. These brochures explain what to expect from a lymph drainage session. Detailed in the brochures are my services, hours, and fees, and directions to my clinic. If my services are of interest to you, please hand these brochures to your patients.

If possible, I would like to schedule 5 minutes of your time to meet you and find out more about your services. I would like to pick up some of your brochures to pass out to my patients, and answer any questions you may have. I will call within the next week to schedule an appointment with you.

Thank you for your time and consideration. I look forward to meeting you.

Yours in health,

Naomi Wachtel, LMT

Figure 2-1.   Letter of introduction.

surgery. Enclosed is an article describing the benefits of presurgery and postsurgery energy treatment. I also enjoy working with individuals looking for a natural, effective way to reduce stress and increase wellness. Please think of me when referring these types of patients for manual therapy.

Include your educational background, years of experience, and professional affiliations. Select one or two of these to enclose: a copy of your license, certifications, professional memberships, Code of Ethics, or Standards of Practice. *I have been a certified Polarity Therapist and a member of the American Polarity Therapy Association for 5 years. My precertificate and postcertificate training includes over 500 hours of class time and 250 hours of supervised clinical time. I studied anatomy, physiology, kinesiology, and Polarity theory and practice, and I have clocked over 1000 hours of patient sessions. Enclosed is a copy of my Polarity Therapy certification and Code of Ethics.*

End the letter with a request for referrals. Provide the necessary information to facilitate referrals: fees, hours, location, services, and contact information. *If you feel I may be of assistance to any of your patients, please pass on my name. I am interested in working with you to serve them. Enclosed are several brochures explaining my treatment style and providing details of service. Please make these available to patients who could benefit from my work.*

Once you have contacted the HCPs you are interested in working with, call to schedule a brief appointment. Five minutes is enough to make an impression and establish a physical connection. Place a smiling face and a firm handshake behind your letter and brochures. Always remember to ask how you can best serve the caregiver—don't focus entirely on yourself. Start the conversation by inquiring about the caregiver's practice. Then ask how you might best fit in and serve. Go to the meeting stocked with additional brochures and prescription pads. Explain how to use the prescriptions (detailed in the next section) and reiterate your request for patients that fit your specialty. This is an effective marketing technique: your name will come to mind first when your type of patient shows up. Of course, let the practitioner know that you are able to treat less specialized cases, but if you are perfect for one or two patients, the ball will be in motion and more referrals will follow.

▼

STORY TELLER 2-1

Marketing

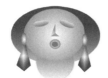

Lucas, the owner of a massage clinic in Seattle, has a unique way of introducing himself and his therapists to chiropractic offices in his neighborhood. The entire massage team takes on-site chairs and healthy box lunches to the chiropractor's office during a pre-arranged lunch hour. Everyone on the chiropractic staff gets a chance to experience 5–10 minutes of each therapists' work and ask questions. Even the busiest doctors find a moment to peek in on the fun their staff is having. Once the doctors have been rubbed and grubbed, Lucas can engage them in a relaxed conversation and make a lasting impression.

PRESCRIPTIONS

Prescriptions are formal referrals for adjunctive services and communicate information from the patient's primary HCP to the manual therapist. (For a blank form, see Appendix: Forms.) A prescription mandates medical necessity and defines treatment parameters.

Sometimes referrals come in the form of a suggestion. A HCP may say, "Try massage for your shoulder pain" or "Have you thought about getting chiropractic care for your back pain?" General referrals such as these are often oral and may or may not include a recommendation for a specific treatment technique or a specific practitioner.

Prescriptions, on the other hand, are very specific. The referral outlines instructions to be followed and is often directed to a particular specialist. Timelines and frequencies are stated, and specific modalities and treatment areas are defined. For example: *10 sessions of neuromuscular therapy with Rafael Hernandez. Complete treatment by June 23rd. Treat the neck and shoulders to reduce pain and restore function. Address other direct and indirect symptoms resulting from carpel tunnel syndrome—including posture, inflammation, and muscle tension—and treat related structures. Treatment should include hydrotherapy and stretching exercises as needed.*

Create your own prescription form[3] and send pads of them to HCPs to expedite referrals. (See Figure 2-2) Their use guarantees you will have the information you need to provide safe treatment and facilitate insurance reimbursement. If a patient has serious health problems or a condition that manual therapy may exacerbate, a prescription provides critical information and peace of mind. A prescription gives permission to treat the condition and sets guidelines for safety.

A prescription is also necessary whenever you or your patient seek reimbursement from an insurance company for medical services. Insurance only covers treatment that is deemed **reasonable and necessary**. A prescription states that the treatment is medically necessary for the patient's health. The prescription also states the patient's diagnosis. Manual therapists without diagnostic capabilities are able to use the diagnostic codes necessary for bill processing when the diagnosis is recorded on the prescription and is on file in the patient's chart. Keep in mind, however, that a prescription does not authorize insurance coverage, but it is necessary to facilitate reimbursement of services that are authorized. (See Chapter 8 for information on insurance billing.)

If a patient schedules an appointment based on an oral referral and later you determine that a prescription is necessary, contact the referring HCP and request the information you need to ensure proper care and facilitate reimbursement. An oral referral for general services or a prescription that simply states "massage" is insufficient documentation for insurance reimbursement. In the event of an oral referral or an incomplete prescription, prompt the referring HCP to write a prescription, state the diagnosis and ICD-10 codes, and direct the frequency and duration of treatment.

Suggest a treatment plan to referring HCPs unfamiliar with manual therapy or with your style of work. If the HCP writes a prescription for a treatment plan inconsistent with your treatment style, discuss the problem with the HCP. The doctor may suggest treatment twice a week for 4 weeks, and you may wish to change the frequency to three times a week for the first week, twice a week for 2 weeks, and once during the last week. Rather than contradicting the prescription, request a change. Most referring HCPs are amenable if the request is substantiated.

A prescription for manual therapy is an indication of medical necessity. Prescriptions must contain the following:

◆ Patient's diagnosis (including ICD-10 codes applicable to manual therapy)
◆ Frequency and duration of treatment
◆ Treatment application (direct and indirect areas of concern)

John Olson, LMP, GCFP

HANDS HEAL

345 Moon River Rd. Ste. 6
Minnehaha, MN   55987
TEL   612 555 9889

PRESCRIPTION

Patient Name _Darnel G. Washington_   Date _2-30-02_

Date of Injury _1-6-02_   Insurance ID# _123-45-6789_

A. Diagnosis

(Include ICD-10 codes that specifically
address Manual Therapy Treatment)

Scoliosis   754.2

Spasm   728.85

Neck Pain   723.1

Thoracic Pain   724.1

Condition is related to

☒ Auto Accident
☐ Work Injury
☐ Illness
☒ Other: _concomittant scoliosis recurrance_

B. Medically Necessary Treatment: Implement Plan as Prescribed Below

Application (Direct & Indirect)

☐ Head _whiplash_
☐ Neck _whiplash_
☐ Chest _scoliosis_
☐ Shoulders _2°—as needed_
☐ Abdomen _2°—as needed_
☐ Back _scoliosis_
☐ Lowback/Hips _whiplash_
☐ Upper extremities _2°—as needed_
☐ Lower extremities _2°—as needed_
☒ All of the above _____
☐ Other: _____

Treatment Type

☒ Manual Therapy _____
☒ Hydrotherapy _____
☒ Self-Care Education _____
☐ Other _____

Treatment Goals

☐ Decrease Pain
☐ Decrease Inflammation
☐ Decrease Muscle Tension/Spasms
☐ Decrease Compensatory Patterns
☐ Increase Mobility
☐ Increase Strength
☐ Restore Function
☐ Restore Posture
☐ Maintain Associated Structures
☒ All of the Above
☐ Other _____

Duration & Frequency

☒ 1× wk for _6_ wks
☐ 2× wk for _____ wks
☐ 3× wk for _____ wks
☐ 2× month for _____ months
☐ 1× month for _____ months

Specific Instructions:
as needed

C. Referring Health Care Provider (HCP)

Contact Information

HCP Name _Sage Redtree MD_
Provider No. _____
Address _87 Old Trail PKWY_
City _Minnehaha_   State _MN_ Zip _55987_
Phone _555-0009_
Fax _555-9000_

Reporting

☐ Send Report After Initial Visit
☒ Send Report at End of Prescription
☒ Send Copies of Chart Notes at End of Prescription
☒ Fax Information
☐ Mail Information
☐ Email Information

HCP Signature: _Sage Redtree MD_   Date _2-30-02_

Revised and reprinted with permission, Adler ♦ Giersch, PS

Figure 2-2. Sample prescription.

Manual therapists who cannot diagnose or prescribe treatment rely on referring HCPs to provide that information. Make sure the prescription specifies areas where treatment should be applied. If the diagnosis only indicates that the neck, for example, is involved in the whiplash injury, treatment to the back and arms may be considered unnecessary and may not be covered by insurance. As a holistic practitioner, you may find it impossible to treat whiplash without treating the back and arms, which are often affected by whiplash injuries. The referring HCP must authorize treatment to indirect areas of concern.

In addition to the diagnosis and basic treatment plan, prescriptions may include further instructions, such as:

◆ Treatment techniques
◆ Treatment goals
◆ Cautions and contraindications

Prescriptions often indicate general treatment approaches; for example, massage therapy, soft tissue manipulation, or movement education. Others may identify specific techniques, such as manual lymphatic drainage, craniosacral therapy, or myofascial release. Avoid requesting authorization for specific manual techniques. Many manual therapists rely on a variety of techniques to elicit the desired response in the patient, and most referring HCPs do not know the difference between muscle energy technique and strain-counterstrain, for example. Prescribing specific techniques limits the practitioner to the techniques identified. As a result, for example, if trigger point therapy is prescribed, the use of drainage techniques may not be reimbursable by the insurance company.

If you seek additional instruction for your treatment plan from the referring HCP, provide a checklist on the prescription form for treatment goals instead of techniques. Include goals such as decreasing pain or increasing range of motion. This approach authorizes the use of any techniques within the practitioner's training and scope to accomplish the specified goals.

Request permission to instruct the patient in self-care exercises. This is helpful in states where rules are vague concerning the manual therapist's **scope of practice**. Although insurance companies encourage teaching the patients stretching and strengthening exercises, some manual therapy professions compete for the right to own this scope of practice. Stay within your governing law, and ask referring HCPs to use this section of the prescription to authorize instructing patients in self-care exercises that you are trained in.

It is always helpful to request information from the referring HCP about cautions and contraindications to treatment. The referring HCP may have information that will assist you in providing safe and effective care.

Use the prescription to determine the referring HCP's preferred style and frequency of communication. For example, find out whether she prefers copies of the SOAP charts with each report, and whether she wants the reports faxed, e-mailed, or mailed to her office. If the referral was oral, send an introductory letter to find out how the doctor would like to receive your reports.

INITIAL REPORT

The initial report thanks the HCP for the referral and reports on the patient's status. This report which typically follows the first session, summarizes the initial findings and recommends a treatment plan. (See Figure 2-3) If the referral did not result in an appointment with the patient, the report explains why: perhaps the patient neglected to attend the scheduled appointment or you are currently unavailable for new patients. (See Figure 2-4)

The initial report is a summary of the **initial SOAP note** written in paragraph form. The initial report contains:

◆ Initial treatment date
◆ Patient's presenting subjective data, if HCP is unfamiliar with data
◆ Objective findings, if HCP is unfamiliar with data
◆ Functional goals for the duration of the prescription
◆ Treatment plan to accomplish the goals
◆ Commitment to report back by a set date

It is not necessary to repeat this information in future reports. Progress reports will follow every 30 days and will only report on the patient's progress (detailed in the next section).

Provided is a standard report form for referrals that do not materialize into patients. (For a blank form, see Appendix: Forms.) It is necessary to inform the referring HCP of the status of the referral. The intent is to be courteous without investing time in a relationship that is not producing income, and at the same time leaving the door open for future referrals. This is one instance in which a hand-written fill-in-the-blank form is appropriate. This can be done quickly and easily by checking off the applicable reason from a list of possibilities explaining why the referral is not resulting in a therapeutic relationship.

If the initial report is your first correspondence with the referring HCP, include a modified introductory letter and brochures. The referral may have come your way because the patient already has a relationship with you, your reputation precedes you, or the patient selected your name from a list of providers. Take the opportunity to educate the referring HCP on your services, the benefits of your techniques, and how to refer to you in the future.

PROGRESS REPORT

Progress reports summarize the patient's progress over a period of time: 30 days or the length of the prescription, whichever comes first. (See Figure 2-5) Progress reports consist of:

◆ Current functional outcomes, or a summary of current subjective and objective progress
◆ Status of the patient
◆ Plan for care

If you are recommending ongoing patient care, include:

◆ Goals for future treatment
◆ Treatment plan for accomplishing those goals

Progress reports focus on **functional outcomes**: the patient's increased ability to participate in daily activities. Functional outcomes are **functional goals** the patient has accomplished. (See Chapter 6 for in depth information on setting goals and charting outcomes.) For example, this statement begins as a goal that Ms. Hostetter is striving to achieve: *Ms. Hostetter is able to stand for 30 minutes cooking, while repeatedly lifting and extending up to 25 pounds over a stove and tossing food, 3 days a week, with moderate pain and fatigue.* Once Ms. Hostetter accomplishes the goal, the statement becomes a functional outcome.

Report changes in symptoms and objective findings if functional limitations were minimal or nonexistent and functional goals were not set. For example, *Mr. Tu's headache pain is mild and occurs weekly, lasting for 2–3 hours.*

Mention the patient's original status in the first progress report. For example, *30 days ago Ms. Hostetter was unable to cook because of pain and fatigue,* or *Mr. Tu initially reported severe migraine headaches lasting for 2–3 days, weekly.* The progress report states the patient's current condition or functional ability. The improvement in the patient's health is noted by comparing the current report to the previous reports. Each consecutive progress report builds on the last, making it unnecessary to repeat the patient's initial condition.

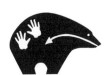

Helena LaLuna, CR
123 Sun Moon and Stars Drive
Capital Hill, WA   98119
Tel   206 555 4446   •   Fax   206 555 4447   •   Email   laluna@email.com

Manda Rae Yuricich, DC

4041 Bell Town Way, Ste. 200

Capitol Hill, WA 98119

Thank you, Dr. Yuricich, for referring Ms. Hostetter to my office. Our first appointment was on April 4, 2001. The results of the sessions are as follows:

Functional goals: Ms. Hostetter would like to return to work as a chef as soon as possible. To facilitate that, our initial goal is to have her cooking for 30 minutes per day, 3 days per week, with moderate pain and fatigue.

Together, we will resolve those findings and accomplish those goals with the following treatment plan: myofascial release for 10 sessions, addressing her shoulder, neck, back and sacral soft tissue injuries, hydrotherapy to reduce the inflammation, and homework exercises to facilitate self-care.

I will report back to you by May 5. Please contact me if you have questions, comments, or feedback.

Yours in health,

Helena LaLuna, CR

Figure 2-3.   Initial report with treatment.

Naomi Wachtel
567 Sunnydale Dr.
Flat Irons, CO   80302
TEL   303 555 8866   •   FAX   303 555 8867   •   EMAIL   wachtel@email.com

Dear ___Dr. Hall:_____ :

Thank you for referring ___Jackie Shenge_____ to my office. Your patient
and I were unable to connect for the following reason(s):

_____ The patient did not schedule an appointment.

_____ The patient did not attend the scheduled appointment.

_____ I am not scheduling new patients at this time. I anticipate my schedule to open back
up again _____ .

___X___ I am unable to benefit the patient for the following reason(s):

___Her condition necessitates intraoral techniques outside my scope of practice. I recommend___

___referring to Sari Goldsmith, LMT, who also has a license in dental hygiene and specializes in___

___craniofacial pain syndromes. Her number is (303)555-5434.___

Thank you for the referral. I hope to work with you again in the future.

Yours in health,

Naomi Wachtel, LMT

Figure 2-4.   Initial report without treatment.

Helena LaLuna, CR
123 Sun Moon and Stars Drive
Capital Hill, WA   98119
TEL 206 555 4446 • FAX 206 555 4447 • EMAIL laluna@email.com

4041 Bell Town Way, Ste. 200

Capitol Hill, WA 98119

Patient: Zamora Hostetter

DOI: 3-31-01

Claim #: C98-7654321

Dear Dr. Yuricich:

Thank you for referring Ms. Hostetter to my office for manual therapy. After 10 sessions of myofascial release, Ms Hostetter has achieved her initial goal. She is able to stand and cook for 30 minutes, while repeatedly lifting and extending up to 25 pounds over a stove and tossing food, 3 days a week, with moderate pain and fatigue.

To facilitate Ms. Hostetter's to return to work, ongoing care is requested. We must extend her cooking time to 90 minutes, 3 days a week, and include 3 hours of additional time at work preparing food. However, Ms Hostetter is able to sit down at work and take frequent breaks during her preparation time. With 3 additional sessions of myofascial release, we should be able to reach the new goal of cooking for 90 minutes, while repeatedly lifting and extending up to 25 pounds over a stove and tossing food, 3 days a week, with mild pain and moderate fatigue. Ms. Hostetter will attend session weekly for 3 weeks, receive additional self-care instructions, and participate in home exercises and hydrotherapy during this time.

Please inform me of your decision to continue Ms. Hostetter's manual therapy. I look forward to working with you in the future.

Yours in health,

Helena LaLuna, CR

Figure 2-5. Progress report.

State the current status of the patient in each report. Here are some common statements explaining the patient's status:

- Patient has achieved identified goals.
- Patient has not achieved identified goals.
- Plateau in patient's progress.

State the current plan of care. Care may be complete, or additional care may be necessary. Suggest changes in the treatment plan, referrals to another type of practitioner, or assistance with self-care education. You may have reached the limits of your abilities and can suggest additional care that will take the patient beyond a plateau. The patient may not have reached their long term goals or preinjury status, and may request ongoing care from you. Common care plans include one or more of these:

- Care is complete:
  –Patient has reached the limits of the referral.
  –Patient met the goals under the referral limits.
  –Anticipate patient will reach long-term goals independently.
- Additional care is necessary:
  –Ongoing care is requested.
  –A change in the treatment plan is suggested.
  –A referral is recommended.
- Patient to return to referring physician.

If the patient could benefit from ongoing care, state the new goals for treatment. Explain how the goals will be accomplished by identifying the proposed treatment plan. Identify which treatment techniques will be used and why; specify the treatment frequency and duration necessary to accomplish the goals.

Send progress reports to adjunctive therapists, as well as to referring HCPs. Keep all members of the health care team apprised of the patient's progress.

All the information in a progress report comes from the SOAP charts, but occasionally referring HCPs need more than a brief summary to create their reports and treatment plans. Send copies of the SOAP notes if requested.

SUMMARY

Communication is expected between referring caregivers and adjunctive therapists. Use familiar pathways and common language to establish relationships with the members of the health care team and share information. Be brief and professional with your communications.

Establish communication with caregivers by sending letters and brochures introducing yourself and outlining your services. Create prescription pads to streamline referrals. Once you have received a referral from a HCP, send an initial report stating the status of the patient. Every 30 days or at the end of every prescription, send a progress report. Use the information recorded on the patient's daily SOAP notes to write the reports.

Progress reports include:

- Current functional outcomes or summary of current subjective and objective progress
- Status of the patient
- Plan for care

If a request for ongoing care is needed, include the following:

- Goals for future treatment
- Treatment plan for accomplishing goals

REFERENCES

1. Hands On, The Newsletter of the American Massage Therapy Association, Vol. XVI, #4, July/August 2000.
2. Polarity Therapy brochure, American Polarity Therapy Association, for information call 1.800.359.5620.
3. Adler RH, Giersch P. Whiplash, Spinal Trauma, and the Chiropractic Personal Injury Case. Seattle: Adler◆Giersch PS, 2000.

CHAPTER 3

Communication and the Legal Team

*U*ncle Darnel was in a car accident on the way to a hockey game. He was riding in the passenger seat, chatting with his nephew, when a large pick-up truck rear-ended them. At first glance, there were no serious injuries, just some fender damage. The guys were eager to get to the game and were ready to leave after exchanging phone numbers, when a police officer pulled up to assist. She asked each of them a few questions. As it turned out, the driver of the truck was uninsured, and a report needed to be filed.

Initially, Darnel was not in pain, just a little shaken up. He and his nephew were able to attend the hockey game after all the paperwork was completed. Later that evening, however, he developed a headache, and stiffness and soreness in his back and neck. A few weeks later, his back pain was getting worse. Darnel finally went to his family physician, who gave him some anti-inflammatories and referred him to a manual therapist. After a month of manual therapy, the neck symptoms were clearing up but the back pain was not. John, the manual therapist, and Darnel were both concerned; and Darnel returned to the doctor. The doctor ordered x-rays, which confirmed what they all suspected: spinal degeneration. Darnel had a history of scoliosis, but with regular exercise, he had been successful in halting the degenerative process early on and had been pain-free until the accident. Now he was in constant pain, and his spinal degeneration was accelerated.

Unfortunately, the scoliosis was not Darnel's only worry. There were financial complications as well. Darnel's private health insurance did not cover manual therapy. The at-fault party had no insurance. Neither the nephew's nor Darnel's car insurance carrier was coming forward to pay the bills. Which one was responsible? Did Darnel have a choice of whom to bill, based on quality of coverage? John wondered whether he could treat the scoliosis and bill the car insurance for the treatments. Darnel was beginning to worry that he was going to be stuck with the medical bills. He was ready to quit therapy, even though the treatments eased his pain and helped him stay active.

John knew just enough about personal injury law from experiences with other patients to know that Darnel needed some professional help. Before the next session, they sat down together and discussed the financial problems. John wanted to help Darnel relieve his financial worries so he could focus on getting well. First, they had to determine whose insurance would pay the medical bills and what type of coverage was available. Second, they needed assurance that the insurance carrier would pay for the scoliosis treatments because the accident caused the flare-up of Darnel's symptoms. John suggested Darnel consult with an attorney specializing in personal injury law about access to health care and financial concerns.

Darnel met with Charma Storro, J.D., and was immediately relieved. Under the laws particular to the state where the accident occurred, the nephew's car insurance was the primary insurance carrier responsible for Darnel's medical bills. The nephew's policy included Personal Injury Protection (PIP) coverage, so Darnel's medical bills should be paid reasonably promptly. The insurance company's staff would be able to track down the driver of the truck from the police report and would handle all communication with him. The attorney instructed the insurance company to put two different adjusters on the case to ensure fair representation for Darnel: one to handle PIP matters and the other to handle issues related to the uninsured motorist claim. Because Darnel's physician had treated him throughout his adult life, he had solid documentation that his scoliosis was asymptomatic before the accident, and the flare-up was related to the accident, the treatment for the scoliosis was covered under the PIP policy.

John noticed a difference in Darnel's health when the stress of managing the claim was removed. Darnel was able to focus on getting well and turn the worry over to the experts.

Introduction

Every manual therapist must have basic knowledge of personal injury law—the rights and obligations of the practitioner and the patient—so as not to burden themselves and their patients with unnecessary risk. Records can be subpoenaed or testimony required years after treatment with a patient has ended, possibly a patient who never mentioned a motor vehicle accident (MVA). It is imperative, therefore, to keep good records on *all* patients and understand your role with the legal team in order to act responsibly in the therapeutic relationship.

The legal team consists of an attorney hired by a person who has suffered injuries as a result of carelessness or recklessness of another person or business. The attorney's staff may include other attorneys, paralegals, investigators, and other support personnel. The legal team and the health care team form the first line of protection between the victim and debilitating physical and financial loss, the potential medical and legal consequences of accidental injury.

MVAs involve collisions between cars, cars and motorcycles, cars and pedestrians, etc. Work injuries that result in disability may also call for legal intervention, as may slip and fall or trip and fall injuries occurring at a private residence or commercial location. For example, Alice suffered a ruptured disc while fighting a fire and was forced into early retirement; Lisa was helping her dad clean the gutters, tumbled off the roof, and broke both feet; and Steven was watching a baseball game at a sports bar when a ceiling tile fell on his head and gave him whiplash. All these injuries might have resulted from someone's negligence. The legal team gathers and preserves evidence proving liability, understands and defends the patient's rights, and negotiates compensation for physical injury, loss of income, pain and suffering, health care expenses, and future health care needs.

The manual therapist is a natural and important part of the medical-legal team. The manual therapist contributes to the team by keeping good patient records, communicating regularly, and understanding personal injury law. (See Chapter 6 for in depth information on record keeping.)

The Role of the Legal Team in Personal Injury Cases

Some patients suffering from personal injury can receive health care benefits even if no fault can be established, if the car or home insurance policy includes Personal Injury Protection insurance (PIP) or **Medical Payments** coverage (**Med Pay**). For example, if Darnel had driven his car into a telephone pole because he fell asleep at the wheel, he would still be eligible for medical benefits up to the limits of his PIP or Med Pay insurance coverage, if the services were deemed reasonable, necessary, and related to the collision. Some states provide **no fault** coverage. This means that health care expenses are covered regardless of who caused the accident. If he had PIP coverage, he might also be eligible for lost wages and household services in addition to medical coverage. Each state has laws, regulations, and rules establishing the mandatory minimum coverage owners of vehicles must carry.

It is critical for each health care professional to have a thorough working knowledge of his state's automobile insurance requirements.

Legal representation can be unnecessary if the injuries are minor, the car repairs are cosmetic, and the insurance company pays the bills promptly, even in situations where negligence can be established.

Some patients understand the benefits of legal counsel in personal injury cases and retain representation when a situation arises that requires it. In these situations, follow the guidelines in this chapter to communicate with the legal team.

Other patients are unaware of the benefits of legal representation and struggle unnecessarily with their insurance carriers or the at-fault-driver's insurer. Perhaps the insurance adjuster is not forthright about the coverage available, or the injuries are complicated and the patient needs assistance in proving that the injuries resulted from the accident. Patients do not always know their legal rights regarding insurance coverage and personal injury law, and health care providers (HCP) want to shy away from answering legal questions or concerns. If the interests of the patient would clearly be served by professional legal consultation, then the manual therapist should say so. For example: the insurance carrier is terminating care even though the patient continues to suffer from flare-ups and coverage is still available; or long-term disability is imminent and the **statutory time limit** is fast approaching for filing a claim and receiving payment for future health care services. Even though manual therapists cannot dispense legal advice, it is important to discuss the need for legal consultation rather than remain silent while the patient's rights slip away. Fair resolution of a legal claim often provides resources for care and bears significantly on the patient's well-being.

These are common scenarios in which the patient could benefit from consulting an attorney experienced in personal injury and insurance law:

◆ The insurance carrier refuses to pay the medical bills or discontinues coverage.
◆ Liability is contested.
◆ Physical injuries are moderate or severe.
◆ Physical injuries are impacting the patient's ability to return to work.
◆ Physical injuries are impacting the patient's earning potential.
◆ **Pre-existing conditions** flare up after the accident.
◆ Additional accidents occur before previous injuries are resolved.
◆ The insurance company schedules an **insurance medical exam** (IME), also known as independent medical exam, (although "independent" is often a misnomer), early in treatment.
◆ The at-fault party has no insurance and the patient needs to present an uninsured motorist claim.
◆ The accident resulted in low property damage yet resulted in injury. It is common for the insurance carrier to argue that a person cannot be injured when the car damage is minimal.

The attorney and his legal team can provide the following services for your patient:

1. *Evidence:* Reviews, retains, and preserves evidence regarding liability and biomechanics of an accident.
2. *Statute of Limitations:* A claimant in an automobile accident must either settle the

claim or file a lawsuit within a specified time governed by state law. For example, in California the time limit is 1 year, in Washington it is 3 years. The legal team is aware of the time limitations and can assist in settling the claim or filing the lawsuit.

3. *Stress:* The legal team can help reduce the patient's stress by lifting away the often daily burdens of monitoring payment of bills, collecting evidence, obtaining records and reports, and dealing with the insurance company.

4. *Negotiation:* The patient has little or no negotiating power with the insurer. For example, if a settlement is not acceptable, the insurance company knows the patient cannot file a lawsuit without an attorney. The claims representative is a trained and experienced negotiator. The claims representative's loyalty and duty is to the insurance company, and he will try to settle a claim for the lowest amount possible. The attorney and her staff are trained in negotiation and will represent the patient's interests.

5. *Knowledge:* The legal team has in-depth knowledge of personal injury and insurance laws and can advocate for the patient's rights. The attorney will ensure that the insurance adjuster complies with "**good faith**" provisions of the law and, if he does not, can take action to remedy the situation.

6. *Protecting the patient when an IME is requested:* The attorney may be able to negotiate with the insurer to ensure the selection of a truly independent medical examiner. Moreover, if the insurance company insists on the IME with a doctor of the company's choosing, then the attorney can accompany the patient to the IME or retain another person to serve as the patient's observer.

7. *Compensation:* The legal team will ensure that the patient receives reasonable and fair compensation for injuries and losses. The patient without an attorney may be harassed, intimidated, or pressured into accepting an unreasonable or unfair settlement and forfeiting his rights.

8. *Contingency Fee:* If there is no recovery, the patient pays the legal team no fee for the time expended.

Be prepared to respond to patients whose circumstances require a legal consultation from an attorney that specializes in personal injury law *and* understands the benefits of manual therapy. To help both the patient and the practitioner, the attorney retained should be knowledgeable and supportive of the manual therapist's role in the patient's care, should encourage compliance with the practitioner's treatment plan, and should not try to compromise or reduce the therapist's bill once the case concludes. Become familiar with who's who in pro-manual therapy personal injury attorneys in your area. Find out which attorneys work as a team with the health care providers and support complementary and alternative medicine (CAM), and which ones frequently ask manual therapists to discount their bills and refuse to sign letters that guarantee payment from the settlement. Know your allies and work with them.

Look for the following qualities in a personal injury legal team:

1. Understands the manual therapist's role in rehabilitation of injuries and ensures the patient's right to CAM care.
2. Encourages compliance with the referring HCP's prescription for manual therapy.
3. Assists in communication about the patient's case with all members of the health care team.
4. Readily knows whether insurance coverage is available, how much PIP coverage is available, when PIP coverage will expire, and whom to bill.

5. Advises the practitioner if there is secondary insurance coverage through the patient's health care plan when PIP is not available or has been exhausted, and provides accurate information on whom to bill.

6. Intervenes when the insurance company is not complying with law, regulations, or the terms of the insurance policy, re: reasonable, prompt payment of bills.

7. Answers the practitioner's questions about deferring payment and waiting for settlement in the event PIP, Med Pay, or secondary insurance is not available or has been exhausted.

8. Honors the patient's written commitment to be responsible for the manual therapist's bill at the conclusion of the personal injury case. (See Figure 3-4 shown later in this chapter for an example of a **Guarantee of Payment** contract.)

9. Challenges the legality of an insurer's request for a medical opinion about the necessity of manual therapy. Alternatively, the attorney attempts to ensure that the IME will be independent.

10. Assists in educating the patient about the effectiveness of manual therapy.

Communication With the Patient's (Plaintiff's) Attorney

ESTABLISH RELATIONSHIP

Send a letter to your patient's attorney and introduce yourself and your practice. (See Figure 3-1) Include an Insurance Status Request form. (For a blank form, see Appendix: Forms) Ask the attorney to complete the form, filling in information about the patient's insurance coverage. The attorney will have the most accurate and current information on whom to bill, whether there is PIP coverage, and how much PIP money is available. This information is critical if you are sending bills directly to the insurance company and the patient has agreed to defer insurance payments to you. If the PIP money has been exhausted on hospital stays, lost wages, household services, or other medical services, you will need to bill the patient directly or decide to defer payment until a settlement has been reached. The attorney can answer your questions ensuring that the patient's access to health care remains open.

In your letter, let the attorney know that you will be in touch monthly to send copies of the bills and update statements. If you bill the insurance company directly, send statements to the patient's attorney as well. This way the attorney can monitor PIP availability, track expenses, and your bill and balance will be known throughout the case. Your statements will also keep the legal team and the patient apprised of the insurance company's payment record. The patient can see how the insurance company is handling the claim and can intervene if bills are not being paid. The attorney can step in when the insurance company does not make payments in a timely fashion.

End the letter by asking the attorney how you can support the patient's case. Find out how the attorney wishes to receive information: fax, e-mail, or mail. Does the attorney want information in addition to the medical bills and statements? Some attorneys want copies of the patient's SOAP charts and progress reports monthly. Others will wait until immediately before settlement to ask for the patient's file. (Remember, patient records are

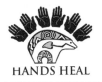

John Olson, LMP, GCFP

345 Moon River Rd. Ste. 6
Minnehaha, MN   55987

Tel   612 555 9889   •   Fax   612 555 9887   •   Email   olsen@email.com

B. Charma Storro, JD

5 Hive Lane

Minnehaha, MN 55987

(612)555-2337

Dear Ms. Storro:

I am treating your client, Darnel Washington, for injuries sustained in a motor vehicle accident on January 6, 2001. I look forward to working with you on this personal injury case. I have enclosed one of my brochures and I am available by phone and e-mail if you have any questions about my work or my practice.

I have been unable to confirm which car insurance carrier to bill for Mr. Washington's treatments. Please advise me of the applicable insurance company, the name of the adjuster assigned to the case, and the claim number. Please include information regarding insurance coverage: is there PIP coverage? Med Pay? Health insurance? Uninsured Motorist coverage? If so, how much is currently available?

Enclosed is a form for your use. If Mr. Washington does not have PIP or Med Pay coverage available, I will forward two copies of a Guarantee of Payment for Health Care Services for you to sign. Please keep one for your records and return the other to me in the envelope provided.

I will update you monthly with the patient's billing statements. Is there any other information you would like me to send in addition to the monthly financial reports? Do you prefer that I send you the information by fax, mail, or e-mail?

Thank you for your assistance. I look forward to your prompt reply.

Yours in health,

John Olson, LMP, GCFP

Figure 3-1. A. Introductory letter.

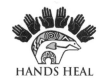

HANDS HEAL

John Olson, LMP, GCFP
345 Moon River Rd. Ste. 6
Minnehaha, MN   55987
TEL   612 555 9889

INSURANCE STATUS—
PERSONAL INJURY

Patient Name __Darnel G. Washington__   Date __2-15-01__

Date of Injury __1-6-01__   Insurance ID# __123-45-6789__

A. Reporting to Attorney
Which information would you like to receive monthly and how do you prefer to receive information:
☐ copies of billing   ☐ fax
☐ monthly statements   ☐ mail
☐ SOAP charts   ☐ email
☐ Progress reports   ☐ upon request

B. Primary Insurance Coverage
Please provide the following information regarding your client's/my patient's insurance status:
Insured _____
Insurance ID# _____
Insurance Carrier _____
Billing Address _____
City _____ State _____ Zip _____
Adjuster _____
Phone _____ Fax _____
PIP policy amount $ _____
Dates of coverage _____
PIP available $ _____
Med Pay policy amount $ _____
Dates of coverage _____
Med Pay available $ _____

C. Secondary Insurance Coverage
Insured _____
Insurance ID# _____
Insurance Carrier _____
Billing Address _____
City _____ State _____ Zip _____
Adjuster _____
Phone _____ Fax _____
PIP policy amount $ _____
Dates of coverage _____
PIP available $ _____
Med Pay policy amount $ _____
Dates of coverage _____
Med Pay available $ _____
If secondary coverage is through the patients' private health insurance, is manual therapy a covered benefit: ☐ Yes   ☐ No   ☐ Don't Know

D. Third Party Insurance Coverage
Insured _____
Insurance ID# _____
Insurance Carrier _____
Billing Address _____
City _____ State _____ Zip _____
Adjuster _____
Phone _____ Fax _____
Liability policy amount $ _____
Dates of coverage _____
Liability available $ _____
Uninsured/underinsured Motorist (UIM)$ _____
Policy Amount $ _____
UIM available $ _____

Figure 3-1. B. Insurance Status Request form.

confidential. All requests for patient information must be in writing and include the patient's written authorization, even requests from the patient's own attorney. (See below for information on requests for medical records.) Most attorneys will tell you that accurate, reliable, and relevant chart notes are the best things you can do to support the patient and the legal team.

MEDICAL RECORDS

The attorney will request the patient's entire medical file at some point in the personal injury case. Everything in the file should be sent, not just SOAP charts and progress reports, but every notation of a phone call or conversation, all intake forms and consent forms, requests from doctors and insurance companies—every piece of paper in the file. Make sure your record keeping is complete, accurate, and organized. A complete manual therapist's file will include:

◆ SOAPs for every treatment date, including extensive SOAP charting of examinations and re-examinations, and brief SOAP notes for daily treatment sessions.
◆ Correct treatment date on every SOAP note corresponding accurately with the treatment date billed.
◆ Prescriptions covering every treatment date, verifying treatment as medically necessary.
◆ Documentation (SOAPs, intake forms, pain questionnaires, etc.) for all information written in progress and narrative reports.
◆ Communication with the health care team, such as progress reports, requests for medical records, copies of other providers' progress reports, and notes from phone calls.
◆ Legend of abbreviations and symbols.

Requests for medical records are made in writing and include the patient's signature authorizing the release of the patient's records to a specific party. *Never* share confidential patient information over the phone unless you have a current and valid legal authorization signed by your patient. Always wait before sending documents until you have a written request with the patient's signature authorizing the release of medical records. After you receive the request and authorization, send copies of the patient's file. The request may specify whether the entire file is requested or simply the SOAP charts and progress reports.

A release form is valid for a set period of time, depending on state law, after which a new release form must be signed to authorize the additional release of medical information. Check the release form for the expiration date and make sure you have a valid one on file before sending out copies of the patient's confidential file.

The attorney may ask the patient to sign a release form that contains a clause negating all previous release forms. (See Figure 3-2) For example, Darnel signed a release form on January 12, authorizing his insurance company to receive copies of his medical records. On March 22, he retains an attorney to represent him and signs an exclusive medical release form voiding the insurance company's release form. Only the attorney's release and release forms signed after March 22 are now valid. Be aware of any exclusive release clauses and honor them.

PATIENT'S RELEASE OF HEALTH CARE INFORMATION

Patient's Name <u>Darnel G. Washington</u>

Social Security Number <u>123-45-6789</u>   Date of Birth <u>4-22-37</u>

Health Care Provider/Facility <u>John Olson, LMP, GCFP</u>

is hereby authorized to release health care information, including intake forms, chart notes, reports, correspondence, billing statements, and other written information to my attorneys, employees, and designated agents of my attorneys, to wit:

Attorney's Name <u>B. Charma Storro, JD</u>   Phone <u>(612) 555-2337</u>

Address <u>5 Hive Lane</u>

City <u>Minnehaha</u>   State <u>MN</u> Zip <u>55987</u>

This request and authorization applies to:

✓ Health care information relating to the following treatment, condition, or dates of treatment: <u>MVA 1-6-01</u>

____ All health care information:

____ Other: _____

Revocation of Prior Authorization: All medical authorizations by the patient or patient's authorized representatives given before the date of this release for any reason whatsoever are hereby revoked.

Information is not to be disclosed to any other person, including insurance agents or adjusters or other attorneys or their employees or agents, without my attorney's prior permission.

Effect of photocopy of this release shall have the same force and effect as a signed original.

Authorization expires 90 days from date of signature. Thereafter, no authorization exists unless an updated release is provided by: <u>B. Charma-Storro, JD</u>

<u>Darnel G. Washington</u>   <u>2-15-01</u>

Signature of Patient or Patient's Authorized Representative   Date

Figure 3-2. Exclusive release of medical records.

The attorney may request **narrative reports** from the patient's health care providers—summarizing the patient's injuries, treatment, and progress from beginning to end—to support the attorney in substantiating the patient's personal injury case. The attorney is ultimately wanting narrative reports from health care providers that contain a diagnosis, examination findings, test results, and a prognosis that will prove significant injury, validate the medical treatments received, and, if necessary, demonstrate disability or the need for ongoing care. Manual therapists without **primary care status** have less to offer in a narrative report than does the referring HCP, because of their inability to diagnose or prognose. However, if the role of the manual therapist is primary in the patient's recovery, a narrative may be requested, but will be modified to include only information found in the treatment notes and progress reports. (See Figure 3-3)

It has been my experience that attorneys rely more on manual therapists' SOAP charts and progress reports than on their narrative reports to substantiate a personal injury case. Good documentation decreases the need for narrative reports from manual therapists, and, when necessary, a good narrative report decreases the need for testimony at depositions or trials. Thorough documentation contemporaneous with treatment minimizes work in the future and is the best support you can provide the legal team and your patient.

In the event that a narrative report is requested, be prepared to write a report that accurately and completely reflects the patient's course of treatment. Because a narrative is written for attorneys and insurers and not for health care providers, use common language and avoid using Latin or formal names for conditions. For example, use the term headache instead of cephalgia. Explain everything so that it can be understood by a layperson. Make sure the report includes all pertinent information without excess. Present the information impartially; do not exaggerate or advocate for the patient. Do not use the narrative as a platform to promote your style of therapy. A narrative report should clearly state the facts of the case from an expert's point of view.

A narrative report includes:

◆ All initial subjective and objective findings.
◆ All current subjective and objective findings.
◆ The manual therapy techniques used and the locations applied.
◆ A summary of progress. Include subjective and objective changes and functional goals achieved.
◆ The status of the patient. Has he reached pre-injury status? Include a suggested course of self-care for the future.

Narrative reports differ from progress reports in several ways:

◆ Narratives summarize the entire personal injury case from beginning to end. Progress reports summarize progress month by month.
◆ Narrative reports include data from all four sections of the SOAP chart: subjective, objective, assessment, and plan. Progress reports only report progress—information found in the assessment section.
◆ Narrative reports are written for the attorney and reviewed by the insurers, are several pages in length, and a fee is customary. Progress reports are written for the referring HCP, are a few paragraphs in length, and are complimentary.

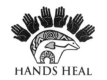

John Olson, LMP, GCFP

345 Moon River Rd. Ste. 6
Minnehaha, MN   55987

Tel   612 555 9889   •   Fax   612 555 9887   •   Email   olsen@email.com

HANDS HEAL

January 20, 2002

Patient: Darnel G. Washington

DOI: 1-6-01

Claim Number: 123-45-6789

Date of Exam: 1-20-02

Mr. Washington was first seen in my office on 2-6-01 for manual therapy treatment to injuries sustained in a motor vehicle accident on 1-6-01. He was referred by Dr. Sage Redtree, MD, with an initial diagnosis of spinal sprain-strain in the neck, mid-back and low back areas, and headaches. Within 2 months of the accident, Dr. Redtree diagnosed Mr. Washington with a flare-up of scoliosis with accelerated spinal degeneration.

Mr. Washington stated: he was a passenger in a Honda Accord and was rear-ended by a Ford F250 pick-up truck. The Honda was stopping for a yellow light, and the Ford was speeding up to go through the intersection. It was a cold and snowy January afternoon and the roads were slick. The car was pushed across the intersection but did not come in contact with any other vehicles or objects. Mr. Washington was turned to his left in his seat to chat with the driver at the time of impact. His head was thrown from side to side.

Initial Subjective Data:

On 2-6-01, Mr. Washington complained of mild neck pain and stiffness, moderate mid-back pain and stiffness, mild low back stiffness, and a moderate headache. The symptoms were constant since the evening of the accident, and increased in severity when he attempted to lift his granddaughter, garden with his wife, or sit for over 30 minutes playing bridge with the club he presides over.

Initial Objective Findings:

I palpated moderate muscle spasms in the right sternocleidomastoid and scalene muscles, left trapezius and rhomboids, and right quadratus lumborum. Trigger points were elicited with light digital pressure in the paraspinal muscles, intercostals, and diaphragm. Muscle tension was mild to moderate throughout the spinal postural muscles. Cervical range of motion was moderately limited with active flexion and extension, and passive lateral flexion bilateraly. Inflammation was palpable in the cervical and thoracic regions: redness, heat, swelling, and loss of function; pain and inflammation seemed to be preventing full range of motion. Mr. Washington's posture showed a moderate left shoulder elevation with internal rotation, mild right hip elevation, mild "hump" or kyphosis in the mid-back, mild curvature of the thoracic spine, and a mild forward head position. He was weight-bearing moderately more on the right, his leg swing mildly closed on the right and arm swing moderately closed on the left when I observed his gait.

Initial Functional Goals:

Mr. Washington is the primary caregiver for his granddaughter during the day. Because of her age, he needed to pick her up to put her into the high chair at meals, and into the car seat, and to put her to bed at nap time. At the beginning of treatment, he was unable to lift or carry her because of pain and stiffness. His initial goal was to be able to lift her 10 times a day with mild pain and fatigue.

–1–

Figure 3-3. Narrative report.

After the scoliosis flared up, his activity level dropped considerably. Simple activities such as getting dressed and driving a car became too painful without assistance or frequent rest periods. His goal was to wash himself, dress himself, and walk around the block every day.

A year later, he was able to accomplish his initial goal.

Current Subjective Data:

Mr. Washington has infrequent and mild episodes of pain and stiffness with mild activity, which increase to moderate episodes of pain and stiffness lasting for several hours if he exceeds the following: 5 minutes of carrying his granddaughter, 1 hour of gardening, and 2 hours of sitting.

Current Objective Data:

Mr. Washington's kyphosis and spinal curvature are more pronounced than they were initially. The muscles around the scoliosis are constantly and moderately tight. His muscles in the mid-back area spasm only with activities in excess of the limitations described above, the rest of the spasms have resolved. The trigger points have resolved except around the scoliosis, the headaches are gone, and his cervical range of motion is normal. His gait is excellent and his posture is compromised only by the scoliosis.

Treatment:

Initially, I used full body lymphatic drainage techniques to reduce the swelling and pain, increase mobility, and strengthen the immune system. Soon I began incorporating movement re-education techniques to find ways that allowed Mr. Washington to move and perform daily activities, such as sitting, standing, and lifting, with more comfort and ease.

Progress Summary:

Within six sessions, the neck pain and stiffness, headaches, and low back stiffness were infrequent and mild. Unfortunately, the mid-back pain and stiffness worsened for several months and were debilitating. After several months, the treatments slowly and steadily diminished the pain and increased Mr. Washington's ability to return to a modified level of activity, but it was more than a year before Mr. Washington's scoliosis stabilized and he could return to his normal activities.

Mr. Washington is able to lift his granddaughter as needed, but can carry her for only 5 minutes at a time. He is able to garden for up to 1 hour, and can sit at a bridge table for 2 hours, after which time the pain kicks in.

Patient Status:

Mr. Washington participates in a daily stretching and strengthening routine, and comes in monthly for group movement classes to maintain his daily activity level. We have attempted to discontinue his treatments and rely solely on his self-care routine; however, after 45–50 days without treatment, his ability to function is compromised and his pain increases to moderate and frequent.

In summary, Mr. Washington responded positively to treatments and adapted to a higher level of self-care responsibilities. Please call if you have questions.

Yours in health,

John Olson, LMP, GCFP

Figure 3-3. (continued)

Guarantee of Payment for Health Care Services

If there is no PIP coverage, or the PIP has been exhausted and you agree to defer payment until a settlement has been reached, obtain a signed authorization from the patient granting permission for your services to be paid directly from the proceeds of the settlement or judgment. (See Figure 3-4) After the patient signs two copies of the contract, submit both copies to the attorney and request she sign them both, keep one on file, and return the other to you. This contract is sometimes called an **Attorney Lien** or Letter of Guarantee. (For a blank form, see Appendix: Forms)

A contractual guarantee of payment is not necessary if the insurance company is making regular payments, but it is highly encouraged otherwise. The contract guarantees that you will be paid before the patient. This ensures you will receive payment in full upon settlement instead of having to collect the money from the patient.

▼

STORY TELLER 3-1

*Guarantee Payment
Upon Settlement*

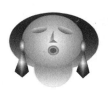

> A patient of mine spent her settlement funds on a vacation. She spent the money that was supposed to pay her medical bills. She eventually paid $100 per month until the bill was retired, but it was 3 years from the last date of service before I was paid in full.

Include a clause restricting the patient from revoking the contractual guarantee once it is signed and stating that the contract follows attorneys in the event the patient decides to change attorneys later in the case.

The same contract that guarantees payment directly from the settlement can prevent attorneys from reducing your bill. State in the contract that payment for health care services will cover the total balance due at the end of treatment. Include payment of interest if you are charging interest and the patient has received written notification of the interest charges 30 days prior to assigning the interest accruement. If the attorney signs the contract, the only way the bill can be reduced without your express permission is if your bill is found to be unreasonable, unnecessary, or unrelated to the injuries in question, as determined by a judge, jury, or arbitrator. An experienced personal injury attorney who supports CAM care will make sure that the settlement is adequate for all the patient's medical expenses.

Communication With the Defense (At-Fault Party's) Attorney
MEDICAL RECORDS

The insurance company and the attorney of the at-fault party are not entitled to the patient's records unless (1) the patient signs a medical authorization giving them permission, or (2) until a lawsuit is filed. Many cases settle successfully before a lawsuit is filed, without the defense attorney having reviewed the patient's medical information. If settlement negotiations fail, and a lawsuit is filed, the at-fault party's attorney begins preparing for the case by gathering medical information from the patient's health care providers. No direct contact is permitted between the health care providers and the at-fault party's legal

CONTRACTUAL GUARANTEE OF PAYMENT FOR MEDICAL SERVICES

I hereby authorize and direct you, my attorney, to pay directly to my health care provider(s), ___John Olson___, the total dollar amount owing for health care services, including applicable interest charges, provided for injuries arising from the motor vehicle accident on ___1-6-01___. I hereby authorize my attorney and the involved insurance companies to withhold sums from any settlement, judgment, or verdict as may be necessary to adequately protect my health care provider(s) and their office. I hereby further consent to a lien being filed on my case by said health care provider(s) and their office against any and all proceeds of my settlement, judgment, or verdict which may be paid to you, my attorney, or myself as the result of the injuries for which I have been treated.

I agree never to rescind this document and that any attempt at recession will not be honored by my attorney. I hereby instruct that in the event another attorney is substituted in this matter, the new attorney shall honor this Contractual Guarantee of Payment for Health Care Services as inherent in the settlement and enforceable upon the case as if it were executed by him/her.

I fully understand that I am directly and fully responsible to said health care provider(s) or their office for all health care bills submitted by them for services rendered to me. Further, this agreement is made solely for said health care providers' additional protection and in consideration of their forbearance on payment. I also understand that such payment is not contingent on any settlement, judgment, or verdict by which I may eventually recover damages.

I specifically request my attorney to acknowledge this letter by signing below and returning it to the office of said health care provider(s). I have been advised that if my attorney does not wish to cooperate in protecting the health care providers' interest, the health care provider(s) will not await payment, but will require me to make payments on a current basis.

Date ___1-3-02___ Patient's Signature ___Darnel G. Washington___

Patient's Social Security Number or Driver's License Number ___123-45-6789___

The undersigned, being attorney of record for the above patient, does hereby agree to observe all the terms of the above, and agrees to withhold such sums from any settlement, judgment, or verdict as may be necessary to adequately protect said health care provider(s) named above.

Date ___1-6-02___ Attorney's Signature ___B. Charma Storro, JD___

Please date, sign, and return one original to
___John Olson, LMP, GCFP___
___345 Moon River Rd. Ste. 6___
___Minnehaha, MN 55987___
___(612) 555-9889___
___fax (612) 555-8998___

THANK YOU.

Revised and reprinted with permission, Adler ♦ Giersch, PS

Figure 3-4. Guarantee of payment for health care services.

team, except to schedule a formal deposition. Requests for medical records by the insurer's attorney is often made through private record collection firms. There are two common types of requests for medical records. One, known as a **stipulation**, contains the consent of the patient and the patient's attorney to authorize the release. The other is compulsory: a **subpoena** demanding access to files.

Before sending medical records to the defense counsel, check the request for signatures and call the patient's attorney to verify that the records may be sent.

DEPOSITION TESTIMONY

The opposing counsel begins formal preparations for a lawsuit by requesting the patient's medical records and scheduling depositions. All health care providers who treated the patient are potential witnesses and can be deposed. As a health care provider and member of the patient's health care team, you possess important information about the patient's injury and treatment. To substantiate the patient's injuries and explain his need for treatment, your expert testimony may be necessary.

A **deposition** is the taking of your testimony under oath. It is conducted out of court, generally in your office. You will be asked questions by the opposing attorney and, in some cases, your patient's attorney. The meeting is recorded by an official court reporter who records every word of every question and answer. The difference between a deposition and a trial is that in a deposition, there is no judge or jury.

The opposing counsel takes your deposition to ascertain how much information you possess regarding the case. He will ask specific questions to assess your abilities as a health care witness and test your credibility. He is looking for:

- Gaps in treatment
- Patient noncompliance
- Patient history that differs from that given by other providers
- Inconsistencies in patient's reporting of symptoms
- Mistakes in billing
- Poor record-keeping
- Unprofessional conduct

The patient's attorney will prepare you for the deposition. Certain questions from the defense attorney can be anticipated. The patient's attorney will go over these with you in advance. Discuss the weak and strong points of the case before the deposition, so that you feel confident answering the defense attorney's questions. Use the preparation time as an opportunity to teach the patient's attorney about your work. She may be able to use some of the information during the questioning. Review all your notes so you can speak confidently about the patient's case. If relevant for the deposition, read the reports of the other practitioners on the patient's medical team, so that you are familiar with all aspects of the patient's treatment.

Follow these guidelines when giving a deposition:

1. Tell the truth.
2. Never lose your temper.
3. Don't be afraid of the attorneys.
4. Speak slowly and clearly.
5. If you don't understand the question, ask that it be repeated or explained.

6. Answer all questions directly, giving concise answers. If you can answer simply "yes" or "no," do so and stop.

7. Do not provide information beyond that which is sought in a specific question. Never volunteer any information beyond that required to qualify the answer as needed.

8. Stick to the facts and testify only to that which you personally know.

9. Describe your patient's injuries clearly and simply, without magnifying them.

10. Testify only to basic facts, not your opinions or estimates, unless you are asked and believe that you are informed and qualified to give such opinions.

11. If you do not know an answer, admit it. Do not think that you have to have an answer for every question asked.

12. Resist requests to interpret or draw conclusions from the records of another health care provider.

13. Do not be drawn into arguing with the defense lawyer.

14. If the patient's attorney objects to a question, stop talking. She will instruct you whether or not to continue with your answer.

15. Demonstrate competence, fairness, and honesty.

TRIAL TESTIMONY

If settlement attempts are unsuccessful after a deposition, the case goes to trial or arbitration. Trial or arbitration testimony is similar to that of a deposition except it is done in a courtroom, in front of a judge, jury, or arbitrator. Again, manual therapists are rarely called to testify because of their inability to offer a diagnosis or prognosis. Usually, the referring HCP or other specialist are called to testify by the patient's attorney to explain treatment approaches, such as, referral for manual therapy. Make testifying on your behalf easy for the referring HCP. Provide documentation she can confidently explain, interpret and defend the reasonableness and necessity of your treatment.

Follow these guidelines if you are subpoenaed to testify at trial:

1. Read over your testimony from the deposition. Be consistent. Review the guidelines for giving deposition testimony.

2. Educate! Everyone in the courtroom can learn a lot from you. Don't hesitate to explain, demonstrate, give examples, and cite authorities.

3. Define and explain all technical terms you use. If jurors do not understand, they will tune you out.

4. Use visual aids when possible. Models, diagrams, slides, and transparencies make strong impressions.

5. Listen to the questions, wait, organize the answers in your head, then speak. Do not try to out-strategize the attorney or anticipate the questions.

6. Face the examiner when answering questions. Do not "play" to the jury.

7. Balance support for the patient with the impartiality of an expert witness. Don't be an advocate, leave that to the patient's attorney.

8. Be familiar with your records. Avoid thumbing through the file.

9. Stay inside your area of expertise.

10. Don't respond to hypotheticals: "If the patient could perform a certain activity, would this change your opinion?"

11. Hold to your position and don't equivocate.
12. Be real, spontaneous, and professional.

Payment for Services

The patient's attorney is responsible for paying for the practitioner's services that the attorney incurs that are related to the preparation and prosecution of the patient's personal injury case. For example, the attorney, on behalf of the patient, covers the expenses associated with prosecuting the case, including:

◆ Copying fees
◆ Narrative reports
◆ Consultations and preparation time for depositions and trials
◆ Testimony at depositions and trials, including travel time

Ultimately, the patient will then reimburse the attorney for the expenses at the end of the case.

Fees for services vary among individuals. Take special consideration to ensure that you are compensated for your time and that your charges are reasonable. Although the attorney pays you directly for litigation services, the patient will eventually pay for all expenses of the case. Here are some guidelines for determining fees for litigation services.

◆ *Medical Records*: Some states regulate access to medical records and set maximum charges allowed for the copying of those records. This often includes a flat fee for clerical searching and handling and a per-page fee. Know the regulations for your state and follow them.
◆ *Narrative Reports*: The value of the report is based on the content and its ability to influence the case. A report is worth more if it provides a diagnosis, conclusive evidence such as x-ray results, and a prognosis that substantiates the case. Research the charges of referring HCPs and other manual therapists in your area to estimate the value of your reports. Check for state regulations that capitate fees for reports.
◆ *Consultation and Testimony*: The hourly rate for consultation and testimony often reflects the practitioner's hourly rates for health care services, as the time you spend being consulted or deposed, or testifying in court is time away from your practice. If your maximum patient load equals five hours of billable time, you may consider capping your fee for testimony at your daily rate.

Prepayment for these services is the norm. Submit an invoice stating the fees for your services, and request payment in advance of providing the service. Be prompt mailing the information upon receipt of the payment.

SUMMARY

Accidental injury has both medical and legal consequences. The legal team can be a valuable asset to the patient and manual therapist. Fair resolution of a legal claim often provides resources for care and improves the patient's well-being. The attorney can:

◆ Gather evidence.
◆ File a lawsuit within a specified time frame governed by state law.
◆ Reduce the patient's stress.
◆ Negotiate on behalf of the patient.
◆ Advocate for the patient's rights.
◆ Protect the patient when an IME is requested.
◆ Ensure that the patient receives reasonable compensation.
◆ Provide immediate access to legal representation under the contingency fee arrangement.

If there is no recovery, the patient pays the legal team no fee for the time expended.

Establish a relationship with the patient's attorney, who has valuable information about the patient's insurance carrier, the type of coverage, and the risks involved in deferring payment. Be prepared to request a Guarantee of Payment from the patient and the attorney if the patient does not have insurance coverage that will pay for medical expenses before the claim is settled.

Keep the legal team apprised of the patient's treatment bills and the insurance company's payment record. Maintain complete, accurate, and organized treatment records to support the patient and the legal team in the personal injury case. Make sure the patient's file contains:

◆ SOAPs for every treatment date
◆ Prescriptions covering every treatment date
◆ Back-up documentation for all information in progress and narrative reports
◆ Copies of all correspondence with the health care team
◆ Legend of abbreviations and symbols

The patient's attorney may request medical records or additional reports such as a narrative report on the patient's entire course of treatment. Check for valid authorization before releasing medical records to the insurance carriers or the attorneys. Look for proper dates and signatures, and check other releases for exclusive clauses.

If a settlement cannot be reached, pretrial activities begin. The opposing counsel begins formal preparations by requesting medical records and scheduling depositions. The patient's attorney will prepare you for testimony. Make sure that your treatment notes are in order and that you present yourself professionally, confidently, and honestly.

SECTION B

Documentation

CHAPTER 4

Why Document?

*S*andee was a middle-aged woman with a history of chronic pain that was becoming a way of life for her. She tried drug therapies and even surgery to rid herself of debilitating back pain. It seemed to be getting worse instead of better. On the advice of a friend, Sandee was exploring manual therapy. She had tried out a few therapists, and was currently seeing Holly, a licensed massage therapist who specializes in chronic pain conditions. Holly thought things were going well, but then Sandee approached her for a referral: she wanted the name of another therapist who might better be able to rid her of pain.

Holly was familiar with this kind of frustration and told Sandee that of course, she knew several good manual therapists in the area. She gently asked Sandee to have a seat, go over her file, and discuss her goals and results together. Holly wanted to clearly understand Sandee's goals for health in order to select a therapist to match her specific needs.

As Sandee sat down, ten pages were laid out in front of her: ten pictures with Sandee's own handwriting on them. As with all her patients, Holly had Sandee draw her pain on a form with human figures on it before each session. Now, seeing all of the pictures together, Sandee found it impossible to deny the changes that had taken place. She could hardly take her eyes off the drawings. Her hand shook in amazement as she retraced the circles of pain she had drawn over the figure's back. On her first visit she had drawn a big circle around her whole low back and hips, a circle larger than the figure itself, numbering nine in pain on a scale of one to ten. Each picture that followed showed the circle of pain shrinking in size and the intensity of the pain diminishing in number. Today's figure showed a circle tightly drawn around the sacrum and marked with the number four.

Softly, Holly asked what living with her condition had been like over the years. Sandee explained that because she woke up every day in pain and went to bed every day in pain, she was frustrated. She felt that her condition was unchanged. She had gone from doctor to doctor, trying various treatments. Once again she found herself repeating the same pattern, going from therapist to therapist, seeking an end to the pain. She had never experienced a cessation of pain and therefore concluded that there was no change in her condition.

Sandee had not experienced the subtle, progressive shifts in her pain. Looking at those pictures, she recognized her healing and began to acknowledge the increase in time spent in her garden and the new-found energy to take her grandson to the park. She smiled at Holly and chose to continue care.

Introduction

Documentation is critical, necessary, and expected, but fun? Not exactly. None of us entered the hands-on healing arts because we loved paperwork. All manual therapists have stories of the patient whose life was changed as a result of their work together. Our work is about relationships and interactions with people—that's what fuels our fire. SOAP (Subjective, Objective, Assessment, Plan) charting doesn't deliver the same emotional satisfaction.

Yet there may be a way for the paperwork to contribute to the success of those healing relationships. If so, we might be motivated to put more energy into the task.

Who Should Document?

Every manual therapist should document every manual therapy session. All licensed health care providers are required by law to document patient visits, insurance provider reimbursement contracts state that documentation is required, and malpractice insurers strongly urge documentation of every patient visit. Yet documentation is a skill and a habit that not all manual therapists have developed. Some manual therapists have not felt the need to document their sessions in the past. Massage therapists, for example, were not considered health care providers until fairly recently. Even today this inclusion is not universal, as evidenced by the lack of consistent licensure in every state. Consumers generally paid cash for their massage sessions and came without physician referrals, and thus massage therapists were accountable to no one but their patients. As a result, it seemed unnecessary to chart massage patients, especially for one-time, palliative visits.

As people are recognizing the benefits of massage, bodywork, and movement therapies, they are receiving manual therapy regularly for the treatment of physical, emotional, and spiritual ailments, as well as for wellness and preventative care. Our patients perceive us as health care providers, regardless of whether the state or insurance company does. We are responsible for the health of others, and we must act accordingly. Good documentation serves as a shield when a patient claims wrong doing and it is a part of our providing safe and effective treatment. Documentation is a necessary skill to master and implement in our practices.

Why Document?

A common misconception among manual therapists, whether we are seasoned paper pushers, is that we chart for someone else. We are driven by the belief that we have to document or we won't get paid. (And therefore we don't chart anyone who isn't an insurance patient.) Maybe we chart for fear of being sued. Or, if a doctor requests a patient's file, we drum up a report based upon memory to maintain the referral flow. We tend to chart for the many eyes that may see our records, including insurance adjusters, lawyers, and doctors. Perhaps we need to chart for our patients.

We have plenty of reasons not to document. Maybe we don't want to bother our patients with so many forms to fill out, especially if they arrive late for their appointments. Maybe we interpret the squirms during the interview to mean, "hurry up and get me on the table," and so we cut our questioning short. Maybe we rush through the assessments because we think the only part of session that the patient values is the hands-on part. Or perhaps we skip the closing interview so as not to disrupt the mood and spoil the work we just did.

The reasons to chart far outweigh the reasons not to chart. We chart because we care about the safety of our patients and we want to provide the best service possible. To avoid medical complications, we have to begin with a health history. To ensure we are using the most effective treatment techniques, we need to track patients' response to the various modalities we are employing. It is difficult to support patients in keeping up on their homework exercises when we can't remember what it is we asked them to do. It is also difficult to convince them of their progress without written proof.

Ideally, serving our patients is the ultimate motivation for documentation. We document to gather and record information that ensures safe treatment and effective care, educates the patient, and clearly states the treatment results so that the patient acknowledges the benefits of the treatment.

The financial and legal motivations exist separate and apart from the primary reason to document our patient's condition. Let's address all the reasons why we should maintain written records on all our patients, regardless of treatment goals or payment method. To tame the paper tiger, let's look through the eyes of all the different parties invested in our documentation.

THE PATIENT
Professionalism

Some patients may consider manual therapies "alternative," meaning riskier, or less scientifically valid than other, more traditional allopathic medical practices. With the integration of complementary therapies into mainstream health care, some people are seeking the care of practitioners they have never considered before. The acts of filling out health history forms, performing assessment tests, and answering questions while the practitioner takes notes can link wary patients to the familiar traditional therapies. This common thread can instill confidence and provide a professional atmosphere, reassuring the patient that you are a health care specialist providing safe and effective health care treatment.

Trust

Manual therapy is intimate. Often the patients remove their clothes and lie on a table with only a sheet covering them. If they are lying face down, they can't see us when we enter the room, and they may feel vulnerable. Even if they don't remove their clothes, we may be touching them in places few people outside of their immediate family touch. Filling out health questionnaires may provide them with a sense of confidence, a feeling that their concerns are our concerns. Interviews focused on gathering and giving information may ease their minds about how we will touch them and why. The act of taking notes demonstrates that what happens in the session is being recorded. All of these things may contribute to building a solid relationship before we put our hands on the person. If we demonstrate concern for the patient's health and take a professional approach, as evidenced through note taking, we may build a strong bond of trust, which can contribute to a successful treatment outcome. The hands-on part of the session may not be the only part that has value after all.

Historical Record

A patient's file is a historical record of wellness and health challenges over time, tracking health patterns and documenting treatment approaches. This is a valuable resource from the patient's perspective for many reasons. Patients may move or change providers, and need to get their new therapists up to speed so as not to waste time or money. Other health care providers may seek clues in our charts regarding progressive illnesses; such information could ultimately help the patient toward recovery. Patient files may provide the proof necessary to validate ongoing reimbursable treatment for awakening dormant pre-existing conditions or aggravating active conditions by recent accidents, allowing patients to get the care they need and deserve without bearing the financial burden.

Safety

Patients need to feel safe in our hands. Repeatedly asking for the same information week after week does not do much to instill a feeling of safety. A written record serves as a data base or memory of pertinent information. In completing a thorough health history, patients are assured that the practitioner has access to information that will assist in determining what treatments are safe and appropriate for them given their condition. Nothing is left up to memory, and patients do not have to repeat information each session to make sure that precautions will be taken.

Proof of Progress

As in the story of Sandee, it is difficult to maintain an accurate perspective of one's condition when one lives with daily pain. It is critical to have an ongoing and periodic account of one's experience and expression of health to supplement subjective memory. Daily charting can serve as a witness to the patient's pain and progress.

Quality Assurance and Value

If progress is evident and goals are being met, patients may rest assured that their money is well spent. Manual therapy is one form of health care that people have traditionally paid for out of pocket.[1] (A true testament to positive outcomes!) This means we are competing with the groceries, mortgage payments, and childcare. Typically, for people to feel good about how they spend their money, the end product must outweigh the expense, or the need must be based in survival. Documentation can express our goal-oriented approach and record the physical results, thus proving the value. Even emotional and spiritual results have a measurable physical expression. If we are not able to demonstrate long-term positive results, we may expect patients to seek better value for their time and money somewhere else.

Education

Documentation done in the presence of the patient may be an educational experience. The intended result is to encourage patients to participate more fully in the treatment. They may experience the results on a deeper level, understand what contributes to positive results, and become motivated to progress more quickly by participating in the documentation process. They learn from seeing what you write down. They understand what is working and what isn't, why, and what your plan is for the future. They know you are going to hold them accountable for their homework because you wrote it down and habitually check in with them about it. Involving them in the treatment process (which includes charting) gets them actively participating and committed to the final outcome. This educational experience can instill a sense of confidence in their own abilities to care for themselves and control their experience of their situation, ultimately the best outcome we can provide for our patients.

THE PRACTITIONER
Financial Security

Patient files that demonstrate positive outcomes can be financially advantageous. Whether you are self-employed or work in a clinic, patient flow depends primarily on your ability to form productive, healing relationships with your patients. Successful results lead to repeat patients and solid referrals. It is helpful to have documented proof of your effectiveness to help patients keep a positive perspective when they lose sight of their progress because they can't see beyond their immediate pain, and to demonstrate subjective and objective outcomes as a result of your care to referring caregivers who have greater access to your charts than to your healing hands. Documentation is often the referring health care provider's (HCP's) only resource for proof of those successful patient relationships. Moreover, not providing updated reports to referring providers goes against documentation protocol.

The fundamental difference between charting for cash patients and charting for insurance patients is that insurance companies can reverse or deny payment or can terminate treatment based on your documentation.[2] To any manual therapist who depends in part on insurance reimbursement for income, documentation is essential for financial security. And not just any documentation. The contract between the insurance company and the insured or the preferred providers requires that treatment be reasonable and necessary. This means that our documentation must demonstrate a need for our care on behalf of the patient's presenting condition, and that the treatment provided must produce documented, measurable results.[2] We may be asked to present this information before payment, or companies may elect to perform periodic audits of patient files. In any case, it is in our best interests to protect our financial investment and chart appropriately.

Those patients who have been injured in an accident because of someone else's negligence may or may not be represented by an attorney. The outcome of the case may determine who pays the bills and how much money is available for those bills. Attorneys typically need to prove that the patient was injured by the accident in order to legitimize financial remuneration. They look to the medical documents for this proof. Our documentation can support the patient's case and contribute to the financial award. Thus, our documentation supports us in getting full payment at the time of settlement.

Legal Assurance

In litigation cases, documentation assists in securing payment for your professional services. In the case of a malpractice suit, documentation may save you more than money. It is rare that malpractice suits are filed against massage therapists (Interview, Marlys Sperger, Executive Director, American Massage Therapy Association, 2000).

▼

STORY TELLER 4-1

Winning and Losing

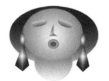

In my experience with a malpractice suit, thorough documentation showed that the symptoms in which the patient accused my colleague's treatment caused, existed months before the care provided at my clinic. Good documentation on behalf of my colleague and the patient's physicians contributed to a positive result for us.

Here is a completely different example, in which the lack of documentation produced a detrimental result. I received a phone call asking for support in a malpractice suit. A person filed for damages as a result of an on-site massage at a health fair. The catch was that the person never really received a massage at the booth. There was no documentation to prove that, however: no sign-in sheet, no signed medical release form, no treatment notes on any recipient at the booth. A favorable outcome for the manual therapist and the company running the booth seemed unlikely. This example is extreme but drives home the point that without written records we have little opportunity to fight for our innocence. Protect yourself with documentation.

Professional Image

Hands-on healing has been in existence for thousands of years. Unfortunately, in our history, massage was sometimes associated with sex for money. To my knowledge, no other health care profession has had to fight that kind of stigma. Other manual therapy professions have had to deal with claims of quackery because of lack of scientific evidence of curative ability. With all this working against us, it may behoove us to stringently apply certain professional practices. The scope of practice or standard of practice for all health care professions requires providers to document. To gain or maintain credibility as a health care profession, all manual therapists must document all treatment sessions. Practitioners that don't consider their modalities "treatment" may consider the possibility that any session that has a health benefit is considered a treatment.

Communication With Health Care Team

The team approach to health care relies on communication for its success. Information is rarely conveyed in person. Most communication—referrals, progress reports, etc.—is on paper. Other members of the team evaluate your effectiveness by reading your documentation, not by experiencing your touch or hearing patient testimonials. The charts and reports must adequately reflect the patient outcomes, or ongoing referrals may not ensue. Regular, brief written communications demonstrate your professionalism and high standards, and substantiate your effectiveness. Referring HCPs are more willing to work with manual therapists who follow familiar lines of communication. Consider this to be the least expensive form of marketing available to you.

Historical Record

Patient charts serve as a memory data base, relieving you of the responsibility to remember all the details of each case. Thus, charts free you up to think ahead instead of backwards. For example, instead of struggling to remember whether the right foot or the left foot had the broken metatarsal, and whether the strain counterstrain technique or the muscle energy technique (MET) produced the quickest result, you can simply reapply the MET to the right foot, reassess, and then move on to another stage of the treatment session.

Safety

A universal vow of health care providers is to do no harm. We are in this profession because we want to help others. We need to educate ourselves appropriately to the depths of our presenting patients, and we need to discover adequate information about them to assist in making safe treatment choices. A health history can provide information about past or current illnesses and pathologies that are potentially aggravated by some modalities. We can track the patient's response to treatments through the daily SOAP charts and reduce the risk of overtreatment. Documentation gives us access to patient information that helps us do our job with reasonable skill and safety.

Efficiency

People on the paying end of health care generally insist that the care received be the most effective available for the least amount of money.[3] To be efficient in the available time, you need to know what has been effective in the past. Health history can provide information about treatments used for past conditions and insight into their effectiveness. Keep a running log of what modalities you have used and the patients' responses to those. Daily SOAP charts record treatments and track the results. This information aids in creating individualized, effective treatment plans. Each session builds on the last, for increased productivity.

SOAP charting provides a system for tracking which treatments are effective for what and for whom. This allows you to make decisions that streamline the care you are providing, both on an individual basis and across the board. You may wish to study the results you have achieved with a given modality or for a particular pathology. Reviewing many patient files allows you to use your own case load as research and to evaluate your own effectiveness as a practitioner.

Clear Boundaries

Patient charts may also serve as a reminder, separating your experience from that of the patient. Transference and countertransference are as real in manual therapy as in psychotherapy. The lines between the patient's experience and the practitioner's experience can become blurred. It is not uncommon to assume the frustration of the patient and mistake that feeling for your own. Use your charts as a reminder of your successes and your patient's progress. Evaluate plateaus in treatment with your self-esteem intact. It is helpful to review patient's files before treatment sessions, to establish your own feelings and prevent being drawn into the patient's feelings.

THE HEALTH CARE TEAM
The Team Approach

Every person is unique, even in expression of trauma and disease. Each person has individual triggers for a condition, unique manifestations, and different combinations of common symptoms. As a result, it is rare that any one treatment cures a given pathology for all patients. Applications of a standard of care can produce varying results. Not every person with stage two lung cancer who receives chemotherapy and radiation ends up with the same prognosis. Some people die, some fully recover, and in others the disease recurs. Life stresses, attitudes and beliefs, and general constitution, to name a few, all contribute to the unique expression of a patient's pathology. We must treat the whole person and consider all options.

A team approach to treatment can lead to the discovery of the most efficacious care for each person. It is in the patient's best interest for us to act as a team, and the team relies on communication for its success. In many situations, direct communication is rare. If we are to function as a team, documentation is essential.

Communication

Communication among members of the health care team may promote complementary treatment plans, ensuring that treatments are not duplicated and that practitioners support each other's efforts and build upon each other's results. The patient may experience the power of the team and feel confident that the combined efforts will produce successful results.

When the patient moves and wishes to continue treatment in a new location, our charts may assist the next manual therapist in maintaining the progress gained. It is important for adjunctive therapists to be able to stand on our shoulders and continue the patient's progress without wasted efforts. If you go on vacation and someone takes over your patients, a well-stated treatment plan can assist your replacement in a successful continuation of care. Solid documentation can ensure the success of the health care team, regardless of who is added to it.

Education

Traditional allopaths may not be well versed in the manual therapies. More and more, however, physicians are eager to educate themselves on alternative therapies. This was prompted by the Eisenberg Study, stating that "in 1990 Americans made an estimated 425 million visits to providers of unconventional therapy. This number exceeds the number of visits to all US primary care physicians (388 million)."[1] In the Follow-up National Survey, Trends in Alternative Medicine Use in the United States, 1990-1997, Eisenberg claims "a 47.3% increase in total visits to alternative medicine practitioners, from 427 million in 1990 to 629 million in 1997, thereby exceeding total visits to all US primary care physicians."[4] Our documentation is a direct and immediate source for educating referring HCPs on how to use our skills, when to refer to us, and why they benefit from working with us.

Relationship and Referrals

Communication is expected. There is a system in place for building relationships in health care. It is common courtesy and the unwritten protocol to report back to referring caregivers on your findings and treatment plan.

Responsibility and Liability

Everyone on the team has the patient's best interests in mind, but few bear as much responsibility for the patient's health as the referring HCP. Referring HCPs are accountable to both patients and insurance companies for the productivity of the specialists they refer to. A referring HCP may be held libel for the actions of another practitioner in the event of a malpractice suit. The presence of familiar documentation can alleviate the weight of that responsibility. Chart every session, send progress reports, and thank HCPs for referrals. Support the HCP's needs for documentation and they will support you with referrals.

THE INSURANCE TEAM
Responsibility for Payment

Insurance personnel are responsible to two parties: the insurance company as an employee, and the insured to honor the terms of the insurance policy. They must provide for the insured within the bounds of their policy, and nothing more. There are several points to consider when determining whether a medical service is the financial responsibility of the insurance company. Our documentation is used by insurance personnel to help determine financial responsibility.

Insurance contracts with the insured and the providers require documentation to support and justify the services provided. Medical reviewers use our charts to determine responsibility for payment. Document the necessary information and protect ourselves and our patients financially.

Proof of Services

Insurance personnel look for proof that the services we are billing for were actually provided. It is not enough to have the patient's name in your appointment calendar. It is helpful to have something with a date and the patient's signature on it. Treatment notes will suffice and must reflect the same date as the billing form. Services itemized on the billing statement must be recorded in the treatment notes. For example, if you billed for hot and cold packs, your treatment notes should reflect that hydrotherapy was applied in the session.

Medical Necessity

Services provided must be medically necessary to qualify for insurance reimbursement.[5] Our documentation can demonstrate medical necessity. The patient files must show that the services provided were consistent with the patient's symptoms and diagnosis. For example, reimbursement could be denied if we received a referral with a diagnosis of lumbosacral strain-sprain and our treatment notes reflected that we treated the patient for tennis elbow.

Insurance personnel rely on our documentation to verify that the modalities we used improved the health of the payment. Progress may be slight or significant, but needs to be measurable over time and documented to validate the legal and insurance standard of reasonable and necessary care.

Safe and Economical

Finally, care must be safe and economical. Manual therapy has few reported complications, but it is difficult to prove that manual therapy is economical. Insurance carriers have standards for determining if fees are **usual and customary**. But more importantly, carriers want to know if manual therapy services are more cost effective than other equally effective services. The cost of treatment is calculated as total dollars spent, but rarely are the manual therapy dollars spent compared to the surgery dollars saved, for example. Insurance representatives at a Complementary and Alternative Medicine (CAM) committee meeting in Washington State, stated clearly that manual therapy dollars are considered to be in addition to other dollars spent, not instead of. "Everyone can benefit from a good rub, but why should the insurance company pay for it? Prove that the surgery won't be necessary in the future, once the palliative care has worn off," they chided. Scientific research on manual therapy is not abundant. The onus is ours to prove our effectiveness in as few sessions as possible and provide the case study statistics necessary to convince the insurance companies that manual therapy produces long-term results with reasonable financial investment. Use documentation to improve efficiency, by tracking functional outcomes and challenging yourself to be more efficient with your treatments.

THE LEGAL TEAM
Winning a Personal Injury Case

Lawyers need evidence. Medical documentation is the primary source of evidence validating a personal injury case.[6] Clear and complete documents contribute to the solidity of the case. Typically, personal injury attorneys work on a contingency fee meaning they are paid a set percentage upon conclusion of a case. Lawyers and their clients have a financial interest in our documentation.

Proof of Significant Injury

Lawyers look to our records for evidence that the patient suffered "bodily injury" as a result of the accident. For the bodily injury to be relevant to the case, documentation must illustrate the patient's pain, location, severity, and frequency. As important is the ability of our paperwork to show how the injury has affected activities of daily living. Medical records are necessary to substantiate injuries resulting from the accident.

In addition to proving that the injury is significant and warrants treatment, the treatment provided must be proven reasonable and necessary before it will be included in the settlement. The attorney can justify treatment that is effective in promoting a change in the condition with your treatment records.

Insufficient documentation may lead to requests for narrative reports or testimony at depositions or in court to clarify or defend care provided. These are costly additions to the patient's out-of-pocket expenses. It is also difficult to recall details of treatment when you are in a stressful, unfamiliar environment such as a court room, or during a deposition with a video camera 2 feet away from you.

Winning a Malpractice Case

To win a malpractice case, the attorney for the manual therapist must prove that the treatment was within the therapist's scope of practice and was provided with reasonable skill and safety. Once again, medical documentation is the primary source of evidence to substantiate the case. Solid documentation resolves claims and lawsuits. Lack of documentation creates evidence holes and has a negative impact on timely resolution and the ultimate outcome of a case.

THE PROFESSION
Positive Image

Manual therapy organizations are invested in the public perception of their profession. Associations provide a professional affiliation; promote education, ethics, and standards; and work as a group to provide public education and increase public awareness. These benefits are highly regarded by members and consumers alike. Among those standards you will often find documentation discussed, defined, and required.

Manual therapy professions value relationships with the health care community. The public may view integration into traditional health care as a stamp of approval that legitimizes the work. Increased public exposure increases the numbers of people receiving manual therapy. The numbers entering into the profession also grow as a result, and membership in professional associations grows accordingly.

Research

Research data supporting the efficacy and cost effectiveness of manual therapy validates its use as a viable treatment modality and promotes public access. No one likes to take risks with someone's health. Insurance companies and physicians rely on research results to help them make informed decisions regarding health care options. With good data, manual therapy becomes increasingly available to all who can benefit from hands-on healing. Traditional methods of research are difficult to apply to manual therapy. Case studies provide qualitative information and are a popular method for drugless therapies. Case study research is only as good as the therapist's documentation.

SUMMARY

Manual therapists who practice documentation display professionalism and high standards, and communicate easily with other health care professionals. Documentation is vital to case study research, which provides statistics supporting health care integration and increased public access.

Manual therapists benefit in a variety of ways when documenting patient relationships. It makes good business sense to protect our investment of time and services by charting the patient's condition, the necessity of care, and the effectiveness of the treatment provided and thus ensure payment. Our own legal difficulties may be avoided or the patient's injury presented successfully with adequate documentation. Patient charts can be used as a communication tool with referring providers, proving patient progress and the effectiveness of treatment, and encouraging future referrals. Communication through documentation establishes rapport within the health care team, promotes a team approach to treatment, and ensures that your patient is well cared for when transition is necessary.

Our patients also benefit from our documentation efforts. We recognize that in their eyes thorough charting demonstrates our professionalism and high standards, provides written proof of their own progress and the value of their time and resources, documents our treatment's efficacy so they can feel confident in their treatment choices, and provides an awareness that they can contribute to a higher quality of life for themselves.

Insurance companies look to our documentation for proof that services were provided, were consistent with the patient's condition and the referring diagnosis, and were medically necessary. The patient files should show that the services improved the patient's quality of life, and used the most effective modalities for the least amount of money.

The legal team depends on medical documentation to win personal injury and malpractice cases. It's as simple as that.

REFERENCES

1. Eisenberg D, Kessler RC, Foster C, et al. Unconventional Medicine in the United States, Prevalence, Costs, and Patterns of Use. The New England Journal of Medicine, #328, 1993.
2. Adler RH, Giersch P. Whiplash, Spinal Trauma, and the Chiropractic Personal Injury Case. Seattle: Adler◆Giersch, PS: 1999.
3. HMO Washington Participating Health Care Provider Agreement, 1996.
4. Eisenberg D, Davis RB, Ettner SL, et al. Trends in alternative medicine use in the United States, 1990-1997. JAMA 1998;280(18).
5. Regence BlueShield Practitioner and Organizational Manual, UM-2, 1999.
6. Adler RH. Medical-Legal Aspects of Soft Tissue Injuries, Handling Motor Vehicle Accidents. Deerfield: Callaghan and Co., 1990.

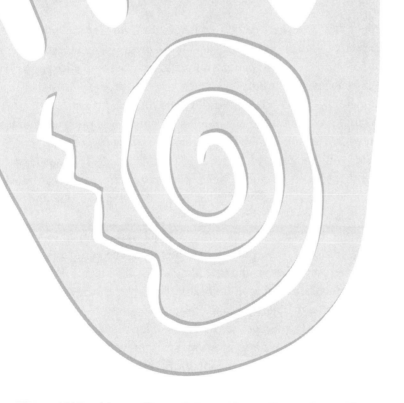

CHAPTER 5

Documentation: Intake Forms

*D*avid was a good student. He performed his duties in student clinic professionally and sincerely. One day, after a 30-minute massage on the elderly patient's neck and shoulders, the patient looked up suddenly and said, "I forgot to tell you, I have blood clots in my neck." As David learned early in school, thrombosis is a contraindication for massage: blood clots could become dislodged and move toward the brain, resulting in a stroke. Luckily, the woman was not harmed by the session and David had a poignant lesson in the importance of taking a thorough health history.

Introduction

Intake forms are the first step in gathering information from the patient. They ask general questions about personal identification, contact information, health history, and current conditions. This chapter introduces a variety of intake forms:

- Health information form
- Fees and policies
- Health report
- Pain questionnaires
- Injury information form
- Billing information form

All of these forms are completed before the initial session, and some are completed before every session or periodically to evaluate progress. Some forms are for all patients to fill out; others are only for patients whose insurance companies pay for their treatment. This chapter explains the purpose of each form and provides assistance in determining its appropriate application for your practice and for each patient.

Intake forms are easy to use and don't require one-on-one attention from the manual therapist. They are self-explanatory and can be filled out by the patient before the initial session without cutting into precious treatment time. It is a good idea to go over the forms with the patient after they are completed to ensure that they are filled out accurately. For example, if an attorney or physician has a question regarding the patient's responses on a form, it is critical that you know the responses are correct.

Once you have reviewed the forms, you are well-equipped to ask specific, personalized questions based on the information provided. These in-depth interviews are important in developing a better understanding of the individuals you are working with and their unique concerns and goals for health. Think of the forms and the ensuing interviews as stepping stones to building healing relationships.

Intake forms serve an additional purpose if the patient is relying on insurance for payment. Record keeping needs to meet two goals for insurance reimbursement. First, there must be justification of care on the specific day the patient is receiving treatment. Second, there must be justification for the patient's overall treatment plan.[1] To justify care, documentation must demonstrate that the injury was significant by recording the patient's symptoms and the effect of those symptoms on daily activities. To justify the treatment plan, the documentation must demonstrate that the treatment provided is reasonable and necessary. In other words, the treatment is justified if it has a positive effect on reducing the symptoms and returning the patient to normal function. The intake forms presented in this chapter will help you record this important information.

Personalize your intake forms with your logo and business information. Space is provided at the top of each form. Place your logo in a position where you won't lose information if your filing system requires you to punch holes in the top of your forms. (See Figure 5-1)

Health Information Form
CONTENT

A health information form is designed for patients to record four basic kinds of information:

- Personal identification and contact information
- Current health information
- Goals for health
- History of injuries, illnesses, and surgeries

Additional information may be included, such as a contract and consent for care, or a statement explaining your scope of practice and treatment goals. (For a blank form, see Appendix: Forms)

Questions in the four categories may vary according to the specialty of the practitioner. For example, a naturopath may include detailed questions regarding the person's diet in the section for current health status. A massage therapist may request more specific information on musculoskeletal dysfunction in the health history section. All basic categories pertain to all patients, regardless of their reasons for the visit.

Personal Identification and Contact Information

The patient's name and a date should appear on every piece of paper in the patient's file. The name connects the data to a living, breathing person, and can be used to organize the files. The date places the information in time, an important reference for tracking the progress of the condition. If multiple entries are made on a single page, each entry should be dated.

Cases involving insurance reimbursement require the claim number assigned to the case or the patient's insurance identification number (ID **#**) and the date of injury (DOI), when applicable, on every form sent to the insurance company. Use the same header on all forms—name, date, insurance ID **#**, and DOI—regardless of the method of payment. If insurance ID **#** and the DOI do not apply to the case, they can simply remain blank. If you omit these identifiers from the header, you risk omitting necessary information and causing a delay in insurance payment. (See Figure 5-1)

Record all possible contact numbers on the health information form. Know how to reach your patient in a timely fashion. Situations arise and appointments need to be changed. You may need to get information to the patient before a session. And don't forget, the patient's address is useful for marketing. Send birthday cards, referral thank-you cards, and discount coupons to stay in touch and show you care.

Be prepared in the unlikely event of an emergency. Have the patient list a contact person who can be reached immediately in case of a sudden illness or accident. At a minimum, a health information form should include the patient's name, date, and emergency contact in the identification and contact section.

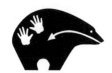

Helena LaLuna, CR
123 Sun Moon and Stars Drive
Capital Hill, WA   98119
Tel   206 555 4446

HEALTH INFORMATION

Patient Name _Zamora Hostetter_   Date _4-4-01_

Date of Injury _3-31-01_   Insurance ID# _C98-7654321_

Figure 5-1.   Personalized header.

Know how to contact the patient's referring health care provider (HCP). Health complications may require additional information or treatment consent. In addition, you may want to apprise other members of the health care team of the patient's progress. Make sure you have their phone, fax, and address. Later confirm how they wish to receive information.

On the health information form, request the permission of your patient to consult with the other health care providers on the patient's team. (See Figure 5-2) This request is courteous and models open communication. Most patients assume you will be in touch with their referring HCP. Others will appreciate being asked. Their doctors may not know they are receiving manual therapy, and the patients may want the chance to tell the doctors first. Some patients may have shared private information with you, and want to limit what can be discussed. Let them know what information you will be sharing, with whom, and why.

Current Health Information

This section asks the patient to list, prioritize, and classify current health concerns, and to identify how those conditions are affecting daily life. (See Figure 5-3) The goal is to identify why the patient is there so you can address the patient's needs and contribute to healing. Specific questions help the patient clarify their reasons for seeking manual therapy.

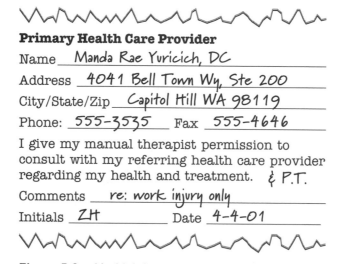

Primary Health Care Provider
Name _Manda Rae Yuricich, DC_
Address _4041 Bell Town Wy, Ste 200_
City/State/Zip _Capitol Hill WA 98119_
Phone: _555-3535_   Fax _555-4646_
I give my manual therapist permission to consult with my referring health care provider regarding my health and treatment. _& P.T._
Comments _re: work injury only_
Initials _ZH_   Date _4-4-01_

Figure 5-2.   Health Information—permission to consult with health care provider.

B. Current Health Information

List Health/Concerns Check all that apply

Primary ___shoulder pain___
☐ mild ☐ moderate ☒ disabling
☒ constant ☐ intermittant
☒ symptoms ↑ w/activity   ☐ ↓ w/activity
☐ getting worse ☐ getting better ☒ no change
treatment received ___ER–x-rays, sling___

Secondary ___back pain___
☐ mild ☒ moderate ☐ disabling
☒ constant ☐ intermittant
☒ symptoms ↑ w/activity   ☐ ↓ w/activity
☐ getting worse ☒ getting better ☐ no change
treatment received ___ER, DC–adjust.___

Additional ___neck pain & Headaches___
☒ mild ☐ moderate ☐ disabling
☐ constant ☒ intermittant
☒ symptoms ↑ w/activity   ☐ ↓ w/activity
☐ getting worse ☒ getting better ☐ no change
treatment received ___ER, DC___

Have you ever received Manual Therapy
before? ☐ Y ☒ N Frequency? _____

List all conditions currently monitored by a
Health Care Provider ___none___

_____

_____

List the medications you took today
(include pain relievers and herbal remedies)
___arnica, calcium, vitamins___

_____

List all other medications taken in the last
3 months ___none___

_____

Figure 5-3. Health Information—current health information.

Unmet expectations are often the product of unspoken desires. Leave little room for interpretation and be clear about goals for the session.

This type of information is useful for insurance cases to prove significant injury and thereby justify treatment. Symptoms and conditions and their effect on normal activities as stated by the patient are considered by the insurance adjusters and peer reviewers to validate care. Subjective documentation—information the patient reports—is critical. Intake forms record this subjective information. Objective information—data the health care provider discovers—confirms the loss of function and further substantiates the injury. The SOAP (Subjective, Objective, Assessment, Plan) chart, used to record objective findings, is covered in depth in Chapter 6.

In addition to recording the patient's concerns, this form also asks what treatment has the patient received for these conditions in the past. Use this information to formulate a treatment plan. You can eliminate techniques that were ineffective, avoid those that other practitioners on the health care team are using, and use or encourage solutions the patient found helpful. Consider the patient's goals for the session, together with your ideas for a treatment approach, and discuss the various options in the interview.

If the patient's condition is recent and the patient has not yet received treatment for this complaint, look to the general health history for information regarding a treatment approach. Something in the patient's history may have contributed to his current health, or the treatment sought for other conditions may provide information that shapes what could be a successful treatment plan for the unique individual before you.

Goals for Health

People don't have to be sick or injured to receive manual therapy. Many patients use manual therapy to stay healthy and reduce stress. Others strive for ease and efficiency while performing athletic and artistic activities. Manual therapy can be used to refine skills you already have, or help you enjoy being active late in life. Ask your patients about their goals for health and work with them to achieve the desired results. (See Figure 5-4)

Health History

This section consists of two parts: (1) a chart listing surgeries, accidents, and major illnesses, and (2) a checklist of symptoms and conditions. The chart allows the patient to identify major health crises and provides quick referencing for the practitioner. This information can provide insight into the origin of current conditions or identify factors that may influence those conditions. (See Figure 5-5)

Naomi Wachtel
567 Sunnydale Dr.
Flat Irons, CO   80302
Tel   303 555 8866

STANDARD HxTxC Chart

Name _Lin Pak_   Date _7-27-01_

Phone _(303) 555-0033 x 253_   Address _IBM 3rd Floor_

1. What are your goals for health, and how may I assist you in achieving your goals? _Limit longterm complications of diabetes through relaxation and stress reduction._

2. Are you currently experiencing any of the following? If yes, please explain.

   pain, tenderness   ☒ No ☐ Yes: _____   stiffness ☒ No ☐ Yes: _____

Figure 5-4. HxTxC Health History—goals for health.

C. Health History

List and Explain. Include dates and treatment
received.

Surgeries ___none___

Accidents ___Broken arm (R) fell out of tree___
___house in 1987, cast for 8 wks___

Major Illnesses ___none___

Figure 5-5. Health Information—health history.

▼

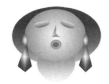

STORY TELLER 5-1

*Health History Affects
Current Condition*

Physical trauma can result in weakness and compensational posture or movement patterns, especially when untreated. These complications may cause concomitant dysfunction or contribute to chronic conditions. In one of our staff meetings, we discovered that the majority of patients with chronic repetitive stress injuries treated at the clinic had a history of previous soft tissue trauma, with whiplash topping the list. Sara, for example, was in a car accident as a teenager. She bounced right back and never thought about the experience again. Twenty years later, she suffers from recurring thoracic outlet syndrome. In the winter she painted every wall and ceiling in her house, in the summer she refinished the hardwood floors, and every spring after long gardening sprees, she was back at the clinic complaining of numbness and tingling in her right arm and hand. It wasn't until we discussed her case as a group that we considered her past history. The accident was so long ago, that no one gave it much thought. Once we determined that Sara had a poorly healed cervical sprain-strain injury, her treatment plan shifted and her condition subsided. Sara's case demonstrates that the chronological chart can help you identify pre-existing conditions that are adversely affecting current conditions. This prompts you to adjust the treatment plan to address the old trauma.

Following the chart is a checklist of symptoms and conditions, organized by body systems. The checklist provides an easy way to identify other factors that may be contributing to the current symptoms and to pinpoint conditions that may require special precautions. You can then apply your knowledge of indications and contraindications to the development of your treatment plan.

The form clearly identifies the pre-existing conditions that are currently symptomatic. (See Figure 5-6) This information is critical in the event of a motor vehicle accident (MVA). In personal injury cases, patients can expect that every attempt will be made to return them to pre-injury status, and that their insurance will cover the health care necessary to the full extent of their benefits. This coverage should include treatment for pre-existing conditions that were exacerbated by the accident.[1]

General

current	past		comments
☒	☐	headaches	MVA
☒	☒	pain	scoliosis
☒	☐	sleep disturbances	can't get comfortable
☐	☒	fatigue	scoliosis
☐	☐	Infectious	
☐	☐	fever	
☐	☐	sinus	
☐	☐	other	

Figure 5-6.   Health Information—checklist.

Contract and Consent for Care

The contract for care is an invitation for the patient to participate in treatment and share the responsibility for the result. It delineates the patient's commitment to the healing relationship. The goal is to empower the patient to become active in the healing process, and to promise goodwill on behalf of the manual therapist.

The consent for care states that the patient is actively choosing manual therapy and giving permission to the practitioner to provide treatment. It may warn of possible risks and limitations of the therapy. Know the limits of your scope of practice and state them clearly here. Include a statement about your practice philosophy and how you intend to assist the patient toward greater health.

▼

STORY TELLER 5-2

Sample Scope of Practice and Treatment Statement

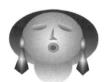

George uses this scope of practice statement as a licensed massage therapist in Washington, a state with a legally defined scope:

I understand that massage therapists do not diagnose medical, physical, or mental disorders, nor do they perform spinal manipulations by the use of a thrusting force. I acknowledge that massage therapy is not a substitute for medical examinations or treatment; massage therapy is complementary to medical services.

George explains the intent of his treatment sessions on his Health Information form this way:

Manual therapy is intended to help you learn more about the dynamics of health that are within your control—increased awareness of your patterns of movement and holding, responses to stress, and accumulation of tension. Manual therapy is a holistic approach to bridging mind and body. Together we will recognize your physical signals of diminishing health and enable you to respond to them in ways that promote vitality, balance, and spirit.[2]

End the health information form with a dated signature confirming that the information provided is complete and accurate, and the patient is consenting to receive treatment. Provide a space for the signature of a parent or legal guardian if the patient is under age 18. This signed statement is sometimes referred to as a treatment disclaimer or waiver. The patient's signature on the form may not legally protect you if something goes awry, but it demonstrates informed decisions regarding safe care. However, the most important element of the contract and consent for care is the verbal discussion that leads to an agreement to engage in a therapeutic relationship. As Jerry A. Green, a malpractice attorney in California and President of the Medical Decision Making Institute, states, "Remember: legal problems begin as disagreements. You prevent legal problems by making meaningful agreements."[2]

TIMING AND APPLICATION

A thorough history takes time to recreate. Instruct the patient to arrive 15–30 minutes before the initial appointment to ensure adequate time for filling out the forms. You may choose to save time by mailing out the health information form and all other applicable intake forms to the patient the week before the first session. People may breeze through the forms in your office because they are eager to get on with the session. When given their own time to think about the questions, to look things up if necessary, or to ask family members for help in reconstructing events, their information tends to be more complete. Occasionally, people forget to bring the forms to the initial session, but most remember and make it worth the trouble of mailing the forms in advance. Even if they forget the forms, filling them out a second time goes much more quickly.

Regardless of individual goals for treatment, each patient should complete a basic health information form annually. If the patient has progressive or degenerative health problems, or if the patient's health changes, the form should be updated semiannually or quarterly.

Use the form as an information database and refer to it for interviewing the patient, designing the treatment plan, identifying possible cautions for care, and contacting the patient throughout the relationship. If an insurance case manager or an attorney request the patient's file, this document may be used to substantiate the patient's injury and to determine the presence of pre-existing conditions.

Fees and Policies

CONTENT

Fees and policies include a **fee schedule**, payment options, and miscellaneous office policies. Determine the policies you need to be financially sound and to set clear boundaries. You can always be more lenient later if special circumstances arise, but it is difficult to get tough after the fact. Ensure your safety by defining the patient behavior necessary for you to relax and enjoy your practice.

Fee Schedules

Fees may be delineated by modalities, stating the various services you offer and the costs associated with each. (See Figure 5-7) Provide a breakdown of the fees in 15-minute in-

A. Fee Schedule

Fees for services are as follows:

- CranioSacral/Lymph Drainage (97140)
  $80 per hour
  ($20 per 15 minute unit)
- Feldenkrais (97112)
  $80 per hour
  ($20 per 15 minute unit)
- Hot and Cold Packs (97101)
  $15 per session
  ($15 per session)
- Therapeutic Massage (97124)
  $60 Per Hour
  ($15 per 15 minute unit)

Figure 5-7. Fees and Policies—fee schedule.

crements. Most **Current Procedural Terminology (CPT) codes**—codes that define standard therapeutic procedures and modalities, and assign time frames for the purposes of insurance billing and reimbursement—assign most physical medicine procedures to 15-minute units. If you provide billing services in your practice, describe your fees for services in 15 minute increments.

Another method for setting your fee schedule is to charge by time rather than by modalities. This method is also known as **bundling** services. A flat fee includes any manual therapy applied that can be billed under one procedural code. For example, you may use Swedish massage, myofascial release, lymph drainage, trigger point therapy, acupressure, and muscle energy techniques in varying combinations, but find it difficult to break it down into time per modality. You may choose to bill using the general massage therapy procedural code and not bother with five different procedure codes and five different rates. Bundling services are common in cash practices and can be used with a billing practice as long as you are not bundling procedures that would be reimbursed at a lower rate than the one you are billing under (a practice known as **upcoding**). Keep in mind that if you have one rate for cash patients, you should use the same fee schedule for your billing patients. If an insurance auditor finds that you used myofascial release and lymph drainage on cash patients but didn't charge them as much as you are charging the insurance company for the same modalities, they may require you to refund them the difference.

State any discounts you offer patients who pay at the time service is rendered. They are allowed within reason as long as they apply to insurance patients as well as cash-paying patients. Check your local laws for requirements and exceptions, if any.

Payment Policies

The payment policies section states the payment methods available and clarifies the type of insurance reimbursement you will accept and under what circumstances. (See Figure 5-8) Insurance reimbursement arrangements vary from manual therapist to manual therapist, from state to state, and from country to country, depending on the scope of practice of the individual therapies and the insurance climate of the region. Be informed of the specific risks and benefits of insurance billing for your unique situation before setting a policy.

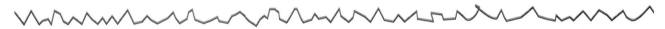

B. Payment Policies

Cash or Check

- A 10% discount is available when payment is made at the time services are provided.
- Pre-payment discounts: 6 sessions for the price of 5.

Billing

I will bill your insurance company directly under the following conditions:

Private Health: verbal verification of coverage
Worker's Compensation: verbal verification of coverage

Auto Accident

- PIP: verbal verification of coverage
- Second Party Coverage: written verification of coverage
- Third Party Coverage: health care lien will be filed and/or letter of guarantee signed by the patient's attorney

All insurance accounts not paid in full within 90 days from date of service will be charged interest. Interest rates are 12% annually and are charged at 1% monthly. Interest is calculated on the principal amount; interest is not compounded.

C. Office Policies

Figure 5-8. Fees and Policies—payment.

It is acceptable to charge interest on past due accounts. Many states have laws regarding interest terms and start dates as they apply to medical services, such as 12% per year simple interest beginning 60 days after the billing date. Know what those are and specify your terms clearly. It is generally mandated that the patient be made aware of interest rates before their accrual.

Office Policies

Provide written statements of your office policies. Make sure your patients read them and agree to abide by them. Require a signature demonstrating that the patient has read and understands your policies. It is easier to enforce something that is in writing, signed, and dated. Keep the signed form in their file. You may have to remind your patients of these policies at a later date.

Cancellation policies are common in practices in which one session makes up a significant percentage of the daily income. Set a standard cancellation fee or charge the full price of the session if the patient fails to cancel within a specified number of hours before the scheduled time. Consider abiding by your own cancellation policy. For example, offer a similar discount to those patients whose appointments you cancel without a 24-hour notice.

Right of refusal is another common office policy. This policy can be helpful for turning away people who are impaired by alcohol or drugs, have an infectious illness, push for treatment outside your scope of practice, or behave inappropriately. It is important to set boundaries, feel safe in your practice, and have permission to take care of yourself. Use this policy any time you have a gut instinct to do so.

TIMING AND APPLICATION

The patient should read and sign your fees and policies before the first session. Include the policy statement with the health information form and any other intake forms completed by the patient at the initial visit. Post your fees and policies to reinforce what you are requiring the patients to read and sign, and to demonstrate your professionalism to potential patients who walk in off the street.

Health Report

CONTENT

The health report provides a snapshot of the patient's health. (For a blank form, see Appendix: Forms) In a few minutes, the patient can chart the location of pain, stiffness, and numbness by writing letters (P for pain, S for stiffness, N for numbness) on the human figures, and can rate his pain and loss of function by placing a dash on the lines of the analog scales. The drawings provide a map of the patient's symptoms that is accurate and easy to read. Below the figures are two analog scales or lines of continuum, one denoting pain, the other activity level. The mark on the line is measured, a numerical score is calculated and recorded, making references to progress a snap.

The health report is the form mentioned in the case study of Sandee in Chapter 4. The benefits of this form are great for the patient and the practitioner. Progress is recorded in the patient's own handwriting, convincing even the most frustrated patients of their health improvements. The manual therapist can use this form to support the health history interview, gathering pertinent information from tentative patients, and streamlining the discussion with the chatty ones.

Human Figures

Learning styles are widely considered in today's classrooms. Visual, auditory, and tactile learners have different ways of processing and storing information. The same is true for patients. Some enjoy filling out forms, others would rather tell you about themselves, and often do so in story format. Still others can draw images more easily than filling in the blanks or talking. Provide a variety of ways to gather information: multiple choice forms, one-on-one communication, and pictures to draw on, such as the ones on the health report. (See Figure 5-9)

Coaxing information from some patients can feel like pulling teeth. Maybe they were taught not to complain, or they are just not comfortable speaking to people they do not know well. For those patients, drawing symptoms on pictures may be easier than having to talk about their pain or disability.

With other patients, trying to keep the interview under 5 minutes is challenging. Some would rather talk about their problems than solve them. Others chatter when they get nervous. Gather the salient pieces of information on a form each session. Once the current information is recorded and reviewed, a few brief questions may suffice to prepare for the session.

Analog Scales

An analog scale is a method of measurement that uses a line of continuum and places one extreme on one end and the opposite extreme on the other end. For example, on this form

A. Draw today's symptoms on the figures.

1. Identify CURRENT symptomatic areas in your body by marking letters on the figures below. Use the letters provided in the key to identify the symptoms you are feeling today.
2. Circle the area around each letter, representing the size and shape of each symptom location.

Key
P = pain or tenderness
S = joint or muscle stiffness
N = numbness or tingling

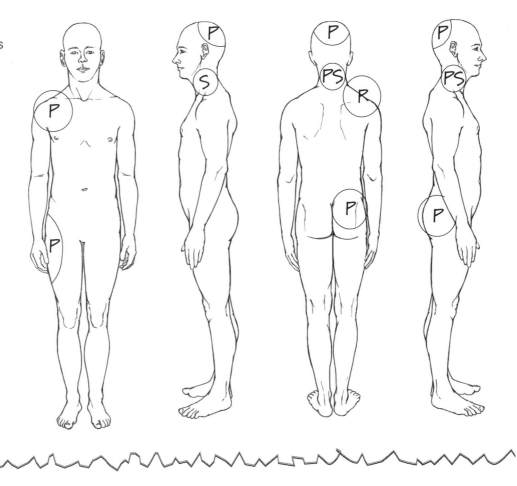

Figure 5-9. Health Report—figures.

we are measuring the patient's pain or loss of function. On the line of continuum, pain free is at one end and debilitating pain is at the other end. The patient places a mark at a point between the two extremes that best represents how they feel at the moment. (See Figure 5-10)

Analog scales are reliable and more accurate than using a numerical rating scale, such as 0–10. The literature suggests that numbers can be remembered from session to session, decreasing the validity of the responses. A malingerer may remember a previous response and manipulate the answer accordingly.[1]

It is cumbersome to use these scales with each subjective complaint or objective finding. A verbal response is indicated during the session; pulling out a piece of paper and a pen is inappropriate. The number scale (0–10) or the word values (mild, moderate, severe) are preferred. Used on the health report, the analog scale is effective and addresses the two primary concerns in health care outcomes: function and pain.

To use the analog scale, the patient simply places a mark on the lines to indicate pain level at that moment. The line represents a continuum ranging from pain free to unbear-

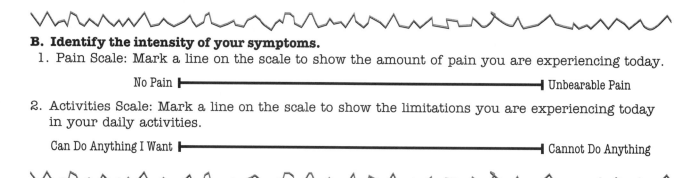

B. Identify the intensity of your symptoms.

1. Pain Scale: Mark a line on the scale to show the amount of pain you are experiencing today.

No Pain ├───┤ Unbearable Pain

2. Activities Scale: Mark a line on the scale to show the limitations you are experiencing today in your daily activities.

Can Do Anything I Want ├───────────────────────────────┤ Cannot Do Anything

Figure 5-10. Health Report—analog scales.

able pain, or from full activity to no activity. The line is 10 centimeters long, making it easy to score the patient's mark on a scale of 0 to 10. On a scale of pain free to unbearable pain, for example, pain free is given the value zero, and unbearable pain is given the value ten. The mark is placed between the two values and the measurement is assigned a value 0–10. The measurement is the score. After the session, measure the mark on the line and record the score in the comments section.

TIMING AND APPLICATION

Patients with injuries or chronic conditions should complete the Health Report before and after each treatment session. If the patient has no subjective complaints, such as pain, loss of function, stiff joints, or neuropathies, simply include the report in the packet of intake forms at the initial visit and the annual updates, to ensure you have all the health information you need.

The health report provides a quick and easy update on how the patient is feeling at each session. Over time it demonstrates progress from session to session. When used before and after each session, it charts the results of the session. These results justify the treatment plan, and document progress.

If motivating yourself to chart is an issue, this form is a simple way to ease into the habit of regular documentation. Have the patient do most of the charting for you! This short-cut is not recommended for insurance patients or for long-term care, but it is a good way to get started. Use the "Comments" section of the form to record your treatment notes, and let the patient do the pre- and post-session subjective documentation for you. As you proceed through this book, you will discover the limitations of using this form for all your daily charting needs, but if necessary, begin with the health report for your daily note-taking. (See Figure 5-11)

Pain Questionnaires

Research shows that pain questionnaires are a reliable and effective tool for measuring the extent and nature of a patient's injury and its improvement with treatment. (See Wise One Speaks 5-1: The Reliability of Pain Questionnaires.) Proof of significant injury is provided through the **disability percentage**. The treatment plan is justified with ongoing use of the questionnaires.

Pain questionnaires consist of questions regarding the patient's ability to sit, stand, wash and dress, walk, sleep, read, drive, travel, work, concentrate, and recreate. The pa-

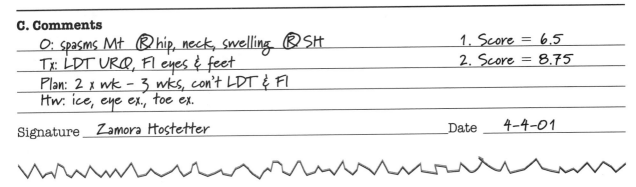

C. Comments

O: spasms Mt Ⓡ hip, neck, swelling Ⓡ SH   1. Score = 6.5

Tx: LDT URQ, Fl eyes & feet   2. Score = 8.75

Plan: 2 x wk – 3 wks, con't LDT & Fl

Hw: ice, eye ex., toe ex.

Signature _Zamora Hostetter_   Date   _4-4-01_

Figure 5-11.   Health Report with treatment notes.

tient answers the questions by checking one of six options provided. The manual therapist collects the form and scores the answers, using a disability percentage scale. Over time, the scores can be compared and progress can be concluded based on the change in scores.

Several pain questionnaires are available. Two are presented in this text: the **Revised Oswestry Low Back Pain and Disability Index** and the **Vernon-Mior Neck Pain and Disability Index**. (For blank forms, see Appendix: Forms) Both indices are backed by strong research and are almost identical in content. Both can be creatively used for other areas of dysfunction—the Vernon-Mior for the upper extremities, and the Oswestry for the lower extremities.

If used throughout a treatment series, pain questionnaires record functional progress. A progressive increase in functional abilities throughout the treatment assists in demonstrating that the treatment is reasonable and necessary. Functional progress reassures the patient, the referring HCP, and the medical-legal team that the treatment is returning the patient to pre-injury status.

▼

WISE ONE SPEAKS 5-1

The Reliability of Pain Questionnaires

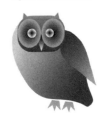

Traditionally, objective measurements of soft tissue injury such as palpable spasm, loss of lordotic curve on x-ray, etc., have been thought reliable as "hard evidence" when measuring the extent of injury and the effectiveness of treatment, while subjective pain and function assessments were criticized as "soft evidence." However, subjective pain assessments as measured through time-tested pain questionnaires have gained substantial acceptance in use and are now considered "hard evidence."[3, 4, 5]

A pain questionnaire, when used together with objective physical measurements, is considered the most reliable assessment of function and disability in the area in which there is no universal norm. One such pain questionnaire is the Oswestry Index, which was developed in 1976 in a hospital unit in Oswestry, Shropshire, England. It scores patients' disability in ten different areas including intensity of pain; ability to lift, walk, sit, and stand; ability for self-care; and impact on social interactions, sex life, sleep, and travel.

Studies have confirmed that the Oswestry Index has good validity (scores improve as patient disability lessens) and reliability (scores are consistent when answered on different occasions by a patient remaining in the same condition).[5] After many refinements, this questionnaire is widely used in both research and clinical

100

HANDS HEAL:
COMMUNICATION,
DOCUMENTATION,
AND INSURANCE BILLING
FOR MANUAL THERAPISTS

practice in Britain. Self-rating disability questionnaires are also in wide use in North America.

As health care providers know, all tools that assist in documenting the nature and extent of a patient's injury and the patient's improvement with treatment are vital. A well-formatted and consistently used pain questionnaire can assist you in monitoring the reasonableness and necessity of your treatment (by showing the day-to day improvements of your patient) for insurance or medical-legal purposes. There is the added benefit that when asked to submit a narrative report or testify at a deposition or trial, you will be invaluably aided in recounting the patient's treatment by the assessment of progress and/or remaining levels of pain and dysfunction.

(Reprinted with permission, all rights reserved. Adler, Giersch, Pain Questionnaire. Article of the Month, Seattle: Adler ◆ Giersch PS, 1991.)

TIMING AND APPLICATION

Pain questionnaires are easy to use and involve a minimal time commitment. You or your staff can provide them to patients on a weekly basis for acute cases, semiweekly or monthly for chronic cases. The patient fills them out before the session begins. You collect the form, check it for completeness, score it, review it, and file it in the patient's chart.

Include pain questionnaires with the initial forms patients complete before the first visit. To use the pain questionnaires, instruct your patient to read the instructions at the top and to fill the form out completely. If a section is incomplete, return it to the patient for completion. Avoid discussing with the patient the reason for using the pain questionnaire. Advising patients on how the process works may influence responses on subsequent questionnaires. Score, review, and look for areas of impaired function. If loss of function is present in any area, repeat the use as suggested above. Or, check the patient's completed health information form for changes in daily activities caused by the patient's current condition prior to handing out the pain questionnaire. If there is no loss of function indicated on the health information form, you may chose to omit the pain questionnaire from the intake forms pack for that particular patient.

SCORING THE PAIN QUESTIONNAIRE

To score the questionnaires, a pain value is assigned to each answer. There are ten sections per questionnaire and six possible answers in each section. The top answer has a pain value of 0. The bottom answer has a pain value of 5. Assign each section a score of 0–5, depending on the answer.

Add all ten scores together. The highest possible score (worst pain) would be 5 for each section, or a total score of 50 ($5 \times 10 = 50$). Multiply this number by two to reach the overall rating of disability, ($50 \times 2 = 100\%$). This number is your disability percentage. (See Figure 5-12)

The rating scale is as follows:

0–20%	Minimal disability
20–40%	Moderate disability
40–60%	Severe disability
60–80%	Crippled
80–100%	Bed bound or exaggerating

Helena LaLuna, CR

123 Sun Moon and Stars Drive
Capital Hill, WA   98119
TEL   206 555 4446

® shoulder   (revised Vernon-Mior)
~~NECK~~ PAIN & DISABILITY INDEX

Patient Name _Zamora Hostetter_   Date _4-4-01_

Date of Injury _3-31-01_   Insurance ID# _C98-7654321_

This questionnaire has been designed to give the health care provider information as to how your neck pain has affected your ability to manage everyday life. Please answer every section and mark in each section only the **ONE** box which applies to you. We realize you may consider that two of the statements in any one section relate to you, but please just mark the box which most closely describes your problem today.

3 Section 1 - Pain Intensity
- ☐ I have no pain at the moment.
- ☐ The pain is very mild at the moment.
- ☐ The pain is moderate at the moment.
- ☒ The pain is fairly severe at the moment.
- ☐ The pain is very severe at the moment.
- ☐ The pain is the worst imaginable at the moment.

3 Section 2 - Personal Care
(washing, dressing, etc.)
- ☐ I can look after myself normally without causing pain.
- ☐ I can look after myself normally but it causes extra pain.
- ☐ It is painful to look after myself and I am slow and careful.
- ☒ I need some help but manage most of my personal care.
- ☐ I need help every day in most aspects of self care.
- ☐ I do not get dressed, I wash myself with difficulty and I stay in bed.

5 Section 3 - Lifting
- ☐ I can lift heavy weights without extra pain.
- ☐ I can lift heavy weights but it causes extra pain.
- ☐ Pain prevents me from lifting heavy weights off the floor, but I can manage if they are conveniently positioned, e.g. on a table.
- ☐ Pain prevents me from lifting heavy weights, but I can manage light to medium weights if they are conveniently positioned.
- ☐ I can lift very light weights.
- ☒ I cannot lift or carry anything at all.

1 Section 4 - Reading
- ☐ I can read as much as I want to with no pain in my neck.
- ☒ I can read as much as I want to with slight pain in my neck.
- ☐ I can read as much as I want to with moderate pain in my neck.
- ☐ I can't read as much as I want to because of moderate pain in my neck.
- ☐ I can hardly read at all because of severe pain in my neck.
- ☐ I cannot read at all.

3 Section 5 - Headaches
- ☐ I have no headaches at all.
- ☐ I have slight headaches which come infrequently.
- ☐ I have moderate headaches which come infrequently.
- ☒ I have moderate headaches which come frequently.
- ☐ I have severe headaches which come frequently.
- ☐ I have headaches almost all of the time.

1 Section 6 - Concentration
- ☐ I can concentrate fully when I want to with no difficulty.
- ☒ I can concentrate fully when I want to with slight difficulty.
- ☐ I have a fair degree of difficulty in concentrating when I want to.
- ☐ I have a lot of difficulty concentrating when I want to.
- ☐ I have a great deal of difficulty in concentrating when I want to.
- ☐ I cannot concentrate at all.

5 Section 7 - Work
- ☐ I can do as much work as I want to.
- ☐ I can do my usual work but no more.
- ☐ I can do most of my usual work but no more.
- ☐ I cannot do my usual work.
- ☐ I can hardly do any work at all.
- ☒ I can't do any work at all.

1 Section 8 - Driving
- ☐ I can drive my car without any neck pain.
- ☒ I can drive my car as long as I want with slight pain in my neck.
- ☐ I can drive my car as long as I want with moderate pain in my neck.
- ☐ I can't drive my car as long as I want because of moderate pain in my neck.
- ☐ I can hardly drive at all because of severe pain in my neck.
- ☐ I can't drive my car at all.

4 Section 9 - Sleeping
- ☐ I have no trouble sleeping.
- ☐ My sleep is slightly disturbed (less than 1 hour sleepless).
- ☐ My sleep is mildly disturbed (1–2 hours sleepless).
- ☐ My sleep is moderately disturbed (2–3 hours sleepless).
- ☒ My sleep is greatly disturbed (3–5 hours sleepless).
- ☐ My sleep is completely disturbed (5–7 hours sleepless).

30 x 2 = 60%

4 Section 10 - Recreation
- ☐ I am able to engage in all my recreational activities with no neck pain at all.
- ☐ I am able to engage in all my recreational activities with some pain in my neck.
- ☐ I am able to engage in most, but not all of my usual recreational activities because of pain in my neck.
- ☐ I am able to engage in a few of my usual recreation activities because of pain in my neck.
- ☒ I can hardly do any recreational activities because of pain in my neck.
- ☐ I can't do recreational activities at all.

Signature _Zamora Hostetter_   Date _4-4-01_

Figure 5-12.   Pain Questionnaire with Disability Percentage.

102

HANDS HEAL:
COMMUNICATION,
DOCUMENTATION,
AND INSURANCE BILLING
FOR MANUAL THERAPISTS

Injury Information Form
CONTENT

The health information form is sufficient for wellness care and most illnesses or injuries. Additional information is necessary when a patient has been involved in an on-the-job injury or a car accident. Different types of insurance cover different kinds of injuries or benefits. Workers' compensation covers on-the-job injuries and illnesses. Private, or group insurance (through an employer), covers general injuries or illnesses. Personal injury protection (PIP) covers injuries related to MVAs. In-depth documentation is recommended to address the specific needs of litigation and of national and state workers' compensation regulations.

As with any insurance case, documentation is vital. The primary difference between record keeping for cash-paying patients and for patients with insurance reimbursement is that care can be discontinued and payment can be reversed or even denied by the insurance company based on the documentation.[1] The injury information form records specific data that may assist in substantiating the patient's claim and in providing information required by insurance companies to continue coverage for your services. (For a blank form, see Appendix: Forms) The mechanics of the injury, symptoms, daily activities affected by the injuries, and any possible health complications resulting from the accident must be documented. The goal is to gather information to substantiate that the injuries are significant and were incurred as a result of the accident and thus justify care.

Personal Identification and Contact Information

The four identifiers—name date, insurance ID **#**, and date of injury—top each form. The address and phone numbers are not included, as this form is used with the health information form.

General Injury Information

Page one of the injury information form is filled out by people with any of the three types of injuries: on-the-job, MVAs, and other personal injuries. Page two is only for people involved in MVAs. For a personal injury case, differentiate between an MVA and other types of injury. Examples of a personal injury case other than a car accident are a patient who was injured falling off the roof of the house while cleaning the gutters, slipping on commercial premises, or being impaled by debris flying from a construction site while walking on the sidewalk.

Type of Injury

On-the-job injuries and MVAs typically result in musculoskeletal dysfunction and therefore are common in manual therapy practices. Musculoskeletal complaints are the number one reason people seek manual therapy.[6] Differentiate between workers' compensation claims and personal injury cases on the injury information form.

Establish whether a record of the incident is on file somewhere other than in your patient's chart. Such records are helpful in substantiating the injury. A person involved in an MVA might have a police report on file, unless there was no significant vehicle damage. Someone injured on the job may have filed an incident report. Both may apply if the person had an MVA while on the job. If a police report has been filed, request a copy.

Description of the Injury

Information provided by the patient about the onset of the injury might explain the presence and severity of symptoms. (See Figure 5-13) On-the-job injuries and personal injuries other than car accidents vary widely, making it impossible to standardize the questions about onset. Prompt those patients to be as specific as possible when describing how the injuries occurred.

Page two of this form asks standard questions and records specific information about the mechanics of MVAs. However, it is important to focus on how the patient got hurt, rather than how the accident occurred. The questions on the injury information form must be stated clearly, and you need to review the answers thoroughly with the patient to ensure the answers are accurate and suitable.

▼

STORY TELLER 5-3

Mechanisms of Injury

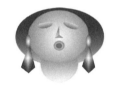

Describing the mechanisms of injury helps explain the type and extent of injury. In the example presented in Figure 5-13, Zamora fell on a hard surface. This injury is more damaging than if she had fallen on grass or bags of rice. As a result, the severity of her injuries may be substantial. Her arms, hips, back, and head all hit an unforgiving tile floor, complicating the overall injury. How she impacted the ground may explain the location of her shoulder injury. Encourage the patient to describe the details about how the injury took place: the environment and the interplay between the body and the objects involved, in addition to the obvious symptoms or physical expressions of the injury.

Describe the details of the injury, but avoid documenting the events that lead up to the injury. At the massage clinic, we treated a patient who was hit by a car while riding her bicycle. She was meticulous in describing the accident on the injury information form. Something that occurred in a fraction of a second seemed to happen in slow motion from the patient's perspective. She described it as it appeared to her, without reference to actual time. Unfortunately, the way in which she recorded her description of the accident made it appear that she had time to prevent it. This impression complicated her personal injury case, making it difficult to receive reimbursement for her health care. Her case went to court.

The lesson in this experience was to let the police report speak to the accident, and use the injury information form to describe the onset of the injury. Had she focused on the mechanics of the injury—for example, how she fell, what body parts hit the pavement—rather than on how the car approached her and what went through her mind leading up to the impact, she might have been able to settle out of court quickly and without disruption in medical payments.

Symptoms

Have the patient record all symptoms since the accident. Establish a timeline for the onset of the injuries. Not all symptoms surface immediately. It may be weeks before the patient seeks manual therapy. The timeline will help chart the progression of the injuries and the healing. (See Figure 5-14)

Effect of Injuries on Daily Activities

An easy way to determine whether an injury is affecting the patient's quality of life is to look at the patient's ability to function in day-to-day activities. (See Figure 5-15) If the

104

HANDS HEAL:
COMMUNICATION,
DOCUMENTATION,
AND INSURANCE BILLING
FOR MANUAL THERAPISTS

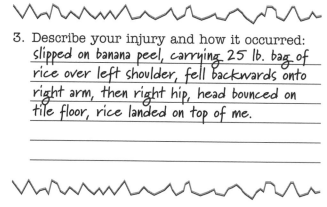

3. Describe your injury and how it occurred:
slipped on banana peel, carrying 25 lb. bag of
rice over left shoulder, fell backwards onto
right arm, then right hip, head bounced on
tile floor, rice landed on top of me.

Figure 5-13. Injury Information—description of injury.

patient's ability to earn a living is impaired, the injury is significant. Such an impairment may include loss of time at work, restrictions of responsibilities (such as assignment to light duty), and loss of productivity. Documentation of changes in work-related activities is critical with many claims, particularly on-the-job injuries.

Activities other than work are also important to one's quality of life. Inability to participate normally in exercise, self-care, and household responsibilities should be recorded. Anything that detracts from the patient's quality of life may be included for personal injuries and for injuries covered by major medical plans. Focus on work-related impairments for workers' compensation cases.

4. Describe how you felt during and immediately after the injury:
shoulder "popped"—immediate pain, head throbbing

Later that same day: backache

The next day: neck stiff, back stiff, can't use Right arm at all

The next week: N/A

The next month: N/A

Describe any bruises, cuts, or abrasions as a result of the injury:
bruise on right hip

Figure 5-14. Injury Information—symptom timeline.

7. What are your work responsibilities?
   cooking, prep, stocking supplies

   Which work activities are affected by this injury? _everything_

   Have your work responsibilities changed as a result of this injury? ☒ Yes ☐ No
   Explain _unable to work_

   What other daily activities are affected by this injury? _everything using my right arm_

Figure 5-15. Injury Information—functional limitations.

Adjunctive Care

Have the patient list all care received for the injury. (See Figure 5-16) This information is helpful for communicating with the health care team, reducing the chance of duplicating treatment, and coordinating treatment plans. Record the primary HCP's diagnosis. You can then refer to the diagnosis in your charts.

Typically, insurance peer reviewers red-flag a case if manual therapy is the only source of treatment, unless the manual therapist has primary care status. The combination of allopathic and complementary care is more acceptable. Noting additional care may help justify the treatment and speed up claims processing.

Pre-existing Conditions

Establish the presence of pre-existing conditions right away. Avoid the unpleasant surprise when the insurance company disallows payment for services because the symptoms treated were present before the accident.

8. Did you go to the emergency room?
   ☒ Yes ☐ No
   Were you hospitalized? ☐ Yes ☒ No
   List the health care providers who have treated you for this injury, the type of treatment provided, and their diagnosis.
   ER—separated shoulder—sling
   DC—whiplash, spinal subluxations, muscle
   spasms—adjust, ice

Figure 5-16. Injury Information—adjunctive care.

106

HANDS HEAL:
COMMUNICATION,
DOCUMENTATION,
AND INSURANCE BILLING
FOR MANUAL THERAPISTS

The information recorded here and on the health information form can help establish that current symptoms, even if associated with pre-existing conditions, are related to the accident. (See Figure 5-17) If the documents state that none of the symptoms were present before, or that the pre-existing symptoms were exacerbated by the current injury, it is easier for the attorney or claims adjuster to conclude that the symptoms were a direct result of the accident or work injury.

Motor Vehicle Accident Information

Mechanisms of Whiplash

Page two of the injury information form highlights the mechanisms that influence the severity of a whiplash injury. (See Figure 5-18) Severity of injury is critical to establish whether extensive, on-going treatment is required to return the patient to pre-injury status. Some research studies suggest that people heal from MVAs in 6–8 weeks, regardless of treatment. This may be true for very minor soft tissue injuries, but not for more complex sprain-strain syndromes or injuries presenting with neurological dysfunction.[7]

Symptoms

Symptoms are gathered on several of the intake forms. The symptoms checklist on this form are specific to head trauma sustained in whiplash injuries and may indicate neurological damage. This information influences the type of care you provide and the type of referrals you suggest, but it generally does not come up in an interview unless specifically asked. Loss of memory is not as obvious as the pounding headache or the bruises. The patient may forget to tell you about them unless prompted on the form.

Other questions about symptoms are more general than the head injury questions above, but also concern symptoms common with whiplash trauma. Breathing difficulties are often associated with seat belt trauma. Sleeping comfort may be used later in the SOAP charts as a tool for mapping progress: track the number of hours of restful sleep, the number of times waking and why, and how the patient feels upon rising, to show the progression of health.

9. Have you ever had this type of injury before? ☐ Yes ☒ No

Explain _____

_____

Did you have any physical complaints before the injury? ☐ Yes ☒ No

Explain _____

_____

Do you have any illnesses or previous injuries that may have been affected by this injury? ☐ Yes ☒ No

Explain _____

_____

Figure 5-17. Injury Information—pre-existing conditions.

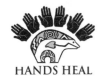

John Olson, LMP, GCFP
345 Moon River Rd. Ste. 6
Minnehaha, MN   55987
TEL   612 555 9889

HANDS HEAL

INJURY INFORMATION page 2

B. Motor Vehicle Accident Information

1. Did the police arrive at the accident?
   ☒ Yes   ☐ No

2. How was your vehicle hit?
   ☒ Rear end   ☐ Head on   ☐ Side swipe
   OR Did your vehicle hit another vehicle/object?
   ☐ Rear end   ☐ Head on   ☐ Side swipe
   If you were hit from behind, was your vehicle pushed forward upon impact?
   ☒ Yes   ☐ No   If yes, how much?
   about 50 feet
   Did your vehicle hit anything else after the initial impact?   ☐ Yes   ☐ No
   Explain _____
   _____
   _____
   _____

3. Were you at a stop or moving at the time of impact?   ☐ Stopped   ☒ Moving
   If you were stopped, was your foot on the brake?   ☐ Yes   ☐ No
   If you were moving, were you:
   ☐ Increasing speed
   ☒ Decreasing speed
   ☐ Traveling at a steady speed
   Was the other vehicle moving at the time of impact?   ☒ Yes   ☐ No
   If yes, was it: ☒ Increasing speed
   ☐ Decreasing speed   ☐ Traveling at a steady speed

4. Where were you seated in the vehicle?
   passenger side-front seat
   _____

5. Which way was your head facing upon impact?
   facing nephew-driver, we were talking
   _____

6. Were you aware of the approaching vehicle or did the impact catch you by surprise?
   ☐ Aware   ☒ Surprise

7. Did you lose consciousness?
   ☐ Yes   ☒ No

8. Were you wearing a seat belt?   ☐ No
   ☐ Lap belt   ☐ Shoulder harness   ☒ Both

9. Is your vehicle equipped with an airbag?
   ☐ Yes   ☒ No
   Did it activate?   ☐ Yes   ☐ No

10. Is the top of your head rest:
    ☐ Above your head   ☒ Below your head
    Does your head touch the head rest?
    ☐ Yes   ☒ No
    If no, how far in front of the head rest is your head?
    a few inches

11. What were the road conditions?
    ☐ Wet   ☐ Dry   ☒ Icy   ☐ Oily

12. What type of vehicle were you in? (make, model, year)
    '82 Honda Accord
    What type of vehicle hit you? (make, model, year)
    '91 Ford F250 Truck

13. Did any part of your body come into contact with the vehicle?   ☐ Yes   ☒ No
    Explain _____
    _____
    _____
    Did any parts of the vehicle break?
    ☒ Yes   ☐ No
    Explain _fender damage_
    _____
    _____
    _____

14. Check all of the following symptoms that you have experienced since the accident:
    ☐ Loss of memory _____
    ☐ Loss of balance _____
    ☒ Visual disturbances _eye strain_
    ☐ Hearing difficulties _____
    ☒ Difficulty breathing _tight & painful_
    ☒ Sleep disturbances _pain keeps me up_

15. Anything else you want to tell me about the accident or how you feel?
    _____
    _____
    _____

Patient Signature _Darnel G. Washington_   Date _2-6-01_

Figure 5-18. Injury Information—MVA.

108

HANDS HEAL:
COMMUNICATION,
DOCUMENTATION,
AND INSURANCE BILLING
FOR MANUAL THERAPISTS

External proof of impact is concrete data. Record any visible trauma. Take pictures of bruises, cuts, and abrasions.

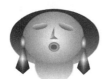
At the massage clinic, we had a patient who, after five car accidents in 8 years, began taking public transportation. She stepped off the bus one day, and the bus hit her. Bruises marking the headlights were imprinted on her chest and abdomen. Some pictures are worth a thousand words.

Space is left at the end of the form for the patient to add comments. It is impossible to cover all possibilities in a standardized form. There is bound to be pertinent information unique to the individual.

TIMING AND APPLICATION

The patient completes this form before the initial session. The injury information form may accompany the health information form in a packet of intake forms sent to the patient the week before the first treatment. The patient fills out the forms at home and brings them to the office. The injury information form needs to be completed only once per incident.

All patients fill out a health information form; all personal injury and workers' compensation patients also fill out the injury information form. Only those involved in an MVA fill out page two of the injury information form. Keep the health information and the injury information forms separate, so as not to burden other patients with unnecessary paperwork.

Injury information is useful in the interview and in the development of a treatment plan. The information recorded is vital to workers' compensation and personal injury cases, and is used to substantiate the injury and justify the treatment.

Billing Information Form
CONTENT

The billing information form gathers all the data necessary to complete the top half of the HCFA 1500, the standard billing form for insurance companies. (See Figure 5-19) (For a blank form, see Appendix: Forms) This information includes:

- Personal identification and contact information—patient and insured
- Insurance information—primary and secondary coverage
- Assignment of benefits
- Release of medical records

(Instructions for filling out the remainder of the HCFA 1500 form are found in Chapter 8.)

Personal Identification and Contact Information

All pertinent contact information is included on the billing information form: the patient, the insurance company and adjuster, the attorney, and the primary care provider. If the pa-

PLEASE
DO NOT
STAPLE
IN THIS
AREA

← CARRIER →

PICA

HEALTH INSURANCE CLAIM FORM

PICA

← PATIENT AND INSURED INFORMATION →

1. MEDICARE (Medicare #) ☐ MEDICAID (Medicaid #) ☐ CHAMPUS (Sponsor's SSN) ☐ CHAMPVA (VA File #) ☐ GROUP HEALTH PLAN (SSN or ID) ☐ FECA BLK LUNG (SSN) ☐ OTHER (ID) ☐

1a. INSURED'S I.D. NUMBER (FOR PROGRAM IN ITEM 1)

2. PATIENT'S NAME (Last Name, First Name, Middle Initial)

3. PATIENT'S BIRTH DATE MM | DD | YY SEX M ☐ F ☐

4. INSURED'S NAME (Last Name, First Name, Middle Initial)

5. PATIENT'S ADDRESS (No., Street)

6. PATIENT RELATIONSHIP TO INSURED Self ☐ Spouse ☐ Child ☐ Other ☐

7. INSURED'S ADDRESS (No., Street)

CITY | STATE

8. PATIENT STATUS Single ☐ Married ☐ Other ☐
Employed ☐ Full-Time Student ☐ Part-Time Student ☐

CITY | STATE

ZIP CODE | TELEPHONE (Include Area Code) ( )

ZIP CODE | TELEPHONE (INCLUDE AREA CODE) ( )

9. OTHER INSURED'S NAME (Last Name, First Name, Middle Initial)

10. IS PATIENT'S CONDITION RELATED TO:

11. INSURED'S POLICY GROUP OR FECA NUMBER

a. OTHER INSURED'S POLICY OR GROUP NUMBER

a. EMPLOYMENT? (CURRENT OR PREVIOUS) ☐ YES ☐ NO

a. INSURED'S DATE OF BIRTH MM | DD | YY SEX M ☐ F ☐

b. OTHER INSURED'S DATE OF BIRTH MM | DD | YY SEX M ☐ F ☐

b. AUTO ACCIDENT? ☐ YES ☐ NO PLACE (State)

b. EMPLOYER'S NAME OR SCHOOL NAME

c. EMPLOYER'S NAME OR SCHOOL NAME

c. OTHER ACCIDENT? ☐ YES ☐ NO

c. INSURANCE PLAN NAME OR PROGRAM NAME

d. INSURANCE PLAN NAME OR PROGRAM NAME

10d. RESERVED FOR LOCAL USE

d. IS THERE ANOTHER HEALTH BENEFIT PLAN? ☐ YES ☐ NO *If yes*, return to and complete item 9 a-d.

READ BACK OF FORM BEFORE COMPLETING & SIGNING THIS FORM.

12. PATIENT'S OR AUTHORIZED PERSON'S SIGNATURE I authorize the release of any medical or other information necessary to process this claim. I also request payment of government benefits either to myself or to the party who accepts assignment below.

SIGNED ______ DATE ______

13. INSURED'S OR AUTHORIZED PERSON'S SIGNATURE I authorize payment of medical benefits to the undersigned physician or supplier for services described below.

SIGNED ______

Figure 5-19. HCFA 1500—patient and insurance information.

110

HANDS HEAL:
COMMUNICATION,
DOCUMENTATION,
AND INSURANCE BILLING
FOR MANUAL THERAPISTS

A. Patient Information

Address 1209 Lake Winnetonka Dr.

City Minnehaha   State MN Zip 55987

Phone: Home (612) 555-1515

Work N/A   Cell/Pgr 555-1155

Date of Birth 4-22-37

[X] Male   ☐ Female

Marital Status: ☐ Single [X] Married ☐ Partnered

Relationship of Patient to Insured:

☐ Self ☐ Spouse ☐ Partner ☐ Child [X] Other

☐ Employed ☐ Student

Employer's Name or School Name:

_____

Phone _____ Fax _____

Is patient's condition related to:

Employment   ☐ Yes   [X] No

Auto Accident   [X] Yes   ☐ No

If Auto Accident, in what state? MN

Other Accident   ☐ Yes   [X] No

Illness   ☐ Yes   [X] No

Primary Health Care Provider

Name Sage Redtree, MD

Address 87 Old Trail Pkwy

City Minnehaha   State MN Zip 55987

Phone (612) 555-0009 Fax 555-9000

Attorney   updated 3-15-01 JO

Has an attorney been consulted? [X] Yes ☐ No

Retained?   [X] Yes   ☐ No

Name B. Charma Storro, JD

Address 5 Hive Lane

City Minnehaha   State MN Zip 55987

Phone (612) 555-2337 Fax 555-7332

Figure 5-20. Billing In-formation—contact infor-mation.

tient was injured in an MVA, an attorney may have been retained. The attorney may monitor the bills, or collect and send bills from all the health care providers to the insurance company at once, or simply wish to stay apprised of the billing status. Know where to send the bills and to whom. A direct contact expedites the payment process. (See Figure 5-20)

Billing Information

The billing information form collects data about the patient, the insured (if other than the patient), and secondary coverage (if any). Here are three examples with the same patient but different insurance scenarios:

Example 1: The patient is Sarah Lobos. She has private health insurance through her work. She is the patient and the insured.

Example 2: Sarah is the patient. Her domestic partner, Jackie Shenge, has insurance for both of them through her city job. Section A of the billing information is for Sarah's information, sections B and C are for Jackie's information.

Example 3: Sarah was injured in an MVA while driving her insured car. She is the patient and the insured, and her car insurance information would be recorded as the primary insurance information. If her car insurance does not cover medical expenses or her injuries require coverage beyond her car insurance plan, the secondary coverage is Jackie's health insurance. (See Figure 5-21) (See Chapter 8 for in depth information on insurance coverage.)

B. Insured (if other than patient) 3-15-01 JO
Name *James Washington*
Insurance ID# *989-76-6789*
Date of Birth *5-31-60*
☒ Male ☐ Female
Address *32 W. Holden Court*
City *Minnehaha* State *MN* Zip *55987*
Phone: Home *(612) 555-7654*
Work *555-4567* Cell/Pgr *555-6574*
Employer's Name or School Name:
Maad Printing and Design
Phone *555-4567* Fax *555-7676*

C. Primary Insurance Coverage 3-15-01 JO
Insurance Carrier *Farmington States*
Contact *Clifford Glens*
Group Number *N/A*
Plan # or Name *N/A*
Billing Address *PO Box 3778*
City *O'Claire* State *MN* Zip *55978*
Phone *(612)555-7887* Fax *555-8778*

D. Secondary Insurance Coverage 3-15-01 JO
Insured *Darnel G. Washington*
Insurance ID# *see patient info*
Date of Birth
☐ Male ☐ Female
Address
City State Zip
Phone: Home
Work Cell/Pgr
Employer's Name or School Name:

Phone Fax
Insurance Carrier *Allied*
Contact *Jarma Jones*
Group Number *G4321*
Plan # or Name *P56789-0*
Billing Address *PO Box 2988*
City *Omaha* State *NE* Zip *68144*
Phone *(402) 555-1991* Fax *555-9119*

Figure 5-21. Billing Information—insurance information.

112

HANDS HEAL:
COMMUNICATION,
DOCUMENTATION,
AND INSURANCE BILLING
FOR MANUAL THERAPISTS

Assignment of Benefits and Release of Medical Records

The upper portion of the HCFA 1500 billing form is for patient identification and insurance information, and for two patient signatures: one to authorize the insurance company to pay the provider directly (assignment of benefits), and the other to authorize the provider to release medical records to the insurance company for the purpose of processing claims (release of medical records). It is acceptable to obtain the patient's signature and keep it on file, rather than have the patient sign every billing form you send out. The signed billing information form serves this purpose. (See Figure 5-22)

An attorney retained for litigation in a personal injury insurance case may ask the patient to sign an exclusive medical release form that restricts the release of health care information to the attorney only. (See Figure 3-2 in Chapter 3 for an example.) This means that the signature on all medical release forms, including the one on our form, are null and void. The intent here is to prevent the insurance company of the at-fault party from obtaining information without the knowledge and consent of the attorney. Verify the date of the patient's signature and compare it with the one on the attorney's form before sending information out.

Financial Responsibility

It is appropriate and legal to remind patients that they are financially responsible for your services, even though the insurance company is expected to pay for the treatments. Ultimately, the patient is accountable for the balance due if the insurance reimbursement is denied or reversed, or if partial payment is considered payment in full. If you have contracted with the insurance company at a discounted rate, then you cannot, by the terms of your contract, seek payment for the remaining amount from the patient. Otherwise, the patient is responsible for the balance. (See Figure 5-22)

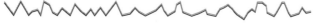

E. Assignment of Benefits
My signature below authorizes and directs payment of medical benefits for services billed to my health care provider.

F. Release of Medical Records
My signature below authorizes the release of my medical records including intake forms, chart notes, reports, and billing statements to my attorneys, health care providers, and insurance case managers, for the purpose of processing my claims. (I will inform my practitioner immediately upon signing any exclusive Release of Medical Records with my attorney.)

G. Financial Responsibility
It is my responsibility to pay for all services provided. In the unfortunate event that my insurance company denies payment or makes a partial payment, I am responsible for the balance. If you have contracted with my insurance company at a discount rate and the agreed-upon fee has been satisfied, the balance will be waived.

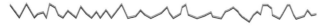

Figure 5-22. Billing Information—patient authorization.

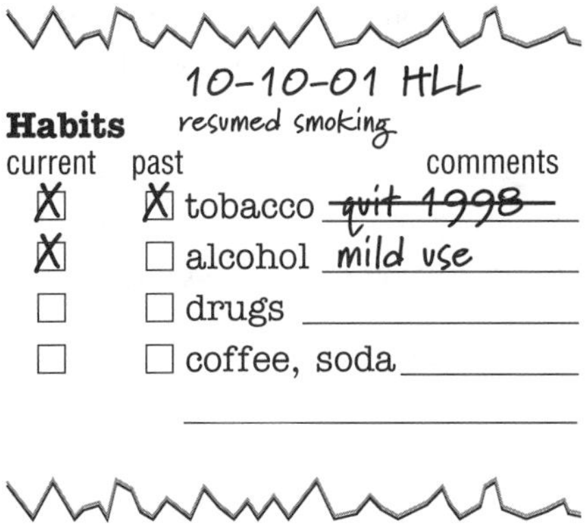

~~~~~~~~~~~~~~~~~~~~~~~~~~

10-10-01 HLL
Habits *resumed smoking*
current   past   comments
  ☒   ☒ tobacco ~~quit 1998~~
  ☒   ☐ alcohol *mild use*
  ☐   ☐ drugs _____
  ☐   ☐ coffee, soda_____

        _____

~~~~~~~~~~~~~~~~~~~~~~~~~~

Figure 5-23. Amending forms.

TIMING AND APPLICATION

This form should be completed and insurance coverage verified before treatment is provided without immediate payment, or as otherwise stated in your payment policies. (Insurance verification is covered in depth in Chapter 8.) Unless the insurance coverage changes, the form only needs to be completed once per incident.

Every patient who wants the insurance company to pay the manual therapist directly for health care treatment fills out the billing information form.

Amending the Forms

You may want to make a slight change, addition, or correction to the information recorded on any of the forms in the patient's file, without asking the patient to complete an entirely new form. The patient's perspective may change or she may wish to include new perceptions. Changes can be made by either the patient or the practitioner, regardless of who originally filled out the form. There are two options for updating the existing form.

1. Write the new information on the original form. If you are replacing existing information, draw a single line through the outdated information, making sure that the previous information is still legible. Date and initial all changes and additions. Never use white-out or erase or discard information. (See Figure 5-23)
2. Attach an amendment to the document. Write the new information on a separate sheet of paper and staple it to the original. Date and initial the attachment.

All medical documents can be amended or updated as needed. Patients have a right to access their files and make sure the information recorded is accurate. Make a habit of record-keeping in the presence of the patient. Avoid misinformation and misinterpretations. Reiterate the information provided to you, and confirm aloud your interpretation of the patient's history and current status.

SUMMARY

There are a variety of intake forms used to document the therapeutic relationship. All of these forms are completed before the first treatment, and some are completed before every session or periodically to evaluate progress.

114

HANDS HEAL:
COMMUNICATION,
DOCUMENTATION,
AND INSURANCE BILLING
FOR MANUAL THERAPISTS

Every patient fills out a health information form, and reads and signs a fee schedule and office policies. Patients who have health concerns and seek treatment for injuries or illnesses fill out a health report and pain questionnaires periodically to document subjective data and assist the manual therapist in evaluating progress. Patients seeking insurance reimbursement complete a billing information form initially and when the insurance coverage changes. The injury information form is completed by patients injured on-the-job or in a motor vehicle accident once per incident.

REFERENCES

1. Adler RH, Giersch P. Whiplash, Spinal Trauma, and the Chiropractic Personal Injury Case. Seattle: Adler ◆ Giersch PS, 2000.
2. Green JA. Holistic Practice Forum, HP–100, Green, Mill Valley, 1990.
3. Deyo RA, Diehl AK. Measuring Physical and Psycho-Social Function in Patients with Low Back Pain, Spine, Vol. 8, Hanley and Belfus: Philadelphia, 1983.
4. McDowell I, Newell C. Measuring Health: A Guide to Rating Scales and Questionnaires. New York and Oxford: Oxford University Press, 1997.
5. Fairbank J, Coupar J, et al. The oswestry low back pain disability questionnaire. Physiotherapy. 1980;66.
6. Cherkin D, Deyo RA, Eisenberg D, et al. National Alternative Medicine Ambulatory Care Study, preliminary findings, 1999.
7. Chelimsky TC. Pain. In Adult Neurology. Mosby, 1998.

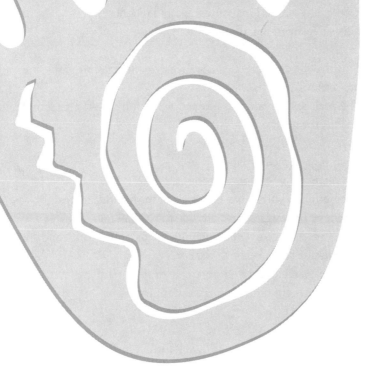

CHAPTER 6

Documentation: SOAP Charting

A medical director of an insurance carrier in Idaho was questioned by a group of massage therapists: "Why isn't manual therapy a covered benefit in any of your plans?" He replied, "If every massage therapist can show me 6 months of SOAP charts on every patient, we will consider it."

Introduction

SOAP (Subjective, Objective, Assessment, Plan) charting is a standard format for documenting treatment sessions in the health care field. It is routinely used by physicians, physical therapists, chiropractors, nurses, massage therapists, and other medical and allied health professionals.[1] The rapid and widespread adoption of the SOAP format is a tribute to its simple structure and inherent flexibility. Any health concern, method of evaluation, and treatment style can be recorded in the SOAP format. The SOAP structure meets the needs of a variety of health care professionals in many settings.

The SOAP chart documents the patient's health information and goals, the practitioner's findings and treatment, and the patient's self-care routine; and records the patient's response to the solutions and progress toward the goals. The information is organized into four categories:

- Subjective—data provided by the patient
- Objective—practitioner findings
- Assessment—functional outcomes and diagnoses
- Plan—treatment recommendations

This structure prompts comprehensive information-gathering and makes data storage and retrieval easy.

The goals and advantages of documentation are discussed in depth in Chapter 4. To summarize, the goals of a SOAP chart are to:[1, 2]

- Organize and record data
- Stimulate the practitioner's recall
- Communicate with other members of the health care team
- Demonstrate progress and provide functional outcomes
- Provide a legal record documenting the patient's health and treatment
- Provide case study research data
- Prove reasonable and necessary care to third party payors
- Prove significant injury in personal injury cases
- Monitor quality

The advantages to using the SOAP format include:

- Consistency across professions
- Common language and communication style
- Demonstration of professionalism
- Proof of progress and functional outcomes
- Brevity and comprehensiveness
- Fast retrieval of information

Many variations of the SOAP format exist. This chapter provides basic information for manual therapists. The **functional outcomes reporting** style of charting—writing notes that address the patient's ability to function in everyday activities, and setting goals and designing treatments to improve function—is emphasized. Some clinics, hospitals, and schools may require a standard of documentation that varies slightly from that presented here; however, the skills acquired through this text can be easily adapted to suit any system of documentation.[1]

Guidelines for Charting

First and foremost, charting should contribute to the therapeutic relationship, not detract from it. Don't let charting be a distraction. Follow the patient's lead in the interview.[2] You do not need to follow the SOAP format in order. The beauty of the SOAP structure is that you can organize your information in a linear fashion without having to think or speak in a linear manner. As information is presented, place it in the appropriate section.

Be attentive and maintain good listening skills, as discussed in Chapter 1. If the patient is emotional and needs your undivided attention, record the information later. It is more important to be attentive to the patient in a moment of need than to write on the chart. Reflect your understanding of the patient's experience after she is composed, and record the data appropriate to her health concern once she verifies the information.

Chart only information applicable to the patient's condition and goals for health. Often a story surrounds pertinent details. Pay attention to the details of the story, but be selective when choosing the information to document. Record only data that substantiate the concern or contribute to the solution. For example, Lin experiences an increase in allergies at work when Sally, a co-worker from marketing, wears heavy perfume. It is not important to mention information about work or the co-worker. What is important to note is that Lin's *allergy symptoms increase when exposed to perfume.*

Be brief. Jot down just enough to jog your memory later: words, dates, or short phrases.[3] It is difficult to discern what information is important to the patient's health as you hear her story. Things often make more sense later, after you have heard the whole story. Take brief notes and fill in the blanks after you summarize the pertinent information to the patient and get confirmation of your interpretation. Make sure you accurately represent the patient's concerns.

As you ask the patient specific questions, for example, to confirm an assessment or rule out a particular pathology, record the positive and negative findings. For example: *No joint deformities. Active range of motion (including hands, wrists, elbows, shoulders, spine, knees, hips, ankles) is normal.*[3]

Consider another example in which "No" answers are as important as "Yes" answers: Jose has shoulder pain. The pain increases when he raises his arm to the side, but there is no pain with any other shoulder movement. Knowing that there is no pain with a particular action, if you are identifying a rotator cuff injury or determining bursitis versus tendonitis, could affect your treatment plan as much as knowing that there is pain with an action. Record all answers that contribute to the case.

Be objective. State everything in a factual manner. Draw conclusions based on factual data and record them in the Assessment section of the SOAP note, if your scope of practice permits it. Leave your opinions off the chart. For example, omit, *I think the patient doesn't want to get better and is avoiding going back to work.* Instead, quote the patient directly in the subjective section. He may comment on their situation in ways that ade-

118

HANDS HEAL:
COMMUNICATION,
DOCUMENTATION,
AND INSURANCE BILLING
FOR MANUAL THERAPISTS

quately represent his state of mind, opinions, or emotions. Chart specific, measurable information and let the lack of progress, for example, demonstrate that the treatment is not producing results. The information should pertain to the patient, not to you.[1] Revisit the discussion in Chapter 1: if the relationship isn't productive, step up the communication and reconsider your approach.

Use consistent terminology and become fluent with standard abbreviations. (See Appendix: Abbreviations) There are common, standardized medical abbreviations used by all types of health care providers (HCP) applicable to manual therapy. For examples of data translated into abbreviations, see Bone Game 6-1: Translation.

▼

BONE GAME 6-1

Translation

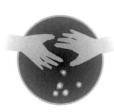

Headache pain, pounding, left frontal, moderate minus, 2 to 3 days, monthly, with menses for 10 plus years.
Abbreviation: HA Ⓟ, pounding, Ⓛ frontal, M-, 2–3 day/mth, c̄ menses 10+ yr

the trigger point was moderately painful with digital pressure at the trigger point site and mildly painful at the referral site.
Abbreviation: TP M Ⓟ c̄ dig. pres. @ TP site & L Ⓟ@ ref. site

cervical flexion passive range of motion was limited moderate minus with mild pain at end range.
Abbreviation: C-flex P-ROM M- c̄ L Ⓟ@ end range

right shoulder active abduction moderate segmented movement with mild compensational shoulder elevation at end range.
Abbreviation: Ⓡsh-abd A-ROM seg c̄ L comp. sh-elev @ end range.

moderate trigger point site pain changed to mild pain, mild referred pain changed to no pain.
Abbreviation: TP site M Ⓟ △ L Ⓟ, L ref. Ⓟ △ Ⓟ̶

moderate segmented movement in right shoulder active abduction changed to smooth movement without compensational shoulder elevation.
Abbreviation: M seg. mvm't Ⓡsh-abd A-ROM WNL s̄ comp. sh-elev

patient supine, anterior-lateral view, deep inhalation, mild plus mobility restriction upper right.
Abbreviation: pt supine, ant-lat view, deep inhal., mob L+ restr. upper Ⓡ

left biceps insertion moderate pain with mild digital pressure, mild plus referred pain into left elbow.
Abbreviation: Ⓛbiceps insert. M Ⓟ c̄ L dig. pres., L+ ref. Ⓟ → Ⓛelbow

1-hour full-body Swedish massage; 30-minute foot reflexology; or 90-minute Hellerwork—inspiration.
Abbreviation: 1 hr FB Sw Ⓜ; 30 min foot reflex.; 90 min HW—inspir.

muscle energy with cervical flexion, direct pressure on scalene trigger point, or myofascial release on diaphragm.
Abbreviation: MET c̄ C-flex, DP scal. TP, MFR diaph.

craniosacral therapy with attention to the thoracic cage, muscle energy for cervical flexion and extension, and lymph drainage for upper quadrants.
Abbreviation: CST T cage, MET C-flex & ext, LDT UQ Ⓑ̶Ⓛ̶

Add personalized abbreviations to the list of standard ones to meet the needs of your practice. Do not use abbreviations that are not on your list, even abbreviated words that you think are common, e.g., quads for quadriceps muscles, hams for hamstring muscles. Others who read the patient file must be able to interpret everything on the chart. Payment of your bill may depend on a claims representative understanding your notes. If you use a series of tests or modalities that do not have standard abbreviations, create your own shorthand and produce a legend to attach to the standardized list. For example, many of Sari's patients have been in car accidents. She finds it helpful to abbreviate information regarding the accident and whiplash-related injuries, but the abbreviations list she uses does not have the medical terms she requires for her practice. Therefore she includes her own shorthand legend with the standard list she sends out when her charts are requested. (See Figure 6-1)

Measure everything. Gather as much detail as possible to document the injury or health concern, and write it down. It is difficult to prove progress if there is nothing to mark progress against. For example, pain may still be present but diminished, occurring less frequently, with a shorter duration and fewer exacerbations than at the previous session. Be thorough.

Avoid vague statements. It is not enough to write: *feeling better, increased pain,* or *limited function.* Be specific. Rate the intensity of pain; describe the activities that are limited. Use measurable data to explain the symptoms, and compare the symptoms to those from the previous session to demonstrate progress. For example: *Moderate pain, constant, increasing to moderate plus pain with sitting for 1 hour or more* expresses an increase in pain when compared with: *mild pain, intermittent, increasing with heavy lifting.* "Feeling better"

Motor Vehicle Accident Treatment and Billing Abbreviations

accel	acceleration
CADS	cervical acceleration deceleration syndrome
CPT	Current Procedural Terminology
G-Force	acceleration force
HCFA-1500	Health Care Financing Administration current billing form
HCP	health care provider
ICD	International Classification for Disease
IME	independent medical examination
MVA	motor vehicle accident
PCP	primary care provider
PIP	personal injury protection
PR	peer review
pre-IS	pre-injury status
pre-XC	pre-existing conditions
+SB	wearing seat belt
SB−	not wearing seat belt
WAS	whiplash associated disorder

Figure 6-1. Addendum to standard abbreviations.

120

HANDS HEAL:
COMMUNICATION,
DOCUMENTATION,
AND INSURANCE BILLING
FOR MANUAL THERAPISTS

is not only vague, but tells insurance companies to discontinue care.[3] If the patient is feeling better, the insurance company could determine that she no longer requires treatment.

Write legibly. Insurance carriers can refuse payment if they are unable to ascertain whether the treatment was reasonable and necessary, or whether the symptoms warranted the type of treatment.[3] Chart notes are the primary source for verifying this information. If the notes are illegible, payment can legitimately be denied. Charting is intended to facilitate communication. Make it easy for others to read the information you are trying to share.

Never use correction fluid or erase information. Cross out mistakes with a single line. Initial and date the error. Do not leave blank spaces where data could be altered.

Sign your legal name or initials to the end of every chart entry. Never use nicknames; SOAP charts are legal documents. Include your health care credentials with your signature. The supervising practitioner signs the chart in addition to student, aide, or apprentice in learning environments or clinic settings.[1]

Functional Outcomes Reporting

The current trend in medical documentation is functional outcomes reporting: setting goals and designing treatments to improve function. This style of documentation addresses the patient's ability to participate in everyday activities. Functional outcomes reporting fits into the SOAP format and shifts the focus of documentation to the patient's quality of life. The practitioner records the patient's functional limitations and works with the patient to develop goals for returning to personally meaningful activities, and together the practitioner and patient implement solutions to reach those goals.

▼

WISE ONE SPEAKS 6-1

Follow the Patient's Lead

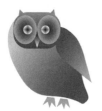

"You should never have expectations for other people. . . . setting goals for others can be aggressive—really wanting a success story for ourselves. When we do this to others, we are asking them to live up to our ideals. Instead, just be kind."[4] This quote from Trungpa Rinpoche reminds us to follow the patient's lead in setting goals. Remember that the patient is in charge in the therapeutic relationship. SOAP notes were designed to help formulate a high-quality treatment plan and promote the practitioner's problem-solving skills.[1] This same format can be equally effective in promoting the patient's problem-solving skills by adding the functional outcomes approach to our information gathering and charting. Focus on the therapeutic relationship and prioritize the patient's goals over our own in every step of SOAP charting.

The functional outcomes style of documentation is increasingly popular[1] and benefits the patient, the practitioner, and all who read the chart, because it addresses directly the basic needs of the patient, monitors effective treatment, and makes the results easily understood—not just to the experts.

As the practitioner, it is important to fully understand the functional outcomes approach before charting data.

FUNCTIONAL OUTCOMES BEGIN AS GOALS

Functional outcomes are written in the form of functional goals, set by the patient with practitioner guidance. Goals are determined through the activities the patient is having difficulty with and is motivated to resume. As the goals are accomplished, they are identified as functional outcomes.

Develop goals that address the needs of the patient and lead to an effective treatment plan—one that will resolve the patient's concerns. Together with the patient, follow these steps:

1. Summarize and prioritize the patient's needs.
2. Summarize the objective findings that are contributing to the patient's condition.
3. Summarize and prioritize the patient's limitations in functional terms.
4. Identify the patient's functional limitations in order of importance.
5. Identify the patient's previous ability to perform these activities.
6. Identify the role these activities play in the patient's current situation.
7. Together with the patient, identify functional goals that will demonstrate the desired outcomes.
8. Create long- and short-term **SMART goals** (LTG, STG).

Functional goals are charted in the Assessment section of the SOAP chart. (See Components of SOAP Format: Assessment later in this Chapter.)

SETTING SMART GOALS

To ensure that the goals will lead to productive treatment plans and produce functional outcomes that serve the patient's needs, follow the SMART[5] criteria. The acronym SMART stands for the following:

Specific—to a daily activity

Measurable—quantified and qualified to note incremental progress

Attainable—able to be accomplished given the patient's condition

Relevant—critical to the patient's daily life

Time-bound—defined to be successful in a specific amount of time

Together with the patient, build functional goals that meet the SMART criteria.

SMART: Specific and Relevant Activity

Select activities that are specific and functional. This could include vacuuming, mowing the lawn, washing hair, lifting boxes onto a conveyor belt, loading and unloading furniture to a truck, rowing a boat, etc. The more specific the activity the better. "Work," "exercise," "child care," or "housework" is not specific enough to base a functional goal on. If house cleaning is the work, explore which activity increases the symptoms. Is it standing at the sink, pushing a vacuum cleaner, pulling sheets off a bed, lifting laundry, scrubbing floors, etc.? If computer programming is the work, is it sitting still, staring at the screen, moving the mouse, etc.? If the exercise is playing tennis, is it the forehand stroke,

122

HANDS HEAL:
COMMUNICATION,
DOCUMENTATION,
AND INSURANCE BILLING
FOR MANUAL THERAPISTS

backhand, serve, lateral moves, etc.? What part of child care is problematic: lifting the child, leaning over to play with her, picking up the toys, etc.?

Reducing pain is a common goal of the patient, but is not functional—based on an activity. Pain is a qualifier, measuring the success of a goal. If a patient states "pain free" as his goal, guide him to a specific activity by exploring activities that cause the pain.

Select the activity that is most relevant to the patient's life. Address work, home, family, exercise, and play activities. The goal should be based on an activity that is critical to the patient's ability to earn a living or care for himself, his family, or his household. If the injury occurred on the job and industrial insurance is paying for the treatment, select a work-related activity.

SMART: Measurable, Time-bound

Once the specific and relevant activity is selected, specify how the success of the goal will be gauged.

1. Quantify the outcome by measuring the activity: number of units, amount of weight, repetitions, duration, or frequency.
2. Qualify the outcome by projecting how the patient will feel upon completion: amount of pain, fatigue, or functional limitations.
3. Schedule a time limit for completion: 30–60 days for LTG, 1–2 weeks for STG.

For example:
Lift 25-pound boxes from a 3-foot high moving conveyor belt and stack them onto hand trucks for 30 minutes keeping pace with the conveyor with mild pain within 6 weeks.

1. Quantify the outcome— *Lift 25-pound boxes from a 3-foot high moving conveyor belt and stack them onto hand trucks for 30 minutes keeping pace with the conveyor*
2. Qualify the outcome— *with mild pain*
3. Time-bound—*within 6 weeks*

Climb up and down four standard steps at a moderate pace three times a day with moderate pain and mild fatigue within 1 week.

1. Quantify the outcome—*Climb up and down four standard steps at a moderate pace three times a day*
2. Qualify the outcome—*with moderate pain and mild fatigue*
3. Time-bound—*within 1 week*

Sleep restfully for 3 hours without waking once each night with mild fatigue upon waking within 2 weeks

1. Quantify the outcome—*Sleep restfully for 3 hours without waking once each night*
2. Qualify the outcome—*with mild fatigue upon waking*
3. Time-bound—*within 2 weeks*

Two standard time frames can be used: long term and short term. LTGs are developed first. Identify the desired end result of the treatment. If it is not possible to reach the goal in 30–60 days, write one or two intermediary LTGs, each one attainable within 30–60 days.

STGs are established to support the LTG and are often written as incremental stages of the LTG. Think of them as baby steps toward the end result. If the end result is to lift up to 50-pound boxes from the floor to a truck up to 100 times a day 5 days a week, write STGs that are fractions of the original goal. For example:

STG #1: Lift 10 pounds from a 3-foot-high shelf 10 times a day within 12 days

STG #2: Lift 20 pounds from a 2-foot-high shelf 10 times, two times a day within 20 days

STG #3: Lift 30 pounds from a 1-foot-high shelf 20 times, three times a day within 12 days, etc.

Write STGs that provide encouragement and motivation for the patient, even if the STG does not appear to be directly related to the original goal. For example: *LTG: pain free and fully functional while swimming the breast stroke for 1500 meters within 30 days.* If the breast stroke is painful because of a neck injury, but the patient is eager to experience success in the water, set a goal that provides a feeling of success in the water. *STG: 1-week goal of 30 minutes of water aerobics with moderate pain.* The aerobic exercises may not require her to extend her neck—the function that causes her pain—and being in the water may be very comforting for the patient. The result is an immediate feeling of accomplishment that may not be realized with long-term goals.

The time limit for LTGs is often dictated by the prescription length. An STG should be written for each session or two. Determine the measurements for the time frames by assessing what is possible for each individual patient, given the patient's condition and constitution.

SMART: Attainable

Be reasonable when writing goals. A goal that is too vast—*pain free and fully functional while swimming the breast stroke for 1500 meters within 30 days*—can be frustrating to reach when the patient is currently unable to swim at all. If we are to eliminate the patient's feelings of powerlessness and inspire her to work hard to achieve her goals, we must develop goals that are not only meaningful but continually within her reach. Evaluate the severity of the injury, the patient's constitution, and functional status, and determine whether the goal as stated is attainable for the patient in the allotted time.

It is helpful to predetermine how the patient's body will respond to treatment. Don't worry if you misjudge this; you can adjust the goal at the following session by renegotiating the time limit or the outcome measurements. Instead of swimming 1500 meters with no pain, adjust the outcome to:

The patient will be able to swim 500 meters with moderate pain within 30 days.

CASE STUDY

Let's use Zamora as an example—the chef who was injured at work when she slipped on a banana peel (see Appendix: Case Studies)—to learn the steps of writing a SMART goal.

1. *Specific activity*: Begin by asking Zamora to select an activity that reflects a prioritized need. Review with her the subjective and objective data. Her symptoms include shoulder, neck, and low back pain. Her shoulder is a priority. Currently, any use of her shoulder is difficult to impossible. ROM tests were severely limited on her shoulder

124

HANDS HEAL:
COMMUNICATION,
DOCUMENTATION,
AND INSURANCE BILLING
FOR MANUAL THERAPISTS

because of the pain and severity of the separation. The subjective section of the SOAP chart lists activities that she can no longer perform because of her shoulder separation—everything from getting dressed to riding a bike. Previously, she was active and fully capable of the heavy lifting required by her job and vigorous exercise, including mountain biking and roller hockey. The priority is that she is unable to work because of her shoulder pain and loss of function.

Zamora wants to be pain free and is eager to get back to work. Neither "pain free" nor "work" are specific activities suitable for a goal; however, work could be if defined further. Assist Zamora in identifying something specific about work that she can formulate a goal around. She identifies cooking. Ask her to be more specific: what does she do when she cooks? She says that, among other things, she is required to stand at the prep counter chopping food for 2 hours, and stand at the stove and ovens for 5 hours. She enjoys sautéing the food better than prepping or baking, but cannot stand for longer than 30 minutes because of pain, nor can she pick up a sauté pan, let alone hold a heavy sauté pan over a flame and toss the food.

The specific activity Zamora identifies for her functional goal is:
stand at the stove and toss food in a sauté pan.

2. *Measurable results*: To monitor progress and determine the success of the goal, the results must be measured. Zamora's goal to cook has been specified to include standing while lifting and extending a pan of food. Now we must identify measurable standards to achieve. Quantify the results by identifying how long to stand, how much weight to lift and extend and how long or how often to lift and extend. Ultimately, Zamora wants to be able to: *stand for 5 hours cooking, while repeatedly lifting and extending up to 25 pounds over a stove tossing food daily, 5 days a week . . .*

Not only must we quantify the results by defining the number of units, amount of weight, repetitions or duration, and frequency, we must also qualify the results. With Zamora, is it a quality achievement if accomplishing the goal causes her so much pain that she is confined to bed rest on pain pills for 3 days? Qualify the results by identifying how Zamora will feel during and after the task. This is most commonly done by defining the level of pain or loss of function the activity causes or by measuring physiological effects, such as an increase in blood pressure, or noting a change in pain medications. Ultimately, Zamora wants to be able to cook as defined above: *. . . without pain or fatigue.*

3. *Attainable*: To determine whether the goal is attainable, we must have a complete understanding of what Zamora can currently do, and what she expects to be able to do. We also need to project the progress Zamora is capable of, given her prognosis. How quickly will Zamora heal? How much recovery is expected? Base your answers on the type of injury, general success rates and recovery rates, Zamora's constitution and attitude, and information obtained from the health care team, to develop goals that are attainable.

Zamora needs to be able to stand for 5–7 hours to work a full shift. Currently she can only stand for 30 minutes. Zamora also needs to be able to lift and extend heavy pans. Currently, she cannot lift any amount of weight with her right arm. She was diagnosed with a separated shoulder which takes time to heal, but Zamora is young and eager to get back to work. Given Zamora's history, injury, general health, and attitude, she will probably reach her goal: *stand for 5 hours cooking, while repeatedly lifting and extending up to 25 pounds over a stove tossing food, daily, 5 days a week, without pain or fatigue.*

4. *Relevant*: Relevance is determined initially, when you and your patient select the specific activity in which to develop a goal. Confirm that the activity selected is relevant to Zamora's daily activities and significant in her life. Otherwise, it will be difficult to motivate Zamora to work hard to achieve her goals. Here we are on solid ground: Zamora enjoys her job and her paychecks are her sole source of income.

5. *Time-bound*: Finally, we need to determine the time Zamora will take to accomplish her goal. Given her current condition, she is unlikely to accomplish her goal within 30–60 days. Take the goal and whittle it down into reasonably attainable long-term goals. When the patient's ultimate goal cannot be achieved in 30–60 days, a series of long-term goals must be developed. Zamora may need two or three long-term goals to achieve her ultimate results. To do this, determine a half-way point to reaching her goal. One simple way is to cut the measurable tasks in half: *stand for 2.5 hours cooking, while repeatedly lifting and extending up to 12 pounds over a stove tossing food, daily, 3 days a week, with moderate minus pain and mild fatigue.*

If this goal is not attainable within 30-60 days, an additional long-term goal can be written. It may be necessary to write a goal that does not involve sautéing; for example: *Stand for 45 minutes slicing kiwis and decorating a cake with mild pain and mild fatigue.*

Zamora's shoulder may not be capable of lifting more than one pound through a limited range for the first 30 days. Kiwis are soft and light-weight. Zamora may be able to lift a knife and slice kiwis as a step toward her bigger goal. We already know she can stand for 30 minutes, so 45 minutes should be feasible in 30 days or less.

This goal may be more appealing if she uses the kiwis to decorate her friend's store-bought birthday cake. She may not be capable of stirring batter, bending and lifting a cake in and out of an oven, but she might feel disappointed if she is unable to use her talents to make her friend's birthday special. Take the time to discover meaningful activities that can become goals and ultimately functional outcomes.

Components of SOAP Format

Subjective, Objective, Assessment, Plan (SOAP) notes are part of a documentation system called the **problem-oriented medical record** (POMR), introduced by Dr. Lawrence Weed in the 1960s. The POMR lists patient problems in the front of the chart, and the practitioner writes a SOAP note to address each problem.[1] This format helps structure the practitioner's efforts to solve the patient's problems. The practitioner records the problems, sets goals for the patient, and develops a treatment plan. Practical and easy to use, the SOAP note has become the charting standard in the health care industry.

1. Subjective—states the health concern, and records the patient's perceptions.
2. Objective—stores practitioner observations, measurable data, interventions, and the patient's response to treatment.
3. Assessment—summarizes the patient's functional limitations and records long-term and short-term goals for health. Also includes conclusions, diagnosis, and prognosis if within the practitioner's scope.
4. Plan—projects future treatments and self-care routines.

SUBJECTIVE

Subjective information provided by the patient includes a health history and current health information. Data collected on the intake forms is considered subjective informa-

126

HANDS HEAL:
COMMUNICATION,
DOCUMENTATION,
AND INSURANCE BILLING
FOR MANUAL THERAPISTS

tion and is used with the SOAP charts to provide comprehensive documentation of the patient's health. Use the subjective section of the SOAP chart to record further details about current health: patient concerns, physical symptoms, emotional complications, changes in functional ability, and impact on the patient's daily routine.

On a SOAP chart, subjective information is divided into three parts:

◆ Health concerns
◆ Symptoms
◆ Activities that aggravate or relieve the symptoms

Health Concerns

Top the SOAP chart with the patient's health concerns. Remain mindful of the reasons why the patient is seeking care. The patient's health concerns may be defined as injuries, health conditions, and symptoms, or as goals for maintaining health or preventing disease. For example, Darnel is seeking care for injuries sustained in a motor vehicle accident; Zamora is anxious to get back to work; and Lin wants to prevent complications of diabetes and learn relaxation skills. Include pertinent information that directly affects the care you provide.

Some of the information may not come directly from the patient. The prescription may provide the diagnosis, or contributing information may come from test results you did not perform. For example, Darnel's x-rays show spinal subluxations and increased progression of scoliosis; Zamora has a diagnosed shoulder separation; and Lin has a family history of heart disease potentially complicating her diabetes. This information is critical to the direction of subjective information gathering and the formation of the treatment plan, but did not originate with the patient. For this reason, the section is technically referred to as the problem section of a POMR, which precedes the SOAP chart. However, with the increased use of SOAP format and the decreased use of the POMR, the problem section is often absorbed into the subjective section of the SOAP chart, or a new section is added (PSOAP).[2]

Prioritize multiple concerns. For example, Darnel has limited neck range of motion, back pain, and headaches. In Chapter 3 we discussed his strong desire to reduce the back pain so he could interact with his granddaughter Madi. His headaches are more distressing than his limited neck mobility. Therefore, we would prioritize his health concerns or needs in the following order: *Treat injuries and symptoms associated with the motor vehicle accident including secondary scoliosis recurrence.*

1. *Reduce low back pain.*
2. *Reduce headache pain.*
3. *Increase neck mobility.*

Symptoms

Obtain a complete list of symptoms from the patient in the initial interview. Subsequent notes may reflect only the symptoms of immediate concern. To obtain a comprehensive list, gather information on the physiological and psychosocial conditions of the patient. Much of this information is recorded on the intake forms. On the initial SOAP, chart additional information and reiterate pertinent information already covered. Inquire about specific areas that have bearing on your treatment applications and are within your scope of practice. Commonly, manual therapists inquire about signs and symptoms in these categories:

◆ General—fatigue, pain, signs of stress, allergies, fever, posture, and general function
◆ Lymphatic—swollen nodes, edema
◆ Musculo-skeletal—tension, weakness, muscle or joint pain, stiffness, swelling
◆ Peripheral vascular—cramps, varicose veins, cold hands or feet, color or pallor
◆ Neurological—numbness, tingling, local weakness, memory, tremors, fainting, blackouts, seizures, paralysis
◆ Psychosocial—lifestyle, home situation, a typical day, important experiences, religious beliefs that may pertain to treatment or illness, perceptions of health, attitude, and outlook for future[2]

Other systems that come into play may not be adequately represented in the intake forms. For further information regarding the systems of the body and examination techniques, consult Bates[2] or Magee.[6]

Once you have identified symptoms—pain, stiffness, weakness, etc.—ask the patient to describe the symptom: its location, intensity, duration, and frequency; and the setting in which it occurred and recurs. Record that information. For example: *Headache pain, pounding, left frontal, moderate minus, 2 to 3 days, monthly, with menses for 10 plus years.*

Description

Once the patient has identified the symptoms, ask her to describe them further. For example, if the symptom is pain it may be described as sharp, shooting, dull, achy, etc. One of my patient's describes her numbness as "cold and wet." Record any information that qualifies the symptom and is helpful in assessing and treating it or in marking progress.

Location

Ask the patient to identify the precise location of the symptom. In addition to locating the symptom, this information can be helpful in identifying the source of the dysfunction and in substantiating progress. As explained in Travell and Simons,[7] the location of the trigger point pain can lead to proper treatment application. For example, if Moira's headache pain is located in the forehead over her right eye, the trigger point is likely to be found in the right sternocleidomastoid.[5] Progress can be demonstrated when the area of pain diminishes in size. In the story of Sandee, her back pain originally covered her entire low back area. Eventually, the location of her pain was reduced to a small area around her sacrum. Be specific about the location to assist with symptom identification, assessment of the condition, and treatment application.

Intensity

Measure all symptoms by quantifying their expression. Ask patients to rate the intensity of their symptoms on a numerical scale of 0–5 or 0–10, a value scale of mild or light (L), moderate (M), and severe (S), or a descriptive scale of normal (N), good (G), fair (F), and poor (P). The value scale can stand alone as a three-point scale, or can be extended into a nine-point scale with the addition of pluses and minuses (L-, L, L+, M-, M, M+, S-, S, S+).

128

HANDS HEAL:
COMMUNICATION,
DOCUMENTATION,
AND INSURANCE BILLING
FOR MANUAL THERAPISTS

Choose the rating scale that works best for you. Be consistent. If you choose a nine-point value scale, use that scale for all patients, every session.

Duration and Frequency

Record how long the symptom lasts when it occurs. Use time to denote the duration: seconds, minutes, days, weeks, months, or years.

Note how often the symptom occurs. Use general terms like seldom, intermittent, frequent or constant; or specific descriptions like twice a day, three times a week, or hourly to note the frequency.

Description of Onset

The description of onset documents the setting in which the injury or condition occurred or the external conditions affecting the injury, and the date of the occurrence. Include the biomechanics of the body positions and movements involved in the injury. Describing the biomechanics of a lift-and-twist injury, for example, requires identifying the side of the body moving the weight and the direction the body was turning to determine which muscles are being overstretched and which muscles are overcontracting. How much weight and the distance the weight had to be moved is also a factor. For example, Moira lifted a box of books from the floor to a shelf above her head. She turned to the left to pick up the box and turned to her right to set the box up on the shelf.

In the case of a fall, it is important to note what body parts contacted what type of surface and in what order. Zamora, for example, was carrying a 25-pound bag of rice and slipped on a banana peel at work. She fell backwards with her arm outstretched to break her fall, landed on a tile floor on her right hand and right hip, and ended up on her back, with her head hitting the floor and bouncing a few times. The heavy bag of rice landed on top of her. This information helps determine the treatment plan by identifying the points of impact and the angles of entry.

In the case of a repetitive movement injury, the onset includes the repeated action and a description of any other contributing data. For example: *Clint hammers repeatedly at shoulder height with right hand, 20-ounce hammer, 8 hours per day, 5 days per week, 5 years at job, carrying heavy nail pouch on left hip.*

Include the date of the onset. In situations involving repetitive movement injuries, the date of the onset may be difficult to determine. As in the scenario above, determine the approximate year the symptoms began occurring. Record a month or a time of year as well as the year of onset. *Summer of `42* or *winter of `83* is more helpful in noting time than simply saying, *for many years.*

The date of onset is easily determined if the symptoms are the result of an accident. For example, Darnel was in a car accident on January 6th, 2001. Both the date and the cause of the injury are noted: *MVA 1-6-01.* If the patient's symptoms are due to a condition that existed before the accident and the symptoms flared-up as a result of the accident, the description of onset should refer to the most recent onset. In Darnel's case, his scoliosis was dormant until the accident. Since the accident, he has been experiencing symptoms associated with a flare-up of the scoliosis. Chart the description of onset of all the symptoms—symptoms directly related to the accident and symptoms associated with the scoliosis flare-up—as *MVA 1-6-01.*

Intake forms are helpful in documenting the onset of an injury or illness. In the case of a motor vehicle accident, the description includes not only physical biomechanics, but also external factors such as size of vehicles, weather conditions, speed and direction of impact, use of seat belts, position of the head rests, etc. This extensive information would be cumbersome to include on a SOAP chart. Use both the Injury Information form and the SOAP chart to document onset. The mechanisms of injury, whether noted on the SOAP chart or an intake form, need only be documented once per incident. All subsequent charts need only briefly identify the incident and state the date of the onset.

Having a clear record of the mechanisms of injury will help justify treating a broader area. For example, with Moira's lift and twist injury, the diagnosis may be a low back sprain/strain. Treatment to her neck and shoulders may seem luxurious and unnecessary to an insurance representative unless you can clearly explain the biomechanical links and compensating symptoms involved. Typically, workers' compensation coverage permits treatment only to the specific location of injury.

Activities—Aggravating and Relieving

Emphasize function—how the patient is able to perform activities of daily living—when charting subjective information. Record the patient's current and prior level of function, how the symptoms affect his ability to function, and how his ability to function affects his life at home and work.

The documentation process—inquiry, discussion, and charting—increases the patients' awareness of their role in exacerbating or reducing the symptoms. Record events of everyday life that aggravate or relieve symptoms to document significant injury, note progress, and educate patients to use activities that relieve rather than aggravate their symptoms.

Apply aggravating circumstances that most affect the patient's quality of life to functional goal-setting. Use relieving activities when planning the patient's homework and self-care regime. Goals are documented in Assessment; homework, in the Plan section.

Activities That Aggravate Symptoms

When documenting activities that aggravate the patient's symptoms, be specific about home and work responsibilities, and include hobbies and play activities. Generally speaking, activities involve basic functions: sitting, standing, walking, lifting, sleeping, etc. Use the Pain Questionnaires to identify the basic functions in which patients experience difficulty. In this section of the SOAP chart, however, explain how each function relates to the patient's daily activities. Include the relevance of the specific activity to the patient's life, how long the patient can perform the activity before the symptoms begin or worsen, and compare with the patient's previous ability. For example: *pain increases from mild to moderate with sitting or standing over 30 minutes. Sits at computer 7–8 hours per day for work, stands in kitchen 1–2 hours per day doing household chores, and reads for recreation. Unable to drive comfortably more than 10 minutes—35-mile commute to work, picks children up from day care, next week a road trip with the family through the Canyon Lands is scheduled—planned for 6 months.*

Include activities the patient can no longer perform because of the symptoms. For example: *unable to lift objects over 25 pounds—job requires lifting objects up to 60 pounds, exercise routine included weight-lifting, small children at home require lifting for care.* Address endurance by describing an activity and stating the amount tolerated before signs of fatigue are exhibited. For example: *must stop reading after 20 minutes, housework after 10 minutes because of pain and fatigue.*

If the patient was injured on the job and workers' compensation benefits cover the treatments, chart work-related activities. Otherwise, be balanced in recording activities that represent all aspects of the patient's life.

130

HANDS HEAL:
COMMUNICATION,
DOCUMENTATION,
AND INSURANCE BILLING
FOR MANUAL THERAPISTS

When daily activities change noticeably but symptoms remain constant, a look at aggravating activities may reveal progress that might otherwise go undetected. Often, when patients are recovering from injuries that have limited them, the better they feel, the more they attempt to do. They are eager to return to work, get out of the house, and feel useful again. The weeds in the garden are nagging them, the stack of laundry is piling up, the kids want to get the flat tire fixed on the bike. When the activity level increases, there may be little to no improvement in symptoms; symptoms may even worsen. Rather than assuming that there is no progress, document the changes in activities. This will explain the lack of progress with the symptoms and show improvement in the patient's health based on activity level.

Activities That Relieve Symptoms

List activities that alleviate symptoms. Include modifying necessary activities, self-care, exercises, or remedies that relieve the symptoms. Changing positions, taking frequent breaks, stretching exercises, self-massage and hydrotherapy techniques are also considered activities that alleviate symptoms.

Investigate closely the steps the patient has taken to care for herself. Uncover as many ways as possible that the patient participates in her health care. Document specific activities that you want to reinforce or that have been particularly effective. For example: *Patient applies ice to low back as needed for pain, sits on a tennis ball to relieve trigger point pain, and squeezes tennis ball throughout day to exercise hands.* You may choose not to record all the information uncovered, but use it to compliment the patient, build her self-esteem, and encourage her to continue to participate in her health care.

OBJECTIVE

This section of the SOAP chart stores objective data: facts the practitioner collects. These include:

◆ Measurable findings
◆ Treatment applications
◆ Patient's response to the session.

State information clearly and concisely. Stick to details within your scope of practice, ones you can confidently prove or support in a peer review or deposition. If you do not have diagnostic license, do not perform or record the results of diagnostic tests in the objective section of the SOAP chart. Do not chart modalities for which you cannot explain the physiological effects clearly and consistently. Avoid data that cannot be measured or reproduced. Third party payors will not reimburse for intervention that "appears" to be needed.[1]

Measurable Findings

Manual therapists primarily gather the following objective, measurable data: visual observations, palpatory findings, and movement and strength tests. Standardized formats can be used for noting posture, palpation, and range of motion and still allow for individual variations. These are presented in the next section of this chapter. Additional assessment tests vary among professions and specialties. Document all tests uniformly and consistently.

Follow these simple guidelines when gathering and charting your objective findings:

◆ Document a full range of data.
◆ Measure every finding.
◆ Measure before and after treatment application.
◆ Perform the post-assessment in the same way as the pre-assessment.
◆ Use consistent terminology and symbols.

The data you record should represent the full scope of your practice. Do not limit yourself by narrowly focusing on one aspect of your expertise. Insurance adjusters or peer reviewers may get the wrong idea and assume that your scope is more limited than it actually is. This can cause problems when others in your profession exercise the full extent of the professional scope.

▼

Recently, I attended a meeting with reviewers and medical directors from a few insurance companies, to defend the scope of practice of massage therapists as a result of a narrowing interpretation of our assessment and treatment abilities. The medical director of one of the health plans claimed she was getting hypertonicities from reading about all the hypertonicities on therapists' SOAP charts. She wanted to know why the providers in her network insisted on listing every tight muscle in the body and nothing else, and whether indeed the therapists were capable of noting inflammation, spasms, trigger points, joint dysfunction, etc. Balance your objective charting by noting a variety of findings.

STORY TELLER 6-1

The Laundry List of Hypertonicities

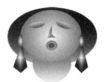

Measure all information. Quantify and qualify data based on deviations from normal. Normal is determined by:

◆ Comparing bilaterally when possible
◆ Defining normal for a general population of similar constitution
◆ Asking the patient to define normal for himself

Quantify data by rating the intensity of its expression. For example: *the trigger point was **moderately** painful with digital pressure at the trigger point site and **mildly** painful at the referral site*; or, *cervical flexion passive range of motion was limited **moderate minus** with **mild** pain at end range.*

Qualify data by describing its expression. For example: *right shoulder active abduction moderate **segmented** movement with mild **compensatory** shoulder elevation at end range*; or, *moderate plus **sharp shooting** pain with movement from prone to supine position while turning on treatment table.*

Assess the condition before and after treatment. It is difficult to document progress or determine the effectiveness of a treatment modality without being able to do a before-and-after comparison. For example: *moderate trigger point site pain changed to mild pain, mild referred pain changed to no pain; or, moderate segmented movement in right shoulder active abduction changed to smooth movement without compensatory shoulder elevation.*

Perform tests identically pretreatment and posttreatment. Data must be comparable. For example, postural analysis in a standing position (weight bearing) provides different

132

HANDS HEAL:
COMMUNICATION,
DOCUMENTATION,
AND INSURANCE BILLING
FOR MANUAL THERAPISTS

information from postural analysis in a supine or seated position (non-weight bearing). Therefore, the patient should be in the same position for both tests. Also, reproduce the test in the original environment. For example, if the patient was sitting in a chair for the pretreatment range of motion assessment, he should be sitting in the same chair, not on the treatment table, for the post-treatment assessment.

Be consistent from session to session. It is difficult to compare data over time if the range of motion testing was done standing initially, seated last session, and supine this session.

Pick qualifying and quantifying terms and use them consistently. *Smooth, segmented,* and *spastic* may describe the quality of the range of motion. *Sharp* and *dull* can be used to qualify pain. Numerical scales (0–10) or value scales (L, M, S) can quantify data. Select terms that adequately represent your assessment test results. Create abbreviations for the terms if necessary and add them to your legend. Most importantly, use the same terms consistently, session to session and patient to patient.

Visual Observations

Visual findings stem from observing movement patterns, posture, muscle atrophy, skin abnormalities, swelling, signs of trauma (such as bruises, abrasions, and scars), etc. Much of the visual data can be recorded on the SOAP chart by drawing symbols on the figures. For example, posture is easily noted on the figures by drawing skewed lines to depict elevations, and arrows in the direction of rotations. Use standard symbols to represent visual findings or add your own to the key. Movement patterns, such as gait or respiration, and comments about general appearance are more easily noted in the space provided for written information. (See Figure 6-2)

Follow these guidelines for documenting posture and movement patterns:

◆ Note the position of the patient (seated, standing, prone, supine, etc.).
◆ Record the angle of the observation (anterior, lateral, posterior, etc.).
◆ Describe the activity being observed (breathing, walking, lifting, standing, etc.).
◆ Follow the guidelines for gathering and charting objective findings (listed previously).

For example: *patient supine, anterior-lateral view, deep inhalation, mild plus mobility restriction upper right.*

Posture can be quantified by rating the amount of deviation from normal.

Chart irregularities: forward head posture, leg length variations, spinal curvatures, etc. Note elevations, rotations, inversions, and eversions. Common sites for observing posture are at the ears, shoulders, superior and inferior angles of the scapulae, anterior and posterior superior iliac spine, knees, and the medial and lateral malleoli.

Breath can be measured by qualifying the pattern and rate of breath, describing sounds associated with breathing, and quantifying the mobility of the ribs with inhalation. Note irregularities such as rattling noise or shallow, rapid, weak, uneven, or inconsistent patterns in breathing. Observe the rise and fall of the ribs and chart the restrictions.

Movement can be qualified and quantified by noting the amount of movement, how well the movement is performed, and how long the patient can sustain the movement before fatigue. Note sensations caused by movement and rate their expression.

Record the full range of data for initial and progress notes. In subsequent notes, focus on data that support the needs of the day.

Palpation Findings

Palpation is an objective test used to locate and assess inconsistencies in various rhythms, pulses, and systems of the body: soft tissue, joints, viscera, lymph, etc. Manual therapists

John Olson, LMP, GCFP
345 Moon River Rd. Ste. 6
Minnehaha, MN   55987
TEL   612 555 9889

HANDS HEAL

SOAP CHART-M

Patient Name   _Darnel G. Washington_   Date _2-6-01_

Date of Injury _1-6-01_   Insurance ID# _123-45-6789_ Current Meds _hydrocodone_

O   Findings: Visual/Palpable/Test Results

v: Primary weight bearing rising and standing-right leg and foot, sits on right pelvis, bends from mid thoracic region, breath moderately shallow and rapid, mild to moderate segmental movement left ribs with deep inhalation

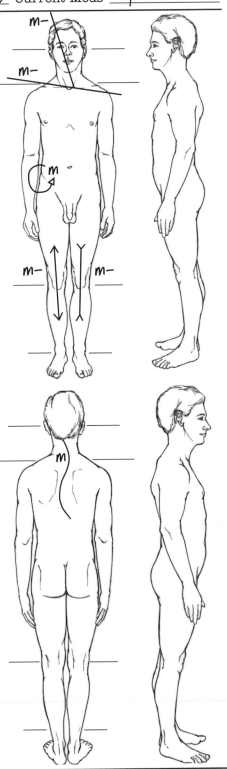

Provider Signature   _JO, LMP, GCFP_   Date _2-6-01_

Legend: ℮ TP   • TeP   ○ ℗   ✳ Infl   ≡ HT   ≈ SP

         ✕ Adh   ≋ Numb   ◯ rot   ╱ elev   ⊱ Short   ↔ Long

Figure 6-2.   Objective: visual observations.

134

HANDS HEAL:
COMMUNICATION,
DOCUMENTATION,
AND INSURANCE BILLING
FOR MANUAL THERAPISTS

tend to be highly trained and adept at sensing subtle discrepancies and changes under their fingers. As a result, detailed palpatory information is a valuable resource for all caregivers involved in the patient's case, and the information can be shared through SOAP charts and progress reports.

Document palpation findings by noting and describing abnormalities and conditions. Terminology varies among professions and specialties. Compile a comprehensive list of evaluative terms for your practice and use the terms consistently. Your list may include:

◆ Muscle tone—tension, hypertonic, hypotonic, spastic, rigid, splinting, contracture, spasm, lines of tension, holding patterns, etc.
◆ Pain—trigger points, tender points, stress points, meridian points, Jones points, sensation, presence or absence of sensation, spasm-pain-spasm cycle, etc. (Note: Pain is usually considered subjective information. Pain becomes objective if it is elicited by the practitioner through touch, testing, etc.)
◆ Scar tissue—adhesions, fibrosis, fibrotic tissue, granulation tissue
◆ Inflammation—swelling, edema, active hyperemia, passive congestion, congestion, stagnation, heat, pitted edema, regeneration or remodeling phase, etc.

Avoid diagnostic terms—Grade II sprain or strain, lymphedema, etc.—to describe findings if you do not have diagnostic scope or if the referring HCP or the patient did not provide you with diagnostic information.

Measure the palpation data by rating the intensity of the finding—i.e. *severe spasm*— or quantifying the size—i.e. *right ankle edema 10-inch circumference.*

Much of the data collected through palpation is easily documented on figures using symbols found in the legend. Write the quantifying or qualifying terms next to the figure with a connecting line. Anything too complicated or cumbersome to draw on the figures can be written out in the space provided. (See Figure 6-3) The figures are intended to increase speed and ease in documentation and to aid in fast recall. This intent is defeated if the figures are overburdened with symbols. If the data are abundant, draw the primary information on the figures, and list the secondary data in the space provided under Objective.

Follow these guidelines when documenting palpation findings:

◆ Identify the specific location.
◆ Rate or describe the type of touch that triggers the finding.
◆ Include any referred sensation, if applicable.
◆ Identify connections or relationships, if any.
◆ Follow the guidelines for gathering and charting objective findings (listed previously).

For example: *left biceps insertion moderate pain with mild digital pressure, mild plus referred pain into left elbow.*

Range of Motion Testing

The most common standardized testing for manual therapists is range of motion (ROM) testing (for a blank form, see Appendix: Forms). It is used in many professions and is familiar to lay people as a means of assessing health. A popular television commercial shows a person bending over and touching his toes, at first with limitation and pain, then—after taking the product—with greater range and ease. The message: greater movement with less discomfort equals better health. As a result, many patients expect ROM testing from any practitioner assessing and treating joint pain.

John Olson, LMP, GCFP

345 Moon River Rd. Ste. 6
Minnehaha, MN   55987
TEL   612 555 9889

HANDS HEAL

SOAP CHART-M

Patient Name _Darnel G. Washington_   Date _2-6-01_

Date of Injury _1-6-01_   Insurance ID# _123-45-6789_   Current Meds _hydrocodone_

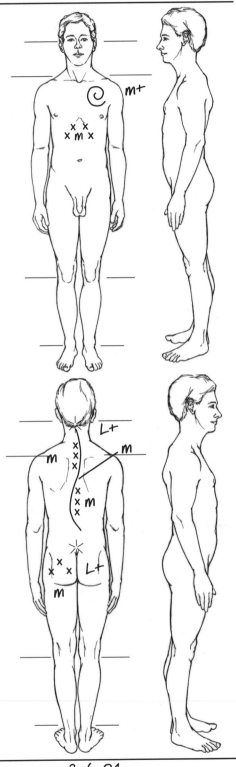

O   Findings: Visual/Palpable/Test Results

P: Moderate right frontal torsion moderate plus, bilateral
sphenoid compression mild plus, adhesion tentorium,
cranial rhythm moderately weak right, mild left

Provider Signature   _JO, LMP, GCFP_   Date _2-6-01_

Figure 6-3. Objective: palpation.

136

HANDS HEAL:
COMMUNICATION,
DOCUMENTATION,
AND INSURANCE BILLING
FOR MANUAL THERAPISTS

ROM testing is a valuable assessment tool for determining the stage of inflammation, the level of severity of sprains and strains, joint trauma, and muscle weakness. Gather and record ROM test results to substantiate dysfunction and validate progress as well as identify conditions. Assessing ROM before treatment substantiates the limitations for the patient. Retesting ROM after intervention demonstrates the effectiveness of the treatment plan and proves progress as a result of the session. Periodic testing pretreatment and post-treatment shows continued progress, and gives the patient, the referring caregivers, and the insurance reviewers evidence that the treatment is working.

Document the test:

◆ Identify the position of the patient—standing, seated, prone, supine, sidelying.
◆ Identify the type of test—active, active assisted, passive, resistive.
◆ Name the joint —right shoulder, left hip, cervical spine, etc.
◆ Name the action—flexion, extension, left rotation, right lateral flexion, etc.

Chart the results of the test:

◆ Identify and rate the deviation from normal—hypermobile, hypomobile, within normal limits (e.g., *moderate decrease in seated active cervical flexion . . .*)
◆ Identify the cause of the limitation—pain, muscle tension, spasm, edema, loose bodies, etc. (e.g., *. . . due to protective muscle contracture and edema . . .*)
◆ Identify and rate the quality of the movement—painful, compensational movement, segmented movement, weak, spastic, rigid, etc. (e.g., *. . . with moderate pain*)

(See Figure 6-4)

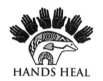

John Olson, LMP, GCFP

345 Moon River Rd. Ste. 6
Minnehaha, MN   55987
Tel   612 555 9889

HANDS HEAL

RANGE OF MOTION

Patient Name __Darnel G. Washington__   Date __2-6-01__

Date of Injury __1-6-01__   Insurance ID# __123-45-6789__

PRE-TEST 1 (circle test parameters)

Position of patient: prone, sidelying, sitting, (standing,) supine, other: _____

Type of test: (active,) active assisted, passive, resistive, other: _____

Joint: C-spine, T-spine, (L-spine,) hip, knee, ankle, shoulder, elbow, wrist, other: _____

Action	Range+Int (R)	(L)	Pain+Int (R)	(L)	Ltd+Int (R)	(L)	Mvmt+Int (R)	(L)
flex	M⁻↓		L		L⁺	1	L	seg
ext	M⁺↓		M		L⁺	1	M⁻	seg
SB	L↓	M↓	L	M	L⁺1	L⁺1	N	Mseg

POST-TEST 1 (circle test parameters)

Position of patient: prone, sidelying, sitting, (standing,) supine, other: _____

Type of test: (active,) active assisted, passive, resistive, other: _____

Joint: C-spine, T-spine, (L-spine,) hip, knee, ankle, shoulder, elbow, wrist, other: _____

Action	Range+Int (R)	(L)	Pain+Int (R)	(L)	Ltd+Int (R)	(L)	Mvmt+Int (R)	(L)
flex	L↓		θ		L	1	N	
ext	M↓		M⁻		L	1	L⁻	seg
SB	A̸	A̸	A̸	L	L1	L1	N	L seg

Figure 6-4. ROM chart.

ROM test results are commonly expressed in degrees or percentages of normal. If you are not trained to use measuring devices such as goniometers and do not have extensive experience in rating ranges of motion, use the value scale of mild, moderate, and severe to rate ROM test results. You will be able to show deviations from normal with enough detail to note progress as changes develop, without putting your credibility at stake should the case go to court and your test results be compared with those of caregivers with more training and expertise in precise ROM measurements. (For information on how to perform ROM tests or use goniometric measurements, see Kendall et al.[8] or Norkin and White.[9])

Treatment

Document the length of the session, the modalities used, and the location the treatments were applied. For ease in insurance billing, this section may record the Current Procedural Terminology (CPT) codes for the modalities, and the length of the session in units. Before using CPT codes on SOAP charts, check your state regulations to verify appropriate use of CPT codes according to your scope of practice, and check with individual insurance plans to verify which CPT codes are reimbursable. (See Chapter 8 for in depth information on insurance verification.)

Record the treatment in two ways. First, provide a big picture of the session: the length of the session, modalities, and general body parts treated. For example: *1-hour full-body Swedish massage; 30-minute foot reflexology;* or *90-minute Hellerwork—inspiration.* Second, fill in the details: particular techniques used to treat specific findings. For example: *muscle energy with cervical flexion, direct pressure on scalene trigger point,* or *myofascial release on diaphragm.* You needn't write down everything you do; just the highlights. Chart enough information to recall the important events of the session at a later date.

Patient's Response to Treatment

Every subjective and objective finding should be reassessed during the session. This may happen as you go—immediately after a specific technique is applied to address a particular symptom—or at the end of the session.

Quantify and qualify the changes. Include positive and negative responses to treatment. Record the updated information on the chart above or along side the original entry. Use the delta symbol (Δ) to distinguish the pre-treatment data from the post-treatment entry. (See Figure 6-5) This is an efficient way to document the patient's response and avoid rewriting in several places on the chart.

Note symptoms and measurable data that did not change. This may help you determine areas of focus for next session. Identify whether the treatment was ineffective or time did not permit addressing the issue. In either case, you will want to address the problem in the treatment plan; make the issue a priority for the next session or select another technique to use. "No change" is easily abbreviated with a line drawn through the delta symbol. ($\cancel{\Delta}$)

ASSESSMENT

Traditionally, the assessment section of the SOAP chart records the practitioner's interpretation of the subjective and objective findings. Conclusions are drawn, the condition is named (diagnosis), and the prognosis—probable course of the disease—is determined and recorded on the SOAP chart. However, practitioners without diagnostic scope are not permitted to assess the patient's condition in these terms.

John Olson, LMP, GCFP

345 Moon River Rd. Ste. 6
Minnehaha, MN   55987
Tel   612 555 9889

HANDS HEAL

SOAP CHART-M

Patient Name __Darnel G. Washington__   Date __2-6-01__

Date of Injury __1-6-01__   Insurance ID# __123-45-6789__   Current Meds __hydrocodone__

S   Focus for Today   ↓ Pain in head, neck, back

Symptoms: Location/Intensity/Frequency/Duration/Onset

Neck, mid, low back pain moderate
constant since car accident Δ L
headache Pain moderate intermittant
daily since car accident Δ ℗̸

O   Findings: Visual/Palpable/Test Results

V: Primary weight bearing rising and standing-
    right leg and foot Δ̸
    sits on right pelvis Δ L ↓ balance
    bends from mid thoracic Δ̸
    breath moderately shallow and rapid Δ L & even
    mild to moderate segmental movement
    left ribs with deep inhalation Δ smooth

P: moderate right frontal torsion Δ L
    moderate plus bilateral sphenoid compression Δ M⁻
    mild plus adhesion tentorium Δ̸
    cranial rhythm moderately weak right Δ L
    mild left Δ Normal

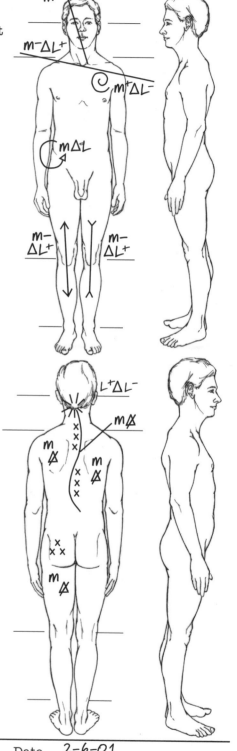

Provider Signature __JO, LMP, GCFP__   Date __2-6-01__

Legend:
    ℮ TP   • TeP   ○ ℗   ✳ Infl   ≡ HT   ≈ SP
    ✗ Adh   ≋ Numb   ↻ rot   ╱ elev   ⊢⊣ Short   ⟷ Long

Figure 6-5. Objective: response to treatment.

In functional outcomes reporting, assessment is also the place to summarize the patient's functional ability: limitations, previous ability, and current situation; and to set goals that, when accomplished, demonstrate functional progress. Every practitioner using the functional approach to SOAP charting will record a functional summary and functional goals in the assessment section. If you have diagnostic scope, include your diagnoses and prognoses as well.

Record the following under Assessment:

◆ The patient's functional limitations in order of importance.
◆ The patient's previous ability to perform these activities.
◆ The role these activities play in the patient's current situation.
◆ The long-term and short-term functional goals that will demonstrate the desired outcomes.

PLAN

The Plan section records the treatment plan and self care exercises. Set the timeline for sessions—frequency and duration—and the reevaluation date. Chart specific instructions for homework suggestions. Document your referrals and recommendations for outside tests.

TREATMENT PLAN

The initial note projects the plans for the first series of treatments. Given the information shared in the extensive initial interview and full body assessment, the practitioner and the patient select treatment modalities to employ. Base your choice of modalities on the goals for the session, what has worked for the patient in the past, and what has worked for others with similar conditions and constitution. List the modalities projected and the general locations for applying the modalities. For example: *craniosacral therapy with attention to the thoracic cage, muscle energy for cervical flexion and extension, and lymph drainage for upper quadrants.*

Record the frequency of the subsequent sessions—*3 times a week, weekly, monthly, etc.*—duration of sessions—*30 minutes, 1 hour, 90 minutes, etc.*—and the reevaluation date. The plan should cover the length of the prescription or the time allotted for the LTG. For example: *45-minute sessions, twice a week for 3 weeks. Reevaluation on 6-15-01.*

Update the plan in subsequent notes if the patient's condition changes or the plan is no longer appropriate based on the patient's response to the previous treatments. Let the treatment plan guide you but not dictate the sessions. Be flexible and respond to individual needs as they arise. Remain mindful of the goals at the same time.

Progress notes reflect the plan for the next series of sessions. Think ahead: how can the two of you accomplish the goals in the allotted time? The plan will help you use the time efficiently.

Self-Care

Record self-care exercises and homework assignments that support the goals. Self-care is a broad term that includes modifying activities to decrease pain and effort and increase safety, stretching and strengthening exercises, and home remedies such as ice packs, Epson salt baths, polstices, ointments, self-massage techniques, etc. Compliment the patient

140

HANDS HEAL:
COMMUNICATION,
DOCUMENTATION,
AND INSURANCE BILLING
FOR MANUAL THERAPISTS

on everything he currently does to improve his condition and reinforce his efforts by charting the self-care exercises that are most productive.

It is common to confuse homework exercises with goals. Goals and homework are intimately related but distinctly different. Homework increases the patient's ability to perform an activity. Homework includes exercises performed repeatedly to strengthen the patient, decrease the symptoms, and help attain the goal. The goals is the intended level of ability to perform the activity. For example, Zamora's goal is to cook. Homework may include lifting light objects to increase her ability to lift a heavy sauté pan and toss food. We might assign homework to Zamora, inviting her to sauté a pan of food every day for an increasing amount of time—5 minutes, 10 minutes, 30 minutes, etc.—until she reaches her goal of 5 hours.

Be specific and provide detailed instructions when assigning homework. Support the patient's self-care routine by recording the homework assignment and the specific instructions or attaching a copy of the instruction sheet to the chart. That is difficult to do if we cannot remember the assignment. For example: *Stand up and stretch for 2 minutes for every hour at the computer. Hold all stretches for 30 seconds. Stretches include: bend over and touch toes slowly, return to standing. Bend over to each side, return to standing. Pull arms behind back using filing cabinet. Before sitting down, walk to the water fountain and drink.*

Keep homework simple. Make sure it fits into their lifestyle. Homework should not be too time-consuming if the patient is very busy, nor too complex if the exercise is new. Assign activities the patient will find familiar and comfortable. Ideally, homework should be the patient's idea, or a modification of something the patient suggests.

Remember, do not provide homework to people who are not ready for it. Some patients do not yet believe that change is possible. Assign awareness exercises for patients who are unaware of their role in the healing process and cannot recognize change when it occurs. Invite them to notice what they feel like when they are performing an activity that exacerbates their condition. For example: *Every hour spent at the computer, stop and take a break. Notice how your neck, back, arms, and hands feel. Make a mental note or jot down a few words that will remind you of that specific feeling. Notice if anything you do makes that feeling better or worse.*

Initial Notes, Subsequent Notes, Progress Notes, and Discharge Notes

Four types of notes are recorded on a SOAP chart:

- Initial notes
- Subsequent notes
- Progress notes
- Discharge notes

(For blank forms, see Appendix: Forms)

The **initial notes** are comprehensive and include extensive information regarding the patient's health and current situation. Much of the information recorded on an initial SOAP chart does not need to be repeated on subsequent notes. Evaluate the full body: how the patient is responding to their current health situation from head to toe, all compensational holding patterns, concomitant dysfunctions, and the impact of the condition on the patient's life. List and prioritize all the patient's health concerns. Determine the treatment goals, discuss and record the plan. Use the extended version of the SOAP chart. (See Figure 6-6)

Subsequent notes are brief and reflect the patient's immediate concerns for the day's treatment session. The notes are less comprehensive and more focused. For example, on Darnel's initial SOAP chart, all cervical actions and ranges of motion were tested and recorded. On a subsequent note, only the cervical active range of motion for lateral flexion was tested, charted, treated, and retested. The intent is to spend more time accomplishing goals than determining the plan. The treatment plan is projected initially and reviewed during reevaluation sessions. Subsequent sessions carry out the treatment plan. The chart should reflect that and not repeat the goals or treatment plans unless changes are necessary. A shorter version of the initial SOAP chart is adequate for recording information between the initial visit and the reevaluation sessions. (See Figure 6-7)

Progress notes are used to chart reevaluation sessions. Reevaluation sessions are nearly as extensive as initial visits. Time is spent assessing progress and creating new treatment plans. Schedule reevaluation sessions every 4–8 visits and document them thoroughly. The notes for these sessions should be comprehensive and include a full-body evaluation. The intent is to present a complete picture of the patient's health and provide summary information for progress reports. Progress notes are recorded on the extended version of a SOAP chart, and are similar to the initial SOAP chart. (See Figure 6-8)

Many facilities also require **discharge notes**: a final summary of the patient's progress, health status and any subsequent course of action. Use the same SOAP chart you used for the progress notes and adapt the plan section to cover discharge data. Write the reasons for discharge—reached limits of referral, patient met goals for care, plateau in patient's progress, etc.—in place of the treatment plan. Ongoing care may be required to maintain the progress established. Document any further action to be taken by the patient. Record the self-care regime you recommend, suggestions for additional care, and any referrals to other caregivers or back to the referring HCP. (See Figure 6-8)

Discharge notes include:

- Summary of treatment, dates, missed or canceled sessions
- Current health status
- Summary of progress
- Reason for ending care
- Recommendations for ongoing care
- Referrals

Timing

SOAP charting may feel time-consuming at this point. You may be just beginning to chart, or you may not have charted this extensively before. Charting may feel burdensome until it becomes habitual and you memorize common abbreviations. In time, you can expect to spend no more than 5 minutes charting outside of each appointment time. Most charting occurs during the session with your patients. Charting in your patients' presence effectively includes them in the healing process. Do this to ensure accuracy and completeness and present an air of professionalism.

Write down subjective and objective information as you gather it from the patient. If you are performing hands-on tests or evaluating data pretreatment and posttreatment,

John Olson, LMP, GCFP
345 Moon River Rd. Ste. 6
Minnehaha, MN   55987
TEL   612 555 9889

HANDS HEAL

SOAP CHART-M

Patient Name   Darnel G. Washington   Date   2-6-01

Date of Injury   1-6-01   Insurance ID#   123-45-6789   Current Meds   hydrocodone

S   Focus for Today   ↓ Pain in head, neck, back

Symptoms: Location/Intensity/Frequency/Duration/Onset
Neck, midback, low back pain moderate
constant since car accident Δ L
headache Pain moderate intermittant
daily since car accident Δ ⓟ

Activities of Daily Living: Aggravating/Relieving
A: sitting (playing bridge) lifting (grandaughter)
    bowling, dancing, gardening
R: rest, heat

O   Findings: Visual/Palpable/Test Results
V: Primary weight bearing rising and standing-
    right leg and foot Δ̸
    sits on right pelvis Δ L ↓ balance
    bends from mid thoracic Δ̸
    breath moderately shallow and rapid Δ L & even
    mild to moderate segmental movement
    left ribs with deep inhalation Δ smooth
P: moderate right frontal torsion Δ L
    moderate plus bilateral sphenoid compression Δ M⁻
    mild plus adhesion tentorium
    cranial rhythm moderately weak right Δ L
    mild left Δ Normal
Modalities: Applications/Locations
97140 Lymph Drainage—trunk
60 min. Craniosacral—head
        Feldenkrais—eyes and feet
Response to Treatment (see Δ)

A   Prioritize Functional Limitations

1. lifting granddaughter—necessary for care: in & out of car seat,
   high chair, bed etc.
2. gardening—vegetable and flower garden, bonding time with wife

Goals: Long-term/Short-term

LTG: Lift granddaughter at least 10 times per day from the floor and
     carry her for 10 minutes with mild pain and fatigue 5 days per
     week in 60 days
STG: Lift light weight toys from floor 10 times per day 3 days per
     week in 2 weeks with mild pain

P   Future Treatment/Frequency

2 times per week for 3 weeks, 60 min. sessions, continue with lymph
drainage, craniosacral and Feldenkrais, focus on ribs, diaphragms, increase
mobility and decrease adhesions
Homework/Self-care
continue using heat on mid back but avoid it on neck and low back—
switch to ice. Deep breathing exercises

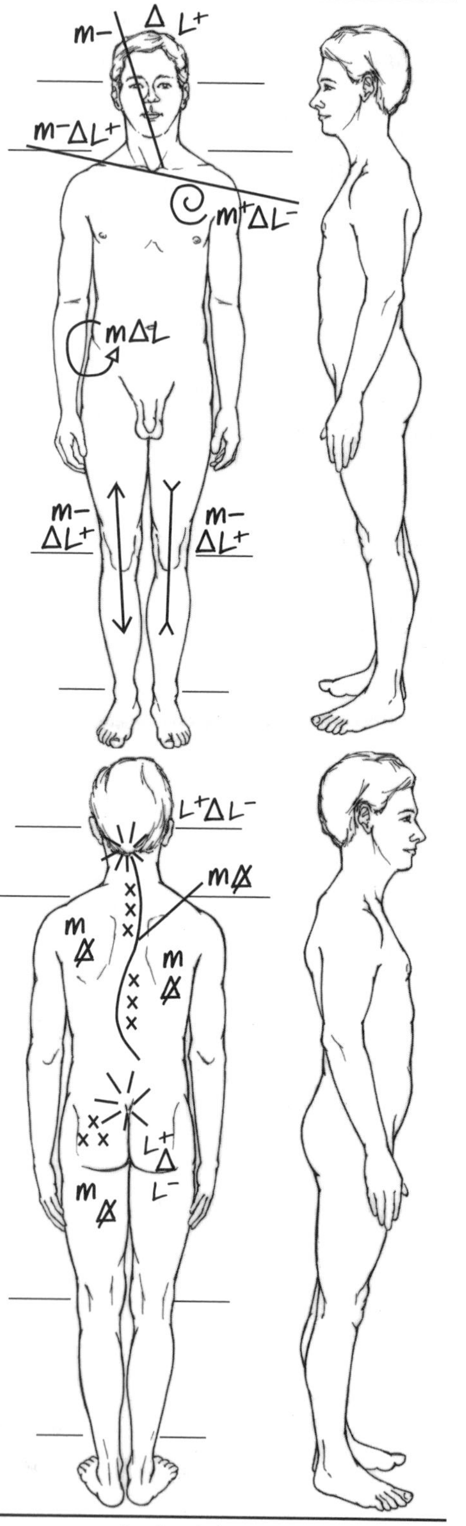

Provider Signature   JO, LMP, GCFP   Date   2-6-01

Legend: ℮ TP   • TeP   ○ ⓟ   ✳ Infl   ≡ HT   ≈ SP
            ✕ Adh   ≋ Numb   ◠ rot   ╱ elev   ⤜ Short   ↔ Long

Figure 6-6. Initial SOAP chart.

John Olson, LMP, GCFP

345 Moon River Rd. Ste. 6
Minnehaha, MN   55987
TEL   612 555 9889

HANDS HEAL

SOAP CHART-M

Patient Name __Darnel G. Washington__   Date __2-8-01__

Date of Injury __1-6-01__   Insurance ID# __123-45-6789__   Current Meds __hydrocodone__

S Focus-decrease pain in head and neck

moderate neck and headache pain   Δ L

moderate stiffness and heat neck   Δ L⁻

O 97140 60 min

Lymph Drainage neck, head

all passive cervical ranges of motion limited-mild-with

mild plus pain at end range due to inflammation

Δ L⁻ with L Pain

A lifting lightweight toys from shelves with moderate

pain

P having good success with ice and breathing exercises

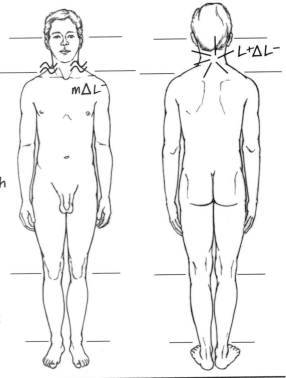

Provider Signature ___JO LMP GCFP___   Date _____

S Focus decrease pain in head & neck

mild plus neck and head pain   Δ L⁻

mild plus stiffness and neck heat   Δ L⁻

O 97140 60 min

Lymph Drainage neck, head, chest, arms, all passive

cervical ranges of motion limited-mild minus-with

mild pain at end ranges due to inflammation Δ N

with L⁻ pain

A con't as above

P con't as above

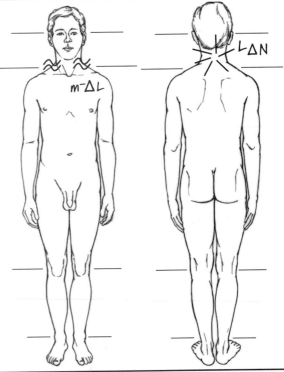

Provider Signature ___JO LMP GCFP___   Date __2-11-01__

Legend: ⊙ TP   • TeP   ○ Ⓟ   ＊ Infl   ≡ HT   ≈ SP

              ✕ Adh   ≋ Numb   ↻ rot   ╱ elev   ⤞ Short   ↔ Long

Figure 6-7. Subsequent SOAP chart.

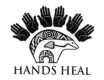

John Olson, LMP, GCFP
345 Moon River Rd. Ste. 6
Minnehaha, MN 55987
TEL 612 555 9889

HANDS HEAL

SOAP CHART-M

Patient Name *Darnel G. Washington*   Date *1-20-02*

Date of Injury *1-6-01*   Insurance ID# *123-45-6789*   Current Meds *Ø*

S Focus for Today   *decrease stiffback*

Symptoms: Location/Intensity/Frequency/Duration/Onset

*Stiff mid back mild constant for 4 days since bridge marathon
last weekend Δ within normal limits*

Activities of Daily Living: Aggravating/Relieving

*A: carrying granddaughter more than 10 minutes sitting or
gardening for more than 2 hours
R: exercises, stretching, rest*

O Findings: Visual/Palpable/Test Results

*moderate weakness with sitting Δ L
moving from mid thoracic instead of hips
rib mobility moderately decreased Δ L
breathing restricted-mild Δ N*

Modalities: Applications/Locations
*97140   Feldenkrais-ribs and thoracic spine
60 min.   Craniosacral-spinal traction and unwinding*
Response to Treatment (see Δ)

A Prioritize Functional Limitations

*has not regained prior functional status since car accident
1-6-01
(note activities of daily living listed above)*

Goals: Long-term/Short-term
*all goals have been reached within the limits of current
health condition*

P Future Treatment/Frequency
*continue awareness through movement classes once per month,
more often as needed, released from care and referred back to
primary care.*

Homework/Self-care

*Remember to breathe and roll ribs when sitting for long periods-
take breaks and do exercises before stiffness sets in*

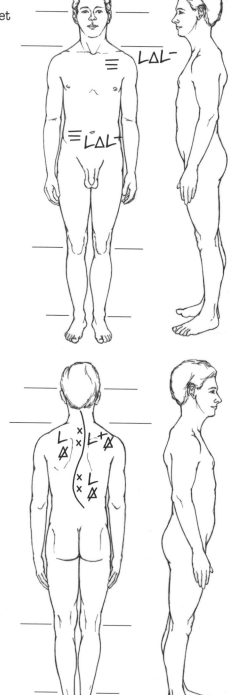

Provider Signature   *JO LMP GCFP*   Date *1-20-02*

Legend: ℮ TP   • TeP   ○ ℗   ✳ Infl   ≡ HT   ≈ SP

✕ Adh   ≋ Numb   ↻ rot   ╱ elev   ⊶ Short   ↔ Long

Figure 6-8. Progress SOAP chart with discharge plan.

take breaks to record information. Recording information as you go will prevent you from forgetting data, and will give the patient time to rest and integrate your treatment.

After the session is over, review the goals and write new ones. Evaluate the progress and share feedback. Speaking the results of the session aloud immediately after the treatment assists the patient in integrating the results, verbalizing his needs for the session, and formulating ideas for future solutions. Discuss homework options and write down all assignments. Record the results of the session and status of the goals, write new goals, and work out the treatment plan together before the session ends.

The only thing left to do after the patient leaves is to review the subjective and objective data and fill in any details that will assist you in remembering information later. Otherwise, all charting is a part of the session and done with the patient present.

SUMMARY

SOAP charting is a standard format routinely used by medical, chiropractic, and allied health professionals for documenting health care sessions. SOAP is an acronym that stands for:

◆ Subjective—states health concerns, records information from the patient
◆ Objective—stores practitioner observations and measurable data, intervention, and the patient's response to treatment
◆ Assessment—summarizes the patient's functional limitations and records short-term and long-term goals for health (includes diagnoses and prognoses if scope of practice permits)
◆ Plan—states the plan for future treatments and the patient's self-care routine occurring between sessions

Documentation guidelines include:

◆ Be attentive and practice good listening skills.
◆ Chart information pertinent to patient's health.
◆ Be clear and concise.
◆ Use consistent terminology and standard abbreviations.
◆ Record positive and negative findings.
◆ Be objective.
◆ Measure everything.
◆ Avoid vague statements (improved, better, less pain, etc.).
◆ Write legibly.
◆ Never use correction fluid or erase information.
◆ Sign or initial legal name and credentials.
◆ Co-sign for students, aides, and apprentices.

Use a functional outcomes style of reporting information. Set long-term and short-term goals that will clearly demonstrate functional outcomes. Follow SMART criteria for functional goal setting. The acronym stands for:

◆ Specific—to an activity of daily living
◆ Measurable—quantify and qualify results to measure progress
◆ Attainable—success is probable given the patient's condition, constitution, and attitude

146

HANDS HEAL:
COMMUNICATION,
DOCUMENTATION,
AND INSURANCE BILLING
FOR MANUAL THERAPISTS

◆ Relevant—activity is critical to patient's ability to earn a living or care for self, family, or household
◆ Time-bound—success within a specified time
  –long-term goals—30–60 days
  –short-term goals—one to two weeks

Describe the symptoms in detail in the subjective section of the SOAP chart:

◆ Describe the symptom.
◆ Note the location.
◆ Rate the intensity, duration, and frequency.
◆ Give a detailed description of the onset.

Record functional limitations:

◆ Identify daily activities the patient can no longer do or cannot do without increasing symptoms.
◆ State the patient's previous ability to perform the activities listed.
◆ State the patient's current situation regarding the activities.
◆ Record activities that relieve the patient's condition.

Follow these guidelines for documenting objective data:

◆ Document the full range of data.
◆ Measure every finding.
◆ Base measurements on deviations from normal.
  –make bilateral comparison when possible
  –define normal for a general population of similar constitution
  –ask patients to define normal for themselves
◆ Measure the data before and after treatment.
◆ Perform the pre- and post-evaluations identically.
◆ Chart posture and movement by:
  –noting the position of the patient
  –noting the angle of the observation
  –describing the activity
◆ Chart palpation by:
  –identifying the specific location
  –rating or describing the touch that triggers the finding
  –including referred sensations
  –identifying connections or relationships between findings
◆ Chart the ROM test by:
  –identifying the position of the patient
  –identifying the type of test
  –naming the joint
  –naming the action
◆ Chart the results of the ROM test by:
  –identifying and rating the deviation from normal
  –identifying the cause of the limitation
  –identifying and rating the quality of the movement

There are four types of SOAP notes:

◆ Initial—comprehensive, prioritized list of concerns or desired results of the sessions, full body evaluation, projected treatment goals and plan
◆ Subsequent—address current concerns and short-term goals, site specific evaluation and treatment
◆ Progress—comprehensive review of concerns, full body evaluation, evaluate progress and re-establish treatment goals and plan
◆ Discharge—full body evaluation, summarize health status, summarize progress and functional outcomes, state reason for discharge, make recommendations for ongoing care

Chart throughout the session in the presence of the patient to prevent charts from piling up on your desk. Memorize abbreviations and in time you will become fast and efficient at SOAP charting.

REFERENCES

1. Kettenbach G. Writing SOAP Notes. 2nd ed. Philadelphia: FA Davis, 1995.
2. Bates B. Guide to Physical Examination. 7th ed. Philadelphia: JB Lippincott, 1999.
3. Adler RH, Giersch P. Whiplash, Spinal Trauma and the Chiropractic Personal Injury Case. 13th ed. Seattle: Adler◆Giersch, 2000.
4. Chödrön P. Start Where You Are, A Guide to Compassionate Living. Boston: Shambhala, 1994.
5. Weaver R. The Touch Factor Foundation Manual. Montana: Weaver, 1997.
6. Magee DJ. Orthopaedic Physical Assessment, 2nd ed. Philadelphia: WB Saunders, 1992.
7. Travell J, Simons D. Myofascial Pain and Dysfunction The Trigger Point Manual. Baltimore: Williams & Wilkins, 1983.
8. Kendell FP, McCreary EK, Provance PG. Muscles: Testing and Function. 4th ed. Baltimore: Williams & Wilkins, 1993.
9. Norkin CC, White D. Measurement of Joint Motion: A Guide to Goniometry. Philadelphia: F.A. Davis, 1995.

CHAPTER 7

Alternative Documentation: HxTxC Charting for Energy Work, On-Site Massage, and Relaxation and Spa Therapies

Jose received massage therapy weekly at the Healing Arts Clinic. He never mentioned to his massage therapists, Annie and Jamie, that he had been in a car accident. It wasn't a secret; he just didn't remember either of them asking. Jose was sure his car insurance would not cover massage because his doctor wouldn't prescribe it. Jose knew he needed something to loosen up his tense muscles and decided to pay cash for his weekly massage therapy.

Jose responded well to his massages. Annie combined Swedish techniques with deep tissue massage and gymnastics to increase mobility, loosen tight muscles, and help Jose relax. Jamie, who specialized in sports massage, used circulatory and drainage techniques. Jose found he had more energy and felt more relaxed. He believed massage was helping him recover from his car accident.

A year into his weekly massage routine, after prompting from his attorney, Jose asked the receptionist at the Healing Arts Clinic for copies of his massage records. His attorney wanted to include the massage records and bills in the settlement package for his personal injury lawsuit. The attorney intended to use the records to substantiate Jose's injuries—strengthening his lawsuit—and the bills for proof of out-of-pocket expenses Jose had incurred as a direct result of the accident. Jose hadn't specified any health complications and wasn't referred by a doctor, and no insurance company was paying for the sessions, so Annie had chosen not to document any of the sessions. Jamie did not chart her sessions either. The receptionist didn't have any records on Jose except cash receipts. Jose's lawyer was unable to establish a connection between the massage sessions and the injuries from the car accident without documentation. Therefore, Jose was unable to get reimbursed for the thousands of dollars he spent on massage, even though the therapy was instrumental in his recovery.

One afternoon, Jamie and Annie were sipping herbal tea at the Sunny Cafe downstairs and commiserating over their misfortune in losing their steady patient, Jose. Jamie told a similar story: Claire had been a patient for many years, coming monthly for relaxation massage. Then, 3 months ago, Claire had been injured at work. Claire's insurance company was refusing to pay for her massage therapy. The insurance adjuster claimed that because Claire had been seeing a massage therapist before the injury, she must have had pre-existing conditions that required her to continue receiving massage treatments. Therefore, the massage therapy was not necessary for treating the recent injury.

Claire asked Jamie for her records so that she could prove to the insurance company that she had been in excellent health until the injury. Jamie had no records of the massage sessions. Even though Claire had been healthy and received massage for relaxation only, there was no way to prove that to the insurance company. Claire was stuck with the bills.

Jamie and Annie shook their heads in dismay. Initially, they had been under the impression that only insurance-paying patients required documentation. Gone were the days when relaxation therapy was an excuse not to do paperwork. They made a pact with each other to better serve their patients and themselves by charting all sessions. It no longer mattered whether the session was for relaxation or injury treatment, or whether payment came from an insurance company or from the patient; they were going to keep records on every patient and document every session.

Introduction

SOAP (Subjective, Objective, Assessment, Plan) charting assists practitioners in solving patients' medical problems. Yet, not everyone seeks manual therapy to treat an injury or care for an illness. People often receive manual therapies in good health for a number of reasons: to relax and reduce stress, for healthy touch, or to detoxify and tone the skin, for example.

If SOAP charting is used to help assess, treat, and cure medical problems and the patient has no pre-existing conditions or current complaints, is the practitioner obligated to keep a medical record?

Yes. Manual therapy is considered a health care modality and practitioners are licensed, certified, or regulated in varying capacities throughout the United States and other countries. In keeping with health care standards, manual therapists must record information about the patient's health and the services provided. Obviously, treatment for healthy or injury-free patients may not require extensive documentation on a SOAP note, as does charting patient symptoms and pathophysiological findings. Documenting manual therapy sessions for healthy patients is brief in comparison, and the format can be tailored to specific environments, such as spas, airport concessions, and sporting events.

HxTxC Format for Documenting Healthy Patients

A simple system for documenting healthy patient treatments is the **HxTxC chart**. HxTxC is an acronym for History (Hx), Treatment (Tx), and Comments (C). An HxTxC chart contains a brief intake questionnaire gathering health history information (Hx) and provides space for recording the treatment provided (Tx). Additional information—such as personal preferences, variations from the routine, or patient progress—can be recorded under comments (C). Three styles of HxTxC charts are provided in this book: Standard HxTxC for relaxation, spa therapies, and energy work, Seated HxTxC for on-site sessions, and Sports HxTxC for sporting events. (For blank forms, see Appendix: Forms)

The HxTxC format meets the three basic needs for alternative documentation:

◆ It is quick and easy to use.
◆ It ensures the patients' safety.
◆ It provides legal protection for the practitioner.

QUICK AND EASY CHARTING

Health history and treatment options in the HxTxC chart are written so the practitioner or the patient can simply check off or circle answers. Narrative charting can be too time-consuming for fast-paced environments with high turnover. One way to speed up charting is to provide your patients with Yes or No questions on the intake and provide yourself with all options for treatment routines. For example: pre-event or post-event might be the only categories for a sporting event; seaweed wrap, mud pack, or herbal moisturizer for a salon; stress buster, smooth and soothe, or energizer for an airport concession. Customize your chart to fit your practice.

PATIENT SAFETY

Intake questions are designed to ensure the safety of the patient. The practitioner must be able to identify health situations that contraindicate treatment or require precautionary measures when providing treatment. For example, inflammation may indicate infection,

152

HANDS HEAL:
COMMUNICATION,
DOCUMENTATION,
AND INSURANCE BILLING
FOR MANUAL THERAPISTS

which contraindicates circulatory therapies. Numbness contraindicates deep pressure. Some symptoms contraindicate locally but not systemically, some techniques are contraindicated but not others.[1]

HxTxC charts have very few intake questions, but the questions are designed to get right to health issues. Any Yes answer to an intake question can require additional information to rule out potential harm.[2] Know how to respond to positive answers to intake questions. Refer to Werner's *A Massage Therapist's Guide to Pathology*, Williams & Wilkins, Baltimore, 1998,[1] for more information on contraindications and precautions for manual therapy.

Adapt the intake questions to the environment. For example, the intake questions for a sporting event cover signs and symptoms of shock, the primary contraindication for treatment after physical stress. Intake questions for a spa environment emphasize allergies to scents, oils, and other products used during aromatherapy and herbal wraps. Questions should identify general health concerns; for example, the patient has colitis, which contraindicates deep abdominal massage.[1] Include information-gathering questions specific to the treatment provided, such as a question about allergy to honey.

LEGAL PROTECTION

Protect yourself in the rare event of a malpractice case by demonstrating that health screening was considered and treatment was appropriate. To do this, have the patient fill out, sign, and date a health questionnaire. If the practitioner completes the form for the patient, require the patient to initial the entries. The HxTxC chart includes a brief health intake that can be used in place of the two page Health Information form. Chart health information on each patient and record the treatment provided. Use the Comments sections for noting anything out of the ordinary. Show that you checked for possible health complications and provided safe treatment.

▼

STORY TELLER 7-1

Review Health History Before Treating

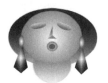

Always look over the health history before proceeding with the treatment. Recently, a malpractice case was filed accusing an on-site massage therapist of harming a patient. Before the session, the therapist handed the intake form to the patient. The patient read the form and handed it back to the practitioner without completing it. The therapist proceeded with the treatment without realizing that the patient had not signed off on the statement of health. As it turned out, the person had one of the conditions listed as a contraindication on the form, and alleged he was injured as a result of the treatment provided. Take the steps to protect yourself, and follow through on them.

SOAP Charting vs. HxTxC Charting

Determine whether a SOAP note is necessary or whether an alternative format, such as a HxTxC chart can be used. The question is not whether or not to document but rather which documentation format to use: SOAP, HxTxC, narrative, etc. It is *always* necessary to chart manual therapy sessions. These are the factors to consider when selecting one style of documentation over another:

- Patient health
- Patient expectations
- Goals of treatment
- Treatment results
- Reimbursement for services

GUIDELINES FOR SELECTING SOAP FORMAT

First, determine whether the SOAP format is appropriate. SOAP charting is your best option any time extensive documentation is necessary. If any one of these statements apply, use the standard SOAP format to document the treatment. (See Chapter 6 for in depth information on SOAP charting.)

- The patient has health problems or symptoms and is seeking treatment to relieve them.
- A doctor referred the patient for treatment.
- Insurance is involved in reimbursement.
- The treatment provided varies from individual to individual, and is based upon patient symptoms, conditions, and practitioner findings.
- The treatment results are significant, specific and measurable.
- The patient considers the treatments to be a regular part of a health care routine.

A SOAP note is appropriate when the patient has health concerns that the manual therapist is expected to address during treatment. Often patients have expectations, sometimes similar, sometimes different than ours concerning treatment. We may think we are providing treatment for relaxation, but the patient may have selected the treatment specifically to heal a whiplash injury, as was the case for Jose. Remember to clarify patient goals and place them above our own, or educate patients on the limitations of the treatment. The key is to reach a mutual agreement regarding goals for health.

All manual therapy treatments should be modified to meet the needs of the patient. The difference between a treatment that warrants a SOAP chart and one appropriate for a HxTxC chart lies in the intent. Sessions where treatments vary based on individual symptoms and findings and are applied in a curative manner deserve a SOAP chart. For example, if cross-fiber friction is applied directly over scar tissue with the intent to decrease adhesions and increase mobility, the treatment has curative intent and should be recorded on a SOAP chart. Modifications to ensure patient safety and comfort, such as adjusting positions or providing a pillow, occur in every session, and do not demand a SOAP chart.

Treatment results that go beyond general therapeutic benefits—such as decreasing pain, increasing postural balance, or increasing mobility—should be substantiated on a SOAP chart. Document progress by measuring significant changes in subjective and objective findings. If initially, you and your patient determined that the treatment was strictly for general health purposes—such as increasing muscle relaxation, increasing circulation, and increasing energy—and you have been using the HxTxC charting method, switch to the SOAP format once you and the patient determine that the goals of the therapy have changed.

If at any time the patient begins receiving manual therapy on a regular basis, use a SOAP chart; as significant changes are probable. Have enough information in the chart to demonstrate the results of regular therapeutic touch.

154

HANDS HEAL:
COMMUNICATION,
DOCUMENTATION,
AND INSURANCE BILLING
FOR MANUAL THERAPISTS

Organize the charts in the patient's file chronologically by date regardless of format. There is no need to keep SOAP notes separate from HxTxC notes. It is acceptable to mix charting formats within a single file.

GUIDELINES FOR SELECTING HxTxC FORMAT

Use HxTxC charting when the patient is healthy, treatment is routine, and sessions are not used as ongoing health care. Follow these guidelines for determining whether a session warrants this style of documentation:

◆ The patient is healthy and has no specific health issues.
◆ If the patient has health issues, the specific health conditions, symptoms and findings are not addressed in the session, other than for patient safety and comfort.
◆ Treatment is provided for general therapeutic benefits (such as improved circulation, relaxation, and energy) without the intent or expectation of altering existing health conditions or symptoms (such as localized pain, numbness, compensatory postural patterns, or limited mobility).
◆ The treatment is routine. The practitioner does not deviate from that routine, other than to ensure patient safety and comfort, regardless of symptoms and pathophysiological findings.
◆ The patient is not using the session as ongoing health care treatment for a specific condition.

RELAXATION THERAPIES: SOAP OR HxTxC?

Either the style or the intent of the treatment can determine the documentation format. Drainage techniques applied as a full-body routine with general circulatory benefits may warrant HxTxC charting; a drainage session designed to treat inflammation resulting from a swollen ankle warrants SOAP charting. Manual modalities, such as Trager, Swedish massage, and Polarity can be applied with either curative or palliative intent. Follow the guidelines outlined above to determine whether to use SOAP charting or HxTxC charting. Use the Standard HxTxC chart for documenting most relaxation therapies. (See Figure 7-1)

In many cases, the guidelines for determining charting format are easy to apply. However, situations exist in which the lines blur. For example, it is nearly impossible for many manual therapists to follow a relaxation routine and not address what they feel underneath their hands. If you find yourself treating specific findings and straying from a routine, note the variations from the routine and the objective findings in the comments section of the HxTxC chart. If the patient returns for additional treatment, and together you make the decision toward a more detailed treatment plan, switch to a SOAP format.

Relaxation is a general health benefit with widespread effects. Simple effleurage strokes can have profound analgesic results. Basic gymnastics can produce dramatic changes in mobility and function. Symptoms have been shown to resolve and illnesses to go into remission from healing touch. The intent in providing an abbreviated format for charting is not to belittle the magnitude of hands-on healing, but to provide an avenue to simplify the paperwork when appropriate. Use the HxTxC format when the treatment is intended to be palliative not curative. If the results are more profound than anticipated, describe them in the comments section.

Naomi Wachtel
567 Sunnydale Dr.
Flat Irons, CO 80302
TEL 303 555 8866

STANDARD HxTxC Chart

Name: Lin Pak   Date: 7-27-01

Phone: (303) 555-0033x253   Address: ____________

1. What are your goals for health, and how may I assist you in achieving your goals? Limit long-term complications of diabetes through relaxation and stress reduction.

2. Are you currently experiencing any of the following? If yes, please explain.

pain, tenderness	☒ No	☐ Yes:	stiffness	☒ No	☐ Yes:
numbness or tingling	☒ No	☐ Yes:	swelling	☒ No	☐ Yes:
allergies	☒ No	☐ Yes:			

3. List all illnesses, injuries, and health concerns you have now or have had in the past 3 years. (Examples: arthritis, diabetes, car accident, pregnancy) diabetes, borderline high blood pressure

4. List medications and pain relievers taken today. insulin

5. I have provided all my known medical information. I acknowledge that manual therapy is not a substitute for medical diagnosis and treatment. I give my consent to receive treatment.

Signature: Lin Pak   Date: 7-27-01

Tx: Full Body Swedish Massage, Lymph Drainage trunk and upper extremities 45-minute session

C: Homework-relaxation exercises, check blood pressure before and after massages at home

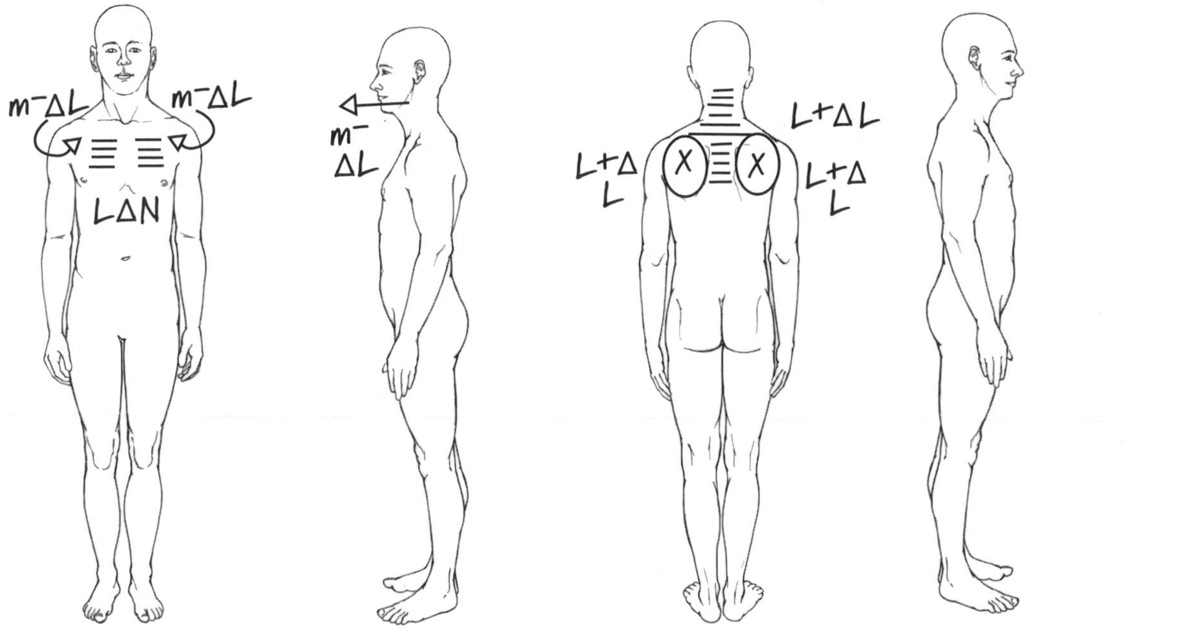

initials: NW, LMT

Figure 7-1. Standard HxTxC—Relaxation.

156

HANDS HEAL:
COMMUNICATION,
DOCUMENTATION,
AND INSURANCE BILLING
FOR MANUAL THERAPISTS

ENERGY WORK: SOAP OR HXTXC?

Energy work, like any other manual therapy, can be charted on either a SOAP note or an HxTxC chart, depending on the condition of the patient and the intent of the treatment. The difficulty in using a SOAP format to record energy work is one of language more than of style. Objective findings are not as tangible to the untrained hand or eye, but are equally valid. The initial challenge is in coming up with a vocabulary to define what you feel and see, and to use it consistently in a way that makes sense to others untrained in energetic modalities on the health care team. (See Appendix: Abbreviations List) The list of abbreviations provided in this book contains standard symbols and abbreviations for energetic findings and treatment techniques. Create an addendum for additional terms to fit your practice.

Guidelines for documenting energy work:

◆ Follow the guidelines for selecting the style of documentation.
◆ If HxTxC charting is appropriate, chart the treatment routine, and note the patient's response to treatment under Comments. (See Figure 7-2)
◆ If SOAP charting is necessary, use the following guidelines:
—S: Note subjective information as defined in Chapter 6.
—O: Note objective findings specific to your energetic training. Emphasize physiological findings. Use common terminology whenever possible.
—O: State treatment duration and modalities used. Highlight specifics.
—O: State measurable changes in the subjective and objective data as a result of the session. Gauge the changes in intensity and quality of expression. Tell how the changes affect the patient's quality of life.
—A: If the patient's ability to function in everyday activities is impaired, set goals based on improving function, as defined in Chapter 6.
—P: Create a treatment plan and provide self-care instructions, as described in Chapter 6.

Energy work is controversial among insurance companies as a reimbursable treatment modality because treatment results have not been adequately substantiated scientifically. This is also the case with other manual modalities. Lymphatic drainage is one of the few manual modalities to date with substantial international scientific evidence of effectiveness.[3] As a result, demonstrating measurable progress based in function, symptoms, and physiological findings is important for *all* manual modalities. When charting energy work, emphasize the physical expressions of the dysfunction in addition to noting the energetic expressions. Emphasize the results of treatment over the modalities used. Use terminology that is easily understood across professions.

Venues Appropriate for HxTxC Charting

There are many venues where HxTxC charting is appropriate. Two common ones are sporting events, in which participants receive pre- or post-event therapy; and spas, in which patients self-select from a menu of treatments designed for relaxation, detoxification, and beautification. The purpose of these sessions is specific to the venue, not to the individual, and the treatment routines do not vary. Patients are not likely to depend on these for ongoing health care because they are not tailored to meet individual needs, but rather to address general therapeutic goals.

Naomi Wachtel
567 Sunnydale Dr.
Flat Irons, CO   80302
Tᴇʟ   303 555 8866

Name   _Lin Pak_ _____   Current Meds _____

Tx: _60 minute Polarity and Somato_ _____
       Emotional Release _____

C: _↑ balance 3rd chakra, shoulder posture,_
      ↓ fascial pull _____

Y _fascial_
  shortening

🗘 _congestion_

↘ _rotation_

date _____ initials _____

Tx: _____
       _____

C: _____
      _____

date _____ initials _____

Tx: _____
       _____

C: _____
      _____

date _____ initials _____

Tx: _____
       _____

C: _____
      _____

date _____ initials _____

Figure 7-2. Standard HxTxC—Energy Work.

158

HANDS HEAL:
COMMUNICATION,
DOCUMENTATION,
AND INSURANCE BILLING
FOR MANUAL THERAPISTS

Each venue has specific documentation needs. The following will be addressed individually:

♦ Events (sporting events, health fairs, etc.)
♦ On-site (offices, malls, airports, etc.)
♦ Spas and salons

EVENTS

A common sight near the finish line at foot races or under a tent at street fairs is a large group of manual therapists lined up with tables or chairs and providing relief for participants. Manual therapy offered at venues like these—sporting events, health fairs, and community events—require HxTxC charting. The pace is fast, the turnover is frequent, the sessions are brief, and the need to document is minimal. The charts will not become permanent records of the patients' health, nor will the information be used for ongoing care. But the charts do assist the practitioner in determining whether treatment is appropriate, and provide a record that will become crucial if the patient claims to have been injured in the course of treatment.

Treatment provided at events meets the guidelines for alternative charting. The patients are healthy enough to be competing or walking long distances. Therapists are there to provide basic services and a routine treatment. People are generally not seeking health care at those venues, and practitioners do not have the time or information necessary to treat specific health conditions. Although many therapists use the event as an opportunity to market their practices, for many it is the only treatment the patient will receive from this therapist. If the patient does seek out the therapist's professional services in the future, a formal intake will ensue and SOAP notes will most likely be appropriate.

Because the pace is fast and distractions are many at an event, you should read the intake questions out loud to the patient. Make eye contact to ensure the patient is paying attention and understands the questions asked. If the patient answers Yes to any of the questions, the practitioner must be prepared to ask additional questions that are not on the intake form to establish the appropriateness of treatment. For example, if the patient says he has swollen feet, rule out infections and heart conditions that could be exacerbated by treatment. If the patient was injured recently, determine whether alternative treatment methods are appropriate and whether treatment to certain areas of the body should be avoided.[1] If the patient has just finished a race and is exhibiting signs of shock, first aid should be administered immediately in the medical tent.

The intake information is brief but critical in event venues. (See Figure 7-3) Compare this to the intake questions for a non-sporting event session recorded on the Standard Hx-TxC chart. (See Figure 7-1). Tailor your event HxTxC chart to the specific venue and the treatment routines you provide.

The nature of manual therapy at events is that there are no repeat visits. The event occurs once, or annually, and the tables or chairs are packed up and gone by the next day. As a result, several patient sessions can be recorded on one form; individual patient files need not be created. The intake questions top the form and are read to each individual, and space is provided below to record the athlete's name, responses to the questions, and the treatment provided.

Provider Name ___Naomi Wachtel, LMT___ Date ___7-4-01___

Event or Race ___Mountain Aid 10K___ Location ___Finish Line Tent___

Ask each athlete the following: (Note individual responses below—concerns only.)

1. Are you currently experiencing any of the following?
   - pain, tenderness, stiffness
   - numbness, tingling
   - cold, clammy skin
   - swelling
   - dizziness
   - shaking

2. How soon do you compete? / When did you finish competing?

3. Have you warmed up? / Cooled down?

4. Have you consumed water since the event?

Athlete's Name ___Janelle Helm___

Hx: (note concerns) ___No water – gave her 12 oz before Tx___

Tx: (check all that apply) _____ Pre-event ✓ _____ Post-event _____ Refer-first aid/med

C: ___gave her 12 oz after Tx___

Initials: ___NW___

Figure 7-3. Sports HxTxC—Intake Questions

ON-SITE MASSAGE

On-site massage is increasingly popular in work environments as an employee benefit. Businesses recognize the detrimental effects of stress on job performance and long-term health[4] and offer on-site massage in an effort to keep productivity high and reduce sick leave.

On-site massage differs from event massage in one important way: the site is often permanent. On-site companies or individual practitioners contract with businesses for regular visits, often weekly. When massage is a regular fixture in the work environment—accessible, non-threatening, and affordable—patients who might not otherwise seek the services of a massage therapist become repeat customers. A permanent site with repeat customers, many of whom have symptoms of repetitive stress conditions, presents some charting challenges, given the time constraints of on-site massage environments.

On-site massage, similar to event therapy, is fast-paced, with high turnover and brief treatments. There is no time for extensive interviews, intake forms, or breaks between sessions for charting. However, the need for documentation is great. Charting must be quick and easy, and must serve the needs of the patient.

In an interview, David Palmer, often called the father of on-site massage, said, "I don't see on-site massage . . . too closely associated with healthcare services because it's not a treatment . . . It's not designed to fix anything. It's merely designed to make people feel better and to produce what I think is the greatest value of massage, which is to simply enhance circulation."[5] In such situations, a brief HxTxC chart is adequate. However, some people in the workplace have carpal tunnel syndrome, chronic headaches, or fibromyal-

159

160

HANDS HEAL:
COMMUNICATION,
DOCUMENTATION,
AND INSURANCE BILLING
FOR MANUAL THERAPISTS

gia. Many of those people use the on-site massage provided in their offices to treat their symptoms and keep them functioning productively in the workplace. A record of their symptoms, physiological findings, and progress could benefit both the practitioner and the patient. Demonstrating tangible results to the business owners and the patients will increase customer satisfaction, demand, and availability.

The Seated HxTxC chart provides an alternative to the Sports HxTxC chart. (See Figure 7-4) The primary addition to the chart are illustrations of a person in a treatment chair. The practitioner draws symbols on figures, quickly charting symptoms and objective findings, and creating an easy reference for demonstrating progress and planning future treatments. The Seated HxTxC chart contains an intake form, records measurable subjective and objective data, notes treatment routines, and provides space for additional comments from the practitioner.

Several treatments for the same patient may be recorded on page two of the Seated HxTxC chart, preventing repetitive health information gathering. (See Figure 7-5)

Other on-site venues—such as airports, convention centers, shopping malls, and grocery stores—are not prone to repeat clientele. The clientele is transient, the desire to receive treatment is spontaneous, and sessions are routine. Do not attempt to record repeat visits on a single form for this type of client. File charts by date, rather than by client name, and have each client fill out a new intake with each visit. Use page one of the Seated HxTxC chart for these venues, or custom design a HxTxC chart that meets your individual needs.

SPAS AND SALONS

Spas are traditionally located in resorts, which cater to a transient population. More and more, however, spas are found in downtown areas and urban neighborhoods, and inside salons. Salons are incorporating massage and hydrotherapy with traditional pedicures, manicures, and facials. With increasing availability, people are becoming regulars of manual therapies in spas.

Spas and salons are ideal environments for HxTxC charting. The need for extensive charting is low, and the turnover is fast. Treatment is routine and consistent, varying little with individual needs. Patients select treatment routines from a menu, based on the general health benefits advertised. The primary role for manual therapy in a spa environment is for pampering, relaxing, cleansing, detoxifying, and toning the skin. Patients rarely consider the treatment as a remedy for illnesses or injuries.

The use of the HxTxC chart in spas and salons is simple and practical. Practitioners use the chart to identify health conditions that contraindicate extreme temperatures or increases in circulation. Skin allergies and sensitivities are also major concerns when gathering health history. Treatment options are checked off, and comments primarily reflect the personal preferences of the patients. Use the Standard HxTxC chart or design a Spa HxTxC chart to meet your individual needs. (See Figure 7-6)

Space is provided for multiple sessions on one chart, as the patients may return. In a curative health care environment, patients visits are weekly or bi-weekly. In a spa environment, monthly or quarterly visits are the norm.

Provider Name _____

Name _____ Date _____

Phone _____ Location _____

1. Are you currently experiencing any of the following? If yes, please explain.

   pain, tenderness   ☐ No ☐ Yes: _____   stiffness ☐ No ☐ Yes: _____
   numbness or tingling   ☐ No ☐ Yes: _____   swelling ☐ No ☐ Yes: _____
   allergies   ☐ No ☐ Yes: _____

2. List all illnesses, injuries, and health concerns you have now or have had in the past 3 years.
   (Examples: arthritis, diabetes, car accident, pregnancy) _____
   _____

3. List medications and pain relievers taken today. _____
   _____

4. I have provided all my known medical information. I acknowledge that manual therapy is not
   a substitute for medical diagnosis and treatment. I give my consent to receive treatment.

   Signature _____ Date _____

   Tx: _____
   _____

   C: _____
   _____

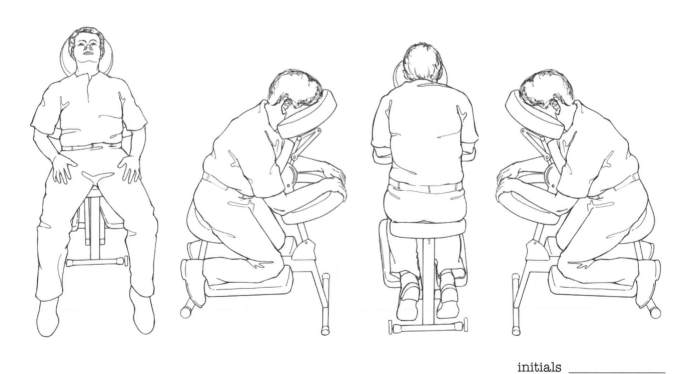

initials _____

Figure 7-4. Seated HxTxC chart—page one.

SEATED HxTxC

page 2

Name ______________________ Current Meds ______________________

Tx: ______________________

____

C: ______________________

____

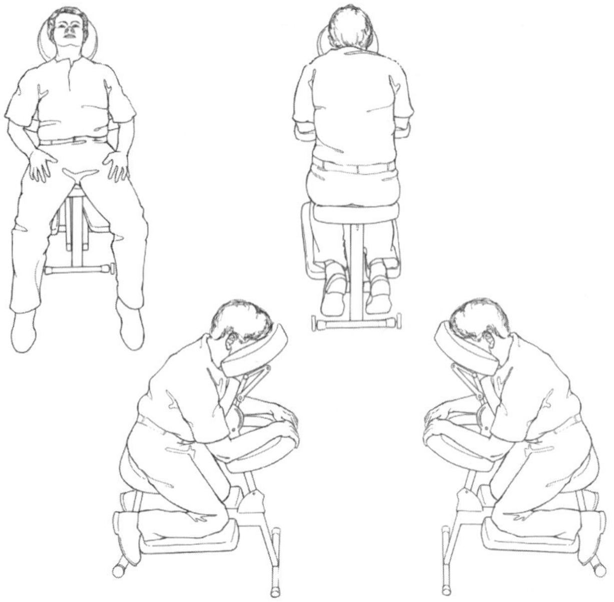

date ____________ initials ____________

Tx: ______________________

____

C: ______________________

____

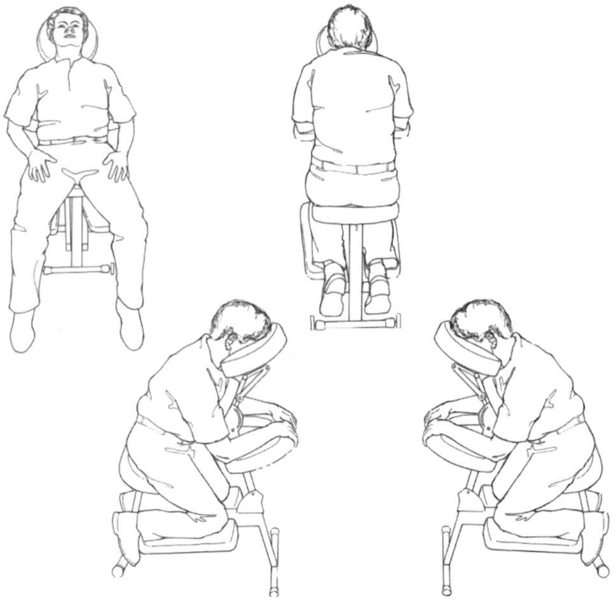

date ____________ initials ____________

Tx: ______________________

____

C: ______________________

____

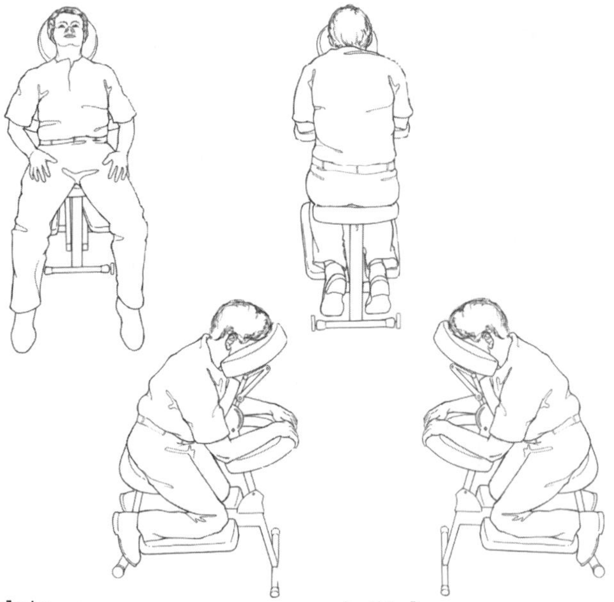

date ____________ initials ____________

Tx: ______________________

____

C: ______________________

____

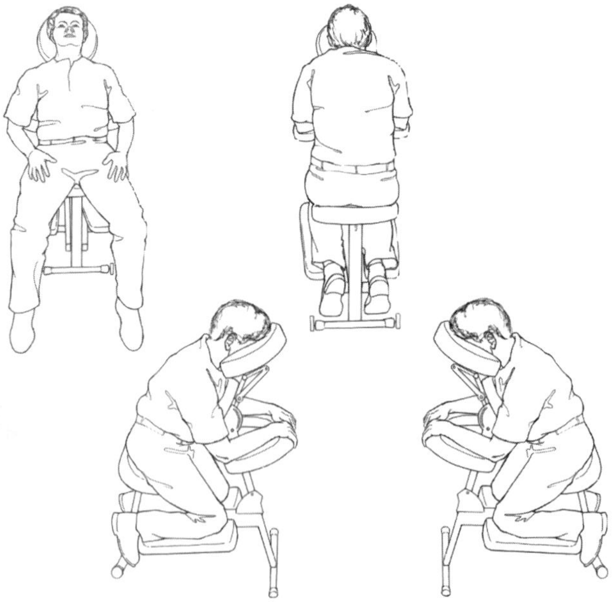

date ____________ initials ____________

Figure 7-5. Seated HxTxC chart—page two.

3. Are you allergic to any of the following? (Please circle all that apply.) Almond Oil, Aloe Vera, Cucumber, Honey, Lavender, Milk, Mud, Olive Oil, Sandalwood, Seaweed.

4. I have provided all my known medical information. I give my consent to receive treatment.
   Signature _____ Date _____
   (for office use only)

Tx: _____ body scrub _____ herbal wrap _____ massage _____ mud pack

_____ seaweed wrap _____ skin moisturizer _____ steam _____ whirlpool

C: _____

_____ initials _____ date _____

Figure 7-6. Customized Spa HxTxC.

SUMMARY

Document all manual therapy sessions. Two options for charting include:

◆ SOAP charting
◆ HxTxC charting

   Use the HxTxC format for the following venues:

◆ Events (sporting events, health fairs, etc.)
◆ On-site (offices, malls, airports, etc.)
◆ Spas and salons
◆ Relaxation treatments and energy work, depending on the health of the patient and the intent of the treatment

   Vary the intake questions and the treatment options according to the venue and the practitioner's treatment style, to ensure the effectiveness of the HxTxC chart.
   Use the HxTxC format for charting sessions that meet the following guidelines:

◆ The patient is healthy and has no specific health issues.
◆ If the patient has health issues, the specific health conditions, symptoms, and findings are not addressed in the session.
◆ Treatment is provided for general therapeutic benefits without the intent or expectation of altering health problems or symptoms.
◆ The treatment is routine.
◆ The patient is not using the session as ongoing health care treatment for a specific condition.

164

HANDS HEAL:
COMMUNICATION,
DOCUMENTATION,
AND INSURANCE BILLING
FOR MANUAL THERAPISTS

REFERENCES

1. Werner R. A Massage Therapist's Guide to Pathology. Baltimore: Williams & Wilkins, 1998.
2. Walton TH. Taking a health history. Massage Therapy Journal 1999;37(4).
3. Chikly B. Lymphatic Drainage Techniques: Advancements in Lymphatic Drainage Disorders, (in press).
4. Hafen BQ, Karren KJ, Frandsen KJ, Smith NL. Mind Body Health: The Effects of Attitudes, Emotions, and Relationships. Boston: Allyn and Bacon, 1996.
5. Mower M. The On-Site Massage Movement: Interviews with David Palmer, Russ Borner, Raymond Blaylock, Massage Magazine, March/April, 1994.

Billing and Ethics

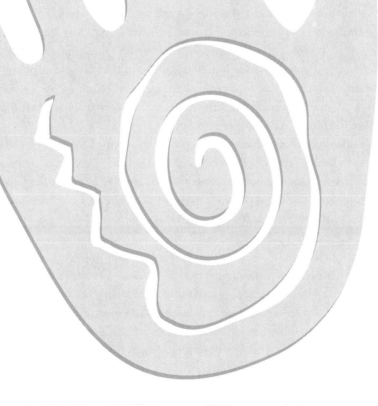

CHAPTER *8*

Insurance Billing

Several years ago I attended a panel discussion on the integration of massage therapy into insurance plans. The panel of physicians offered advice on participating in health care teams and billing insurance companies. The massage therapist mediating the panel opened her introduction with this joke: "I have some good news and some bad news. The good news is that we can now bill insurance for our services. The bad news is that we can now bill insurance for our services."

So far, the good news appears to outweigh the bad. Inclusion in insurance plans carries many benefits. As insurance consumers, we have fought for the right to choose our health care providers and our preferred treatment modalities. The widespread inclusion of Complementary and Alternative Medicine (CAM) into a variety of insurance plans proves that consumers can affect the health care industry. As health care providers, we have the opportunity to improve the lives and health of more people by participating in insurance programs.

Not only does this inclusion acknowledge our impact on patients' health, but it also permits us to promote change from inside the insurance and health care arenas. Manual therapists are hands-on, relationship-based practitioners who educate patients to ask questions and participate in their own care. All aspects of health care delivery shift as these newly empowered patients demand the same respect from other practitioners.

We also change the insurance industry by participating in insurance administration. A group of CAM providers was recently hired as consultants by an insurance company to assist with integrating acupuncture, massage, and naturopathy into the company's health plans. The goal was to educate staff and medical personnel on when and why to refer for complementary services. A massage therapist spoke at length to the medical director about the company's policies for treating lymphedema. She explained that lymphedema is a chronic condition that requires long-term treatment and self-care education, and should not be treated as an acute condition with a 2-week limit on care. By the next monthly meeting, the company had rewritten its entire policy on lymphedema treatment to reflect her suggestions.

Manual therapy is an industry that relies on word-of-mouth referrals. Opening our practices to health care referrals and insurance networks invites patients who may never have sought our services before: those who are not yet aware of the benefits of manual therapy, those who cannot afford to pay out-of-pocket for our services, and those who would not normally seek out CAM care unless recommended by a doctor they trust. Each of these populations are large and can have an immediate impact on a manual therapist's practice.

Patients with acute conditions respond quickly to treatments. Health care referrals can offer an unparalleled learning environment. Patient files become a source for identifying effective and efficient treatments for a variety of conditions.

Accepting health care referrals and providing billing services can expand your patient load and your income. For example, I began offering insurance billing services in 1985. Before that, I had a modest practice in the evenings and on weekends. Immediately, I needed to hire three therapists just to service all the referrals. In a year and a half, my clinic had 15 manual therapists working full-time to meet the demand for services.

The panel mediator was right, however. There is bad news. Insurance billing can be complicated, costly, and time-consuming, and payment is not 100% guaranteed. It requires frequent communication with insurance carriers and referring health care providers (HCP). The paperwork associated with insurance billing takes time in addition to the time we spend treating patients. You must be willing to maintain clear paper pathways, remain flexible and pleasant in response to the demands of each carrier's protocols and procedures, and persistent enough to see your way through to the end: payment in full.

Unfortunately, you must also be willing to discount your fees and sign restrictive contracts to participate in many health insurance plans. On the other hand, research shows that people are willing to pay out-of-pocket for our services,[1] but given the possibility of financial support from the insurance carriers, they will seek out manual therapists who are providers under their plans. If we do not open our practices to insurance, we risk losing patients who go in search of a manual therapist willing to provide insurance billing services.

Colodia Owens, author of *Managed Care Organizations, Practical Implications for Medical Practices and Other Providers*, asks, "Is health care a right, a privilege, or a rationed commodity?"[2] I believe that health care is a right, and with a little tenacity and organizational skill, I can provide health care to my patients under their insurance plans. My participation in the insurance industry is a choice, and it makes me feel glad every time I look into a patient's grateful eyes: the police officer with the broken neck, the poet with lymphedema from a double mastectomy, and the professor with a closed-head injury. Together we nod knowingly. This is care they don't get anywhere else.

Introduction

Insurance regulations and procedures vary from plan-to-plan, from state-to-state, even among health care professions. Just when you think you have it all figured out, billing procedures change or a new CPT code is introduced and a familiar one deleted. Luckily, there are ways you can prepare for the fluctuating demands of insurance billing. This chapter provides guidelines for staying on top of the shifting information and decreasing the risks associated with accepting insurance reimbursement as payment for services.

Before you begin, ponder these questions to determine whether insurance billing services are appropriate for your practice:

1. Are peers in your area billing insurance companies? Are enough of them successful at it? Are they getting paid? Are their practices full as a result? If few of your peers are successful, you must be very creative and determined to break new ground for your profession. If many of your peers are billing insurance, you might find it difficult to compete if you choose not to participate.
2. Do you turn people away because you are unable to accommodate them? Or would you like more patients? Have you ever lost a patient because you were unwilling to bill an insurance company? Have people changed their minds about scheduling with you when they found out that you do not accept insurance patients?
3. Can you afford to wait 30–90 days to get paid—the typical turnaround time for insurance reimbursement? Do you have adequate cash flow to meet your monthly expenses as you establish a consistent flow of insurance payments?
4. At what point will you feel motivated to offer insurance billing services? Many networks credentialing providers fill up quickly and close their doors to new providers within a year of offering manual therapy coverage in the plans. Will the insurance networks be closed when you are finally ready to join? Or will you retire before insurance billing is standard for your profession in your area?

170

HANDS HEAL:
COMMUNICATION,
DOCUMENTATION,
AND INSURANCE BILLING
FOR MANUAL THERAPISTS

If you choose not to provide billing services for your patients, and are legally able to request payment up front for your services and provide a superbill with instructions on how patients can seek insurance reimbursement on their own, you must educate yourself thoroughly so as not to burden your patients with unnecessary risk. [2]

Use the guidelines provided in this chapter together with information you gather that is specific to your state or region, and to your scope of practice. Collecting this information requires some effort on your behalf: making phone calls to peers, governing bodies such as the Department of Health or Education, insurance representatives, and attorneys; reading current research materials specific to your location and practice, professional journals, insurance provider newsletters, and billing texts; and taking local workshops and seminars. Because of regional and professional differences in insurance billing and because licensing laws are in flux in many areas, it is critical to stay abreast of trends in insurance reimbursement.

Playing "ostrich-in-the-sand" is not a viable option if an insurance review determines you have received payment for services that were not within your scope of practice or that the fees charged were in excess of your usual fees. You can be forced to pay back money that was paid to you; violations can be retroactive for several years. Follow the strategies suggested for managing insurance reimbursement, and fill in the blanks with information specific to your local and professional laws and regulations. Be well-informed and prepared to meet the demands of insurance billing.

Know the following information before providing billing services to your patients.

◆ If you are a licensed health care provider, what services are within your legal scope of practice? Can you bill directly for your services? Do you need a prescription from a referring HCP, or do you have diagnostic scope? Which type of HCP has primary care status and can refer patients for manual therapy treatments?

◆ If you are not licensed, do regulations exist that permit you to provide health care services under the license or supervision of a HCP with primary care status? Can you bill directly, or must the supervising HCP bill for you? Do you need direct supervision, or will a prescribed treatment plan and a referral suffice?

◆ Which types of insurance will reimburse for manual therapy services in your state (for example, health insurance, worker's compensation, or personal injury coverage)? If the plan covers manual therapy, who can provide the manual therapy treatment (for example, a physical therapist, massage therapist, or nurse)?

◆ Which manual therapy treatments or modalities are covered under each plan (for example, massage, exercise, neuromuscular reeducation, or hydrotherapy)? What Current Procedural Terminology (CPT) codes correspond with the acceptable treatments?

◆ Which conditions warrant manual therapy treatment under each plan (for example, pain, musculo-skeletal dysfunctions, or cancer)? Know the corresponding **International Classification of Diseases-10th edition (ICD-10) codes** acceptable to the insurance plan for each patient, and whether the ICD-10 codes must be identified on the billing form.

In this chapter, forms are provided for identifying and recording information on your patients according to each individual plan. The accompanying guidelines assist you with communication and organizational skills to make the insurance billing process flow smoothly and to decrease the risks involved.

Types of Insurance Coverage

Three common types of insurance offer medical coverage: personal injury insurance, workers' compensation, and private health insurance.

Manual therapists, licensed and unlicensed, are often able to bill personal injury insurance because of the litigation process. If injuries are sustained because of the negligence of another, the at-fault party is ultimately financially responsible for the injured party's reasonable and necessary medical treatments at the conclusion of the case. These treatments generally include services to return the patient to preinjury status or to reach a maximum medical improvement. If manual therapy is medically necessary, is prescribed by a primary HCP, and is performed by a HCP or under the supervision of a primary HCP, it is covered under the at-fault party's liability insurance.

Many workers' compensation plans cover manual therapy services because in-house statistics support it as an inexpensive and effective way to return patients to work quickly. These state plans provide for manual therapy treatments for most on-the-job injuries, and lead the way for inclusion in other health plans. [3]

Private health insurance, on the other hand, tightly defines which treatments and modalities are reimbursable for which conditions. Insurance plans that cover manual therapy will often reimburse the treatment only if it is provided by physical therapists, nurses, or chiropractors. Few cover manual therapy provided by licensed massage therapists or certified bodyworkers. However, consumers are demanding that insurance carriers include CAM care in their plans—massage therapy, acupuncture, naturopathy, etc. In addition, states such as Washington are benefiting from legislative action indicating that insurers must contract with every category of health care provider. (In this example, health care providers must be licensed or certified under the Department of Health and contracted by the insurance carrier, the patient's condition must be within the HCP's scope of practice to treat, and treatment must be within the provisions of the patient's insurance policy.) Before long, manual therapy will be a standard modality covered in health plans across the US.

Manual therapists in some states can bill all three types of coverage successfully, in other states, success may be found in only one or two of the three. Do your homework before providing the service.

PERSONAL INJURY INSURANCE

Personal Injury insurance is bundled into insurance policies such as car insurance, homeowners insurance, and commercial building insurance. Commonly, policy holders purchase medical coverage within these plans for Personal Injury Protection, Medical Payments, and **Liability coverage** which includes bodily injury and property damage.

The most common type of personal injury insurance claim is for injuries sustained in a motor vehicle accident (MVA). Each year, 3–5 million MVAs are reported to the police and hospitals in the United States, and countless more go unreported.[4] Because of these staggering numbers, we will most frequently find ourselves billing car insurance carriers.

There are five types of insurance coverage that a manual therapist needs to be aware of when treating a patient who has been involved in a MVA:

- Personal Injury Protection (PIP)
- Medical Payments (Med Pay)
- Secondary PIP or Med Pay Insurance

This section is revised and reprinted with permission, all rights reserved. Adler, Giersch. Whiplash, Spinal Trauma, and the Chiropractic Personal Injury Case. Seattle: Adler◆Giersch PS, 2000.

172

HANDS HEAL:
COMMUNICATION,
DOCUMENTATION,
AND INSURANCE BILLING
FOR MANUAL THERAPISTS

◆ Third Party Coverage or Liability Insurance
◆ Uninsured Motorist (UM)

Personal Injury Protection

Personal Injury Protection (PIP) is one component of automobile coverage that can be purchased as part of the auto policy. In some states, it is a requirement for drivers to purchase PIP, in other States it is optional. In Washington State, for example, insurers are required to offer PIP to their policyholders. The policyholder has the right to refuse such coverage by signing a formal written "waiver" recognizing their understanding of the coverage and decision to reject it. Benefits may include medical and hospital fees, loss of wages and loss of services (household help, for example), and funeral services. Payment of these benefits does not depend on determining who is at fault.

Various levels of PIP coverage can be purchased, and every company has different options within those levels ($5,000, $10,000, $25,000, $35,000). A standard time provision on PIP coverage varies from 1 to 3 years. Therefore, it is important to know the provisions specific to each patient's plan before agreeing to bill directly to the insurance carrier to ensure the time limit has not expired or that coverage has not been exhausted by bills from other health care practitioners (HCP).

PIP is the most attractive type of coverage from a reimbursement standpoint. You do not have to wait for fault to be determined or deal with health insurance policies that may not cover your treatment modalities or provide for your profession. The primary requirement is that your documentation must prove that your care is reasonable and necessary, treatment is for injuries sustained in the accident, and a referring HCP has prescribed the treatment as medically necessary.

Medical Payments

Medical Payments (Med Pay) is also a provision that can be purchased under the auto insurance policy. Again, the amount of coverage differs from state-to-state and insurer to insurer. If there is no PIP coverage, Med Pay may be available to cover manual therapy services. Med Pay is generally for a lower dollar amount than PIP and covers medical expenses only. Like PIP, payment does not depend on determining who was at fault.

Secondary PIP or Med Pay Insurance

One or more PIP or Med Pay policies may cover your patient for the same accident. For example, if Darnel was a passenger in his nephew's car, the nephew's PIP pays for Darnel's medical expenses as the **primary insurer**, even though Darnel has car insurance. Once the nephew's PIP is exhausted, Darnel's PIP insurance coverage can kick in as the secondary PIP insurer if additional medical services are needed.

If Darnel does not have PIP or Med Pay and the nephew's PIP is exhausted, Darnel's health insurance becomes the **secondary insurer**.

Third Party Coverage or Liability Insurance

Third party coverage refers to the liability insurance coverage of the at-fault party. The driver of the truck that rear-ended Darnel is the at-fault party, and his insurance plan is the third party or liability insurer. It is not productive to bill the third party insurance until fault is determined. If the truck driver's insurance carrier paid for Darnel's treatments, it would be admitting fault. Generally, payment is not made by the third party coverage until a settlement is reached or until fault is determined by a court of law.

End-of-settlement cases are those in which the patient was not at fault; the patient's PIP coverage, Med Pay coverage, or secondary coverage is insufficient or nonexistent; and the provider must wait until the claim against the at-fault party settles or a judge or jury issues a verdict before receiving payment for services. End-of-settlement cases can be risky. Will the patient be able to prove that he was not at fault? If Darnel has an attorney who is convinced fault can be established on the truck driver, for example, the risk is lessened. Can you afford to wait until the case settles before getting paid? In many cases, years pass before a settlement is reached, depending on the statute of limitations and whether the case goes to trial. If the patient and the lawyer are willing to sign a contract guaranteeing your payment from the settlement, the risk is reduced. A **health care lien**, filed in accordance with the requirements of your state, can lower the risk further.

The positive side of an end-of-settlement case is that it becomes a savings account gaining simple interest monthly. Interest can be applied within the legal limit for health care services if you notify the patient at the beginning of treatment that interest begins to accrue 45 days after no payment is made. Some states also regulate how much time must pass before interest can accrue, such as 60 days. If you ensure adequate cash flow by limiting the number of end-of-settlement cases you carry at a time and if you take precautions to reduce your risk, the occasional end-of-settlement case can enhance your cash flow.

In the event that the patient's insurance carrier pays for expenses up front, it will rely upon the subrogation provisions in the patient's insurance contract with the insurers. Under subrogation, the insurer will seek reimbursement from the third party coverage for expenses after the case settles. Subrogation is a complicated legal principle that has many exceptions and differences in implementation from state-to-state.

Uninsured Motorists

Uninsured motorists coverage protects the policyholder against MVA injuries inflicted by someone who does not have any insurance, or who flees the scene and remains unidentified. It is also activated when the person who causes the accident has insurance but the injured person does not.

WORKERS' COMPENSATION

Workers' compensation (comp) is insurance that employers are mandated to purchase for all employees. The plans furnish medical and disability benefits for illnesses, injuries, disabilities, and death that result from job-related conditions and activities.

The primary intent of the coverage is to return the employee to full-duty work quickly without recurrence of injury. Benefits vary from state-to-state. Often there are limits on the services that are reimbursable, who can perform those services, and how many sessions are available. Restrictions apply, for example, fees allowed must be accepted as payment in full; and providers must agree to contracted provisions. Request a copy of the provider regulations for your profession and an application for a provider number, if applicable. Read the regulations thoroughly before determining whether you want to provide this service to your patients. (See Appendix: Contact Information—Workers' Compensation.)

Each state has an insurance plan available to employees through its Department of Labor and Industries or workers' compensation program. Employers pay fees according to

174

HANDS HEAL:
COMMUNICATION,
DOCUMENTATION,
AND INSURANCE BILLING
FOR MANUAL THERAPISTS

job description, and funds are collected quarterly. Employers have the option of using the insurance provided by the State or, if their business is large enough, remain self-insured. These **self-insured** plans must meet or exceed the coverage mandated by state law. For example, the US Federal Government is self-insured. Rather than managing different plans covering employees in each state, the Federal Government has created its own plan that meets or exceeds the requirements in every state. All Federal claims, regardless of which state the employee works in, are submitted to the same workers' comp insurance carrier.

PRIVATE HEALTH INSURANCE

Health insurance provides payment of benefits for covered illness and injury. There are many types of health care reimbursement plans, with an array of companies that supply them, including:

- Managed Care plans
- Indemnity plans or fee-for-service
- Major medical
- Medicare and Medicaid

The most widespread type of health insurance plan today is **Managed Care**. Managed Care is on the opposite end of the spectrum from traditional **Indemnity** or **fee-for-service** insurance plans.

Traditionally, we would go to our own doctor whenever we felt it was necessary. The doctor would do whatever she deemed necessary for our health, and submit a bill to the insurance company for that visit. The insurance company would pay the doctor for the services provided. This is known as an Indemnity plan, or a fee-for-service type of health care.

Because of an increase in accessibility of health care, unrestricted use of reimbursement, and rising health care costs, insurance companies were driven to search for ways of managing health care costs. Managed Care was created to limit:

- Coverage of services
- Who supplies those services
- Fees for those services

Major Medical insurance covers the expense of major illness and injury. There are usually high benefit maximums and high deductibles, and the insurance company reimburses a percentage of the costs after the deductible.

Medicare and **Medicaid** provide public assistance to the aged and the financially challenged. These types of health insurance restrict which modalities are reimbursable.

Managed Care Plans

Managed Care organizations manage costs by contracting with a selected group of providers for a predetermined payment. An administrator manages the patient's access to health care, assessing the patient's case from a financial and clinical perspective, developing a plan of care in conjunction with the referring HCP and other health care providers, determining medical necessity, and evaluating the quality of care provided. Managed Care

This section is revised and reprinted with permission, all rights reserved. Owens C, Managed Care Organizations: Practical Implications for Medical Practices and Other Providers, Los Angeles: PMIC, 1996.

integrates the financing and delivery of health care services to covered individuals. Significant financial incentives are offered for members to use providers and procedures associated with the plan.

Health Maintenance Organizations

Health Maintenance Organizations (**HMOs**) are a type of Managed Care organization. HMOs combine insurance reimbursement with the delivery of health care services. An HMO provides specified medical services to a defined group of individuals during a defined period of time at a fixed price.

HMOs vary in structure and in reimbursement methods. Some vary in their contracts with providers. For example, a group model contracts with a group of providers. An **independent practice arrangement** (**IPA**) contracts with providers in private practice. The point-of-service model allows the insured to use the contracted providers or receive services from outside the network. There are financial incentives to stay within the network of providers, however.

Reimbursement arrangements in HMOs include:

◆ Discounted fees for services
◆ Capped fees for services
◆ Bundling fees for all services provided
◆ Capitation

A **discounted fee** arrangement is a system in which the provider contracts with the insurance carrier to offer the insured a discount. This is also known as an **affinity plan or affinity network**. The patient pays the provider the discounted fee directly, and the provider accepts this fee as payment in full.

With a **capped fee**, the provider contracts with the insurance carrier for services at a reduced amount. The insurance carrier reimburses the provider for services at the capped rate—payment comes from the insurer—and the provider accepts this fee as payment in full.

Bundling, or a **global fee** schedule, lumps all services provided into one fee. For example, Helena, Zamora's manual therapist, provides several services: Rolfing, hydrotherapy, and Polarity Therapy. She bills each one at a different rate. With this reimbursement arrangement, all of her services are lumped into one CPT code—97124—and billed at the same rate.

Capitation is a set fee for a patient paid monthly regardless of the number of visits or the type of service received. Capitation is nearly impossible to apply to manual therapy practices because of the time required for delivering the service and the physical inability of the practitioner to provide more than a predetermined number of sessions per day.

Preferred Provider Organizations

Preferred Provider Organizations (**PPOs**) are similar to HMOs, except they primarily contract with independent providers and they share similarities with the traditional fee-for-service health plans. PPOs were developed as a bridge between Managed Care plans and Indemnity plans as a response to concerns that the HMO's services might become inflexible, that patients' choice of providers might be eliminated, and that accelerating costs would make indemnity plans too expensive for employers and policyholders.

176

HANDS HEAL:
COMMUNICATION,
DOCUMENTATION,
AND INSURANCE BILLING
FOR MANUAL THERAPISTS

Becoming a Preferred Provider in a Managed Care System

Credentialing

Some insurance plans have a credentialing process for contracting with preferred providers. Other insurance carriers buy contracts from an insurance network. Networks credential providers and sell their contracts to insurance carriers for a user fee. The credentialing process varies among carriers and networks, but generally consists of the following:

- Review of company standards, such as years in the profession, accessibility, etc.
- Completion of an application and professional references
- Signed contract agreeing to company policies and provider services, such as a "**hold harmless**" clause if the carrier becomes insolvent, preventing you from seeking payment from the patient
- Proof of licensure/certification/registration
- Proof of business license
- Proof of liability insurance
- Proof of education certificate, continuing education hours, current CPR training
- Proof of professional affiliations with organizations enforcing a Code of Ethics
- Background check for complaints and disciplinary actions

Plans often hire a consultant from the profession to assist them in developing credentialing criteria and procedures as plans integrate manual therapy. However, once the criteria are in place, credentialing and peer reviews are usually done by someone familiar with several professions, not just the one being reviewed. For example, a nurse might be hired to conduct peer reviews for massage therapists, physical therapists, and occupational therapists.

Site inspections and reviews of patient records are common components of credentialing. Many insurance carriers will not credential practitioners who work at home, who do not provide handicapped accessibility, or who do not maintain adequate patient records.

Specific continuing education courses (such as courses in documentation or billing) may be required as part of the credentialing process. Similar **Quality Improvement Programs** may be mandatory for recredentialing annually. The manual therapist also agrees to comply with **Utilization Management Programs**, which randomly audit practitioners to ensure the effectiveness, appropriateness, and quality of services provided.

Contracts

Contracts vary among plans and among providers. Read all contracts carefully, for they are legally binding. An article in The Journal, A Publication of the American Massage Therapy Association–Washington Chapter mentions paying close attention to the following sections of a contract (revised and reprinted with permission from Grigsby and Rosen[5]):

- Fee schedules
- Patient access
- Contract termination
- Records and documentation

By contracting with an insurance carrier, you exchange discounted services for marketing. Marketing can be expensive and time-consuming. Many manual therapists are unprepared for the demands of self-employment and the responsibilities of marketing in addition to providing services. Becoming a preferred provider may be a great boon to your business. Before agreeing to a discount, calculate your expenses, including additional office expenses for handling billing services, and determine your bottom line for each patient visit. Make sure the discount supports your business and does not become an unnecessary burden.

A contract may require you to keep a specified percentage of your practice open to their insureds. This can limit your ability to hold appointments open for cash patients. Other contracts require you to provide the agreed-upon discount to patients paying cash for wellness care if they are members of the plan, even though you are not billing the carrier for treatments. Some plans extend the discounted rate as payment in full to insureds involved in MVAs or on-the-job injuries, even if the worker's comp or personal injury insurance reimburses at a higher rate. Read the patient access provision carefully and sign a contract only if you are willing to abide by it.

Consider how many days it takes to terminate a contract. Plans may require written notice from 30 to 120 days before the contract can be terminated without cause. If a plan reserves the right to revise the pay scale at any time, you may be bound to a rate that is unacceptable to you for months before you can terminate your contract. Most plans increase the fee schedule over time, but if the rates are reduced, it could cause you financial hardship.

The contract will specify reasons for immediate termination. Read these carefully. Something as simple as not providing copies of patient records within 3 days can breach the contract and result in immediate termination. Again, know what is expected of you and determine whether you are able to comply before signing the contract.

Inadequate documentation, as defined by some contracts, can allow the plan to refuse to pay you for your services. Find out the plan's definition of adequate documentation. Follow the guidelines presented in this book, and you will most likely meet or exceed the requirements.

Many contracts stipulate that copies of patient files must be provided upon request free of charge within days of receiving the request. Contracting with an insurance plan may mean that you need to purchase a copy machine. Figure that expense into your bottom line when determining whether providing billing services for your patients is cost-effective for you.

Contracts may be amended, if both parties agree to the changes. If the original contract is unworkable for your practice, but several of your patients are policyholders, request changes to the contract. The insurance carrier *may* be willing to negotiate with you. Your chances of successful negotiation are greater if a number of you approach the company in an organized and professional manner to make your requests heard. Use your membership affiliations to join forces, pay for counsel, and shape your relationships with carriers. Take care not to violate Federal anti-trust laws prohibiting providers from joining together to boycott a contract or set fees. Hire legal counsel to ensure all laws are followed. For example, the AMTA-WA Chapter hired counsel to review insurance provider contracts and advise them of changes to request as a group. The reviews were published in The Journal and benefited hundreds of massage therapists considering the contract.

Approach the carriers from a position of cooperation and education, rather than animosity. You may feel insulted when they offer to pay you 75% of your customary fee, but an adversarial approach will not win you respect or give you an edge in negotiations. All types of health care providers are struggling with contracts, fee schedules, and reimbursement arrangements; all are trying to negotiate a living wage. Be professional, educate the

178

HANDS HEAL:
COMMUNICATION,
DOCUMENTATION,
AND INSURANCE BILLING
FOR MANUAL THERAPISTS

carriers about your profession, and try to understand the insurance company's position as well as your own during the negotiations.

Guidelines for Insurance Documentation

PATIENT INFORMATION

Documentation for insurance personnel carries the same requirements as other forms of patient documentation. Everyone is interested in information that accurately reflects the patient's health and the treatment provided. The only thing to consider is that care can be discontinued and payment reversed or denied based on the documentation.[6] Ensure that you have adequate documentation, including:

◆ Intake forms
◆ Prescription
◆ SOAP notes
◆ Progress reports

Record-keeping must meet two goals for insurance reimbursement. First, you must justify care on that day. Second, you must justify the overall treatment plan.[6] To justify care on the day of service, document:

◆ Symptoms consistent with the condition covered by the insurance plan at the time treatment was provided
◆ Alteration of the patient's daily routine because of his condition
◆ Positive objective findings within your scope of practice
◆ Patient's response to the treatment provided

To justify that the patient needs ongoing care:

◆ Identify functional goals that the patient, with the assistance of the proposed treatment, will strive to accomplish.
◆ Create a plan to accomplish the goals and justify the number of sessions, the length of each session, and the modalities you will use.
◆ Perform periodic progress evaluations to assess the effectiveness and efficiency of the treatment plan and identify the patient's progress.
◆ Adjust the treatment plan to respond to the individual needs of the patient, as determined by the progress evaluations and the goals accomplished.

Follow the guidelines presented throughout this book and feel confident that your documentation meets insurance requirements for reimbursement.

INSURANCE INFORMATION

Make sure you have all the information necessary for insurance reimbursement before filing claims. The primary cause of delays in payment of claims is lack of information or inaccurate information on the billing form.[7] Because each type of insurance, each company, and each plan has its own requirements for billing and reimbursement, you may need to confirm the billing and reimbursement information for each new patient and for each new occurrence or condition.

Two forms will help you identify the information necessary for insurance billing and reimbursement. The first, the Billing Information form, is one of the intake forms the patient filled at the initial visit. (For a blank form, see Appendix: Forms.) This form provides information about the type of claim, contact information for the insurance company, and contact information for the patient's attorney and referring HCP, if applicable.

The second, the Insurance Verification form, is completed by the practitioner, based on information recorded on the Insurance Information form and details provided by the patient's referring HCP, attorney, and insurance representative. (For a blank form, see Appendix: Forms.) The form verifies the insurance coverage, identifies limitations or restrictions on the benefits, and verifies that reimbursement is authorized for your services. Completing this form greatly reduces the risk of accepting insurance reimbursement as payment for services.

Any time information is verified over the phone, record the date, time, and name of the person you are speaking with in a phone log, and include notes on the conversation. Use a phone log in addition to filling out the information directly onto the forms. It is easier to confirm information with the insurance carrier, should something go awry, if you can provide specific information about the date and time and the name of the person with whom you spoke.

Billing Information Form

Refer to Chapter 5 for details on filling out the Billing Information form. Use the form for every patient who requests insurance billing services. The information provided by the patient on the Billing Information form identifies whom to call to gather additional information necessary for verifying insurance benefits. Four phone calls may be required once the Billing Information form is completed: to the referring HCP, attorney, Human Resources representative, and insurance representative. A phone call to the attorney is necessary only if the patient has retained counsel for a personal injury claim. A phone call to Human Resources may be necessary if the insurance is provided through the patient's work. When making the phone calls, have the Billing Information form and the Insurance Verification form in front of you. When calling the referring HCP, have the prescription handy.

Insurance Verification Form

The Insurance Verification form prompts the necessary information-gathering and records the information from the referring HCP, attorney, Human Resources representative, and insurance representative. (See Figure 8-1) Complete the form for every patient who requests insurance billing services. Update the form with each request for ongoing services. Complete a new form for each recurrence of a previous condition and for each new condition.

Referring Health Care Provider Information

The first section of the Insurance Verification form confirms the information on the referring HCP. Identify whether the referring provider is the attending provider. Sometimes the referring provider is not the provider who sees the patient regularly. For example, Zamora's referral came from her physician, whom she saw immediately after her on-the-job injury, but whom she did not see thereafter. Her chiropractor is the attending provider she sees regularly. If the attending provider is different from the referring provider, send

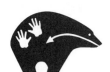

Helena LaLuna, CR

123 Sun Moon and Stars Drive
Capital Hill, WA   98119
TEL   206 555 4446

INSURANCE VERIFICATION

Name _Zamora Hostetter_   Date _4-4-01_

Date of Injury _3-31-01_   Insurance ID# _C98-7654321_

A. Patient Information

Employment
Employer __Howling Moon Cafe__
Phone _555-4444_   Fax _555-3333_
Currenty Employed? ☒Y ☐N
Effective date of benefits _6-24-00_
Expiration date of benefits _6-24-01_
Contact name _Betty_
Date/Time verified _4-4-01   4:00 pm_

Attorney
Name _N/A_
Phone _____ Fax _____
Guarantee of Payment filed? ☐Y ☐N
Medical Lien filed? ☐Y ☐N
　Date _____ Expires _____
　Renewed _____ Expires _____
Copies of patient file requests
　Date requested _____ Date sent _____
　Date requested _____ Date sent _____

Primary Health Care Provider
Name _Manda Rae Yuricich, OC_
Phone _555-3535_   Fax _555-4646_
Attending provider for this injury/illness? ☒Y ☐N
Referring provider for manual therapy services? ☒Y ☐N
Prescription received? ☒Y ☐N
Prescription date _4-1-01_   # of Tx _10_
　Tx duration/frequency _2x wk/5 wks_
　Diagnosis (ICD-10 codes) _724.2, 723.1, 840.9,_
　_728.85, 784.0_
　First Renewal date _5-12-01_   # of Tx _3_
　Tx duration/frequency _1x wk-3 wks_
　Second Renewal date _____ # of Tx _____
　Tx duration/frequency _____

B. Insurance Information

Workers Compensation Insurance
Contact _Aziz Amaden_
Phone _(360) 555-6655_ Fax _555-5566_
Date/Time verified _4-5-01   9:30 AM_
　Is claim open? ☒Y ☐N
　Date Opened _4-1-01_ Date Closed _____
　Date Reopened _____

Private Health Insurance
Insurer _N/A_
Contact _____
Phone _____ Fax _____
Date/Time verified _____

Personal Injury Insurance
Primary Insurer _N/A_
　Adjuster _____
　Phone _____ Fax _____
　Date/Time verified _____
　　PIP policy amount $ _____
　　Dates of coverage _____
　　PIP available $ _____
　　Med Pay policy amount $ _____
　　Dates of coverage _____
　　Med Pay available $ _____

Secondary Insurer _____
　Adjuster _____
　Phone _____ Fax _____
　Date/Time verified _____
　　PIP policy amount $ _____
　　Dates of coverage _____
　　PIP available $ _____
　　Med Pay policy amount $ _____
　　Dates of coverage _____
　　Med Pay available $ _____

C. Verify Benefits/Authorize Services

Ask the insurance representative the following questions
　regarding the patient's coverage:

1. Is manual therapy a covered benefit? ☒Y ☐N
2. Is the patient eligible for the manual therapy benefit for this
　condition (supply diagnosis/ICD-10 codes)? ☒Y ☐N
3. Am I eligible to provide manual therapy services (supply
　professional license/certification)? ☒Y ☐N

If the answer to any one of these questions is No, bill the patient
　for manual therapy services.
If the answer to all three questions is Yes, continue verification
　on page two, and bill the insurance company for manual therapy
　services.

Figure 8-1. Insurance Verification form.

C. Verify Benefits/Authorize Services, cont.

Record the answers you get to questions 4, 5, and 6 in this table. In the first column list the services you provide. In the second column, record the corresponding CPT code. Complete the table with the answers you get to questions 4, 5, and 6.

4. Which manual therapy services are authorized? (Go through each one listed below.)
5. Are there any restrictions or limitations to each authorized service?
6. What is the maximum allowable reimbursement rate for each authorized service?

Service Item	CPT code	4. Authorized?	5. Restrictions?	6. Max Rate?
1. myofascial	97140	☒Y ☐N	4 units max/tx	28.78
2. Polarity	97139	☐Y ☒N		
3. hot/cold packs	97010	☐Y ☒N	bundled	
4.		☐Y ☐N		
5.		☐Y ☐N		
6.		☐Y ☐N		
7.		☐Y ☐N		
8.		☐Y ☐N		
9.		☐Y ☐N		
10.		☐Y ☐N		

Complete 7-17 as applicable

7. Does a deductible apply? ☐Y ☒N Amount $ _____
   Paid to date $ _____
   Policy year dates _____
8. Does a Co-Pay apply? ☐Y ☒N Amount $ _____
9. Does a co-insurance apply? ☐Y ☒N Amount % _____
10. Is there a limit on the # of sessions per policy year?
   ☒Y ☐N Total per year 12 per incident
   Number available to date 12
11. Is there a limit on the total $ spent on these services or similar services per policy year? ☐Y ☒N Amount $ _____
   Amount available to date _____
12. Treatment dates authorized 4-1 → 5-1
13. Number of sessions authorized 6
14. Preferred billing method/form:
   ☒HCFA 1500 ☐Electronic ☐Other _____
15. Send with each bill:
   ☒Prescription ☐SOAP notes ☒Progress Reports
   ☐License/Certification ☐Other _____
16. What is the expected turnaround time on claim reimbursement? 30 days
17. Are you able to authorize payment? ☒Y ☐N
   If Yes, authorization # 47329
   If No, can you connect me with someone who is able to authorize payment? ☐Y ☐N
   Name _____
   Phone _____ Fax _____

Send a copy of this form to the insurance representative with a letter confirming the information gathered.
Date sent 4-6-01

Re-Authorization/Verification

Contact Terry Farr
Phone (360) 555-6655 Fax 555-5566
Date/Time verified 4-24-01   10:00 AM
Treatment dates authorized 4-25-01 → 5-25
Number of sessions authorized 6
Is payment authorized? ☒Y ☐N
   Authorization # 47499
Confirmation sent? ☒Y ☐N Date sent 4-24-01
Verify remainder of policy year, if applicable:
1. Deductible paid to date $ _____
2. Total # of sessions to date _____
3. Total $ spent to date $ _____

Re-Authorization/Verification

Contact _____
Phone _____ Fax _____
Date/Time verified _____
Treatment dates authorized _____
Number of sessions authorized _____
Is payment authorized? ☐Y ☐N
   Authorization # _____
Confirmation sent? ☐Y ☐N Date sent _____
Verify remainder of policy year, if applicable:
1. Deductible paid to date $ _____
2. Total # of sessions to date _____
3. Total $ spent to date $ _____

182

HANDS HEAL:
COMMUNICATION,
DOCUMENTATION,
AND INSURANCE BILLING
FOR MANUAL THERAPISTS

a copy of the prescription to the attending provider. It is critical for the attending HCP to have knowledge of all adjunctive care. The attending HCP may choose to write any additional prescriptions to ensure the adjunctive care complements the patient's treatment plan.

The form verifies a prescription has been obtained, as required for all adjunctive services. Record the details of the prescription on the Insurance Verification form to ensure the information is available when you speak with insurance representatives.

Attorney Information

The second section of the verification form is for attorney information and personal injury insurance information. These apply if the patient has sustained a personal injury, regardless of whether an attorney has been retained. If the patient has hired counsel and you have corresponded with the attorney (as suggested in Chapter 3) and received information about the patient's insurance status, you will have the information necessary to complete this section. If the patient has not retained an attorney, ask the patient to provide you with a copy of the car insurance policy. The insurance claims adjuster assigned to the case can verify the information the patient provides. If the secondary coverage is the patient's health insurance, fill out the benefit authorization section in addition to this section. If the MVA occurred while the patient was on the job, fill out the employer information. Otherwise, the employment and benefit information does not apply to personal injury cases.

Identify the primary and secondary coverage available. For each, note the existence of PIP and Med Pay coverage, the benefit amount, the dates the benefit is available, and the amount currently available. The insurance carrier may not be willing to provide available dollar amounts as the patient's attorney can. For example, if the patient was hospitalized from the injury, the benefit may have been depleted and you will need further research into available funds for your services. In that case, find out from the patient how much care has been provided to date and estimate the benefit available. The patient has a right to accurate information on his insurance benefits from the insurer. The patient may need to call the insurer to get this information.

Document information regarding health care liens and attorney liens. If PIP, Med Pay, or any secondary coverage is exhausted or nonexistent, file liens on the patient and the attorney as per the requirements of state law. Health care liens may need to be renewed prior to expiration dates; note the date filed and the dates renewed. Note the date the contractual guarantee was requested from the attorney and the date it was returned and filed.

Note the expiration dates of authorizations on the Insurance Verification form; confirm that requests for records fall within the authorized dates. Note the date the requests were received and the date the information was sent.

Employment Information

The third section verifies employment. If the insurance coverage is provided through the patient's job—workers' compensation or a group health insurance plan—it is important to verify that the patient is employed and eligible for coverage. For example, even if the patient is employed, coverage might not be activated yet because the probationary period has not been satisfied; or the patient might have quit recently, and the insurance coverage will expire soon. Verify eligibility through the patient's insurance representative first. This may prevent the need for an additional call to the patient's employer. If you are unable to verify eligibility through the insurance representative or there are discrepancies in information, contact the human resources personnel or benefits administrator at the patient's work place to verify whether the patient is currently employed, how long she has been at the company, when the insurance coverage became effective, and when it expires.

Benefit Authorization

The fourth section verifies coverage, benefit eligibility, and authorizes services. For workers' compensation and private health insurance cases, fill out all applicable information. Some of the information requested in this section does not apply to both types of coverage. For example, workers' comp plans do not require deductibles and co-pays. Mark a line through information that is unnecessary for the patient's insurance type.

First, identify whether manual therapy is a benefit in the patient's plan. Be specific about your health care license: if you are a massage therapist, ask whether massage therapy is covered. If you are a physical therapist, ask whether physical therapy is covered. If you are not a licensed health care provider with a designated title, ask whether manual therapy is covered and who can provide the service.

Confirm that you are eligible to provide the service. You may be required to have **preferred provider status** or to have an assigned provider number to be eligible. The manual therapy benefit might be available only if a nurse or a doctor provides the service. If you are not a licensed health care provider and you are billing under the license of a primary HCP, you will need to ask the question specific to your situation. For example, "Is manual therapy a covered benefit for Zamora Hostetter if provided by an employee of the chiropractor under the chiropractor's immediate supervision?"

Next, confirm that the patient is eligible for the manual therapy benefit for the current condition. Provide the ICD-10 codes or the diagnosis from the prescription to the insurance representative to verify eligibility. Confirm whether an ICD-10 code is required on the billing form or whether the bill can be processed with a description of the diagnosis instead. The referring HCP may have written "low back pain" on the prescription, for example, without providing an ICD-10 code. If the insurance company insists on an ICD-10 code identified on the billing form for reimbursement, call the referring HCP and ask her to provide the proper code for the diagnosis.

Ask for clarification if a diagnosis code is denied. Sometimes a code is too specific and as a result is not listed in the insurance manual as an authorized diagnosis for your service. Instead, a general ICD-10 code describing the same diagnosis will authorize the treatment. For example, at HealthCo lumbar pain is an acceptable diagnosis (724.2) for manual therapy reimbursement but lumbar subluxation (839.20) is not covered for manual therapy services. If a code is denied, ask the insurance representative for a list of the allowable codes for the condition. Then call the referring HCP and request that a different diagnosis code be recorded on the prescription. This practice is acceptable as long as it does not misrepresent the patient's diagnosis.

Verify that the specific services you provide are covered. For example, if you are a massage therapist in New York, several manual therapy procedural codes fall within your scope of practice. However, the patient's insurance plan may not reimburse for all the codes available to your profession. Check out each CPT code individually with every insurance plan. If you are a contracted provider for the plan, the reimbursable codes will be specified in the fee schedule. If so, fill in the spaces provided in this section according to your contract. If not, compile a list of the techniques and modalities you provide in your treatment sessions. Find the corresponding CPT codes and write them beside the description of each service. CPT codes for manual therapy are listed in CPT code books and updated annually. Ask the insurance representative the following questions about each CPT code you list:

184

HANDS HEAL:
COMMUNICATION,
DOCUMENTATION,
AND INSURANCE BILLING
FOR MANUAL THERAPISTS

◆ Is the code reimbursable under the patient's plan?

◆ Am I eligible to provide the service?

◆ Are there any restrictions or exclusions for this code? Is there a limit to the reimbursable amount for each segment of time the service is provided (fee cap per unit)? Is there a limit to the amount of time I can bill for each session (unit cap)?

For example, manual therapy is a benefit in Zamora's plan, and she is receiving manual therapy for a lumbar sprain/strain, a covered condition. Helena, Zamora's manual therapist, is a certified Rolfer, and needs to verify that the CPT code for her modalities and techniques are reimbursable. Helena uses myofascial release therapy, hot and cold packs, and Polarity therapy in her sessions. 97140 is the current CPT code for manual therapy techniques, such as myofascial release, manual lymphatic drainage, and manual traction. 97139 is the current code for miscellaneous physical medicine often used for energy modalities, and 97010 is the current code for hot and cold packs. Helena goes down her list, asking the insurance representative whether each code is included in the manual therapy benefit for Zamora, whether she can provide the service as a certified Rolfer, whether there is a limit to the number of units for each session, whether there is a limit on the dollar amount per unit, and whether there are any other restrictions or exclusions for each CPT code. As it turns out, 97140 is included as a benefit, Helena is approved to bill for the service, and the code is reimbursable at a maximum of $28 per unit with a maximum of four units per day. 97139 is not reimbursable in Zamora's plan, and 97010 is a bundled service. Helena now knows her sessions with Zamora are limited to four units (1 hour), she cannot bill for time spent treating Zamora with Polarity Therapy, and she can apply hot and cold packs but she will not be paid an additional fee for that service. (See Figure 8-1)

Note if there is a limit on the total number of sessions allowed and a total dollar limit for the manual therapy benefit for a policy year. For example, Lin's plan limits chiropractic care to 20 visits per year and massage therapy coverage to $500 per year. The policy is renewed yearly from the date purchased, at which time the benefits are renewed.

Generally, Managed Care plans stipulate a **deductible**—a set dollar amount the patient pays out-of-pocket before coverage for designated services begins. Some services—such as annual physicals—may be covered even if the deductible has not yet been satisfied. Find out whether a deductible applies to your services, how much the deductible is, and how much has been paid to date. If the deductible has not been satisfied, the patient should pay at the time services are rendered. Submit the patient's bills to the insurance carrier, showing the amount paid so the payments can count toward satisfying the deductible. Once the deductible is satisfied, defer payment to the insurance company.

Find out when the policy is renewable. For example, John may have satisfied his deductible, but his policy is up for renewal and the deductible will need to be satisfied over again, beginning next month. If this is the case, request payment at the time of service after the specified date of renewal. Submit the bills showing payments made, to help the patient satisfy the deductible again.

Health plans usually require the insured to pay a portion of each health care visit in the form of a standard fee or **co-pay**. For example, every time John sees a preferred provider within his health care plan, he pays $10. Co-pays must be collected from the patient at the time of service and will not be paid by the insurance carrier. Some preferred provider contracts state that failure to collect the co-pay is a breach of contract and can result in termination.

Other plans may stipulate that the patient pays a percentage of the service fee rather than a co-pay, called a **co-insurance**. This is common if the provider is outside the network and is not a preferred provider of the carrier. Record the co-insurance percentage and collect it from the patient at the time of service.

Ask the insurance representative for verbal authorization to provide your services to the patient. Request an authorization number for the services, and verify the number of sessions authorized and the dates for providing the service. If possible, request authorization for payment of services as well. However, many insurance plans will authorize services but will not authorize payment until the bills are submitted. Verify the re-authorization date: if ongoing treatment is necessary, when must re-authorization occur to avoid a break in service?

Before ending the call, confirm that bills will be submitted on a HCFA 1500 billing form. If you are capable of complying, find out whether the carrier prefers electronic billing. Carriers that prefer electronic billing provide the software necessary to comply with their systems. A few companies prefer forms customized with their own bar code tracking system. Insurance carriers that require a special form generally provide them to you free of charge.

Find out whether copies of the patient's file should accompany the bills. If so, which records should be copied: SOAP notes, progress reports, prescriptions? If you are contracted with the insurance plan, your contract may stipulate that you send copies of the patient's file upon request. The patient's signature authorizing the release of the file is not necessary in this case. If you are not under contract to provide the patient's information, make sure you have the patient's written authorization before sending confidential information.

Ask about the expected turnaround time for payment. Inform the insurance representative of your fees, if not already determined by contract. Find out whether any further information would assist in ensuring timely payment. You might want to ask about common mistakes that delay payment, and how to avoid making those mistakes.

Send a confirmation letter verifying verbal authorization of benefits and services. Include a copy of the Insurance Verification form demonstrating that you have gathered all the necessary information. (See Figure 8-2) Verbal authorizations are sufficient for reimbursement, provided the claim is complete and accurate, but the confirmation letter ensures that the insurance carrier has the authorization documented and on file. Record the date the letter was sent on the verification form immediately before sending the copy. Both you and the insurance carrier can refer to the date if complications arise.

Once you have verified the insurance information and coverage, you are ready to provide treatment and to bill for the services. Repeat the verification process with each request for ongoing services beyond the number of sessions and dates of service previously authorized.

Guidelines for Insurance Billing
THE HCFA 1500 BILLING FORM

The **Health Care Financing Administration form** (**HCFA 1500**) is the standard billing form approved by the American Medical Association (AMA). (See Figure 8-3) The Insurance Information form and the Insurance Verification form provide information necessary to complete the HCFA 1500 billing form. The form is divided into two parts: patient and insured information, and provider information. It is fairly self-explanatory, but some sections can be confusing or do not apply to manual therapists. Each section is numbered and corresponds with the explanation that follows.

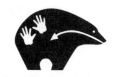

Helena LaLuna, CR

123 Sun Moon and Stars Drive
Capital Hill, WA   98119
Tel   206 555 4446   •   Fax   206 555 4447   •   Email   laluna@email.com

Dear __Aziz Amaden_____ :

Thank you for the opportunity to provide services to __Zamora Hostetter_____.

This letter confirms that:

1. Manual therapy is a covered benefit for the following diagnosis: __724.2_____
   __723.1, 840.9, 728.85, 784.0_____

2. The following CPT codes are authorized for the following rate: __97140_____
   __@ 28.78 per unit maximum 4 units per tx_____

3. __6_____ sessions are authorized to be completed between __4-1 → 5-1-01_____.

4. The patient's co-pay/co-insurance amount of $ __0_____ will be collected from the patient at the time of service.

5. ☒ Prescription   ☐ SOAPs   ☒ Progress reports   ☐ License/Certification

will accompany each billing statement.

6. Payment is anticipated within __30___ days of receipt of a clean claim.

7. If ongoing care is deemed necessary by the referring HCP, re-authorization will be requested by __4-24-01__ to ensure no break in care for the patient.

8. All claims will be sent to: __WA. Dept. of L & I_____

Attn: __claims department_____   Address __PO Box 323 Olympia WA 98055___

If you have any questions, please call. If I do not hear from you within 24 hours of receipt of this letter, I will assume that reimbursement for services is confirmed.

Sincerely,

Helena La Luna, CR

Figure 8-2. Confirmation letter.

186

HEALTH INSURANCE CLAIM FORM

PICA | PICA

1. MEDICARE	MEDICAID	CHAMPUS	CHAMPVA	GROUP HEALTH PLAN (SSN or ID)	FECA BLK LUNG (SSN)	OTHER	1a. INSURED'S I.D. NUMBER (FOR PROGRAM IN ITEM 1)
(Medicare #)	(Medicaid #)	(Sponsor's SSN)	(VA File #)			☒ (ID)	C98-7654321

2. PATIENT'S NAME (Last Name, First Name, Middle Initial)
Hostetter Zamora

3. PATIENT'S BIRTH DATE MM DD YY: 05 22 80 — SEX M ☐ F ☒

4. INSURED'S NAME (Last Name, First Name, Middle Initial)
Same

5. PATIENT'S ADDRESS (No., Street)
63 18TH Ave W

6. PATIENT RELATIONSHIP TO INSURED
Self ☒ Spouse ☐ Child ☐ Other ☐

7. INSURED'S ADDRESS (No., Street)

CITY: Capitol Hill STATE: WA

8. PATIENT STATUS
Single ☒ Married ☐ Other ☐
Employed ☒ Full-Time Student ☐ Part-Time Student ☐

CITY STATE

ZIP CODE: 98119 TELEPHONE (Include Area Code): (206) 555-1221

ZIP CODE TELEPHONE (INCLUDE AREA CODE): ( )

9. OTHER INSURED'S NAME (Last Name, First Name, Middle Initial)
Same

10. IS PATIENT'S CONDITION RELATED TO:

11. INSURED'S POLICY GROUP OR FECA NUMBER

a. OTHER INSURED'S POLICY OR GROUP NUMBER
555-63-1819

a. EMPLOYMENT? (CURRENT OR PREVIOUS)
☒ YES ☐ NO

a. INSURED'S DATE OF BIRTH MM DD YY SEX M ☐ F ☐

b. OTHER INSURED'S DATE OF BIRTH MM DD YY SEX M ☐ F ☐

b. AUTO ACCIDENT? PLACE (State)
☐ YES ☒ NO

b. EMPLOYER'S NAME OR SCHOOL NAME
Howling Moon Cafe

c. EMPLOYER'S NAME OR SCHOOL NAME
Howling Moon Cafe

c. OTHER ACCIDENT?
☐ YES ☒ NO

c. INSURANCE PLAN NAME OR PROGRAM NAME
WA Dept. L & I

d. INSURANCE PLAN NAME OR PROGRAM NAME
Health Co Selections

10d. RESERVED FOR LOCAL USE

d. IS THERE ANOTHER HEALTH BENEFIT PLAN?
☒ YES ☐ NO If yes, return to and complete item 9 a-d.

READ BACK OF FORM BEFORE COMPLETING & SIGNING THIS FORM.
12. PATIENT'S OR AUTHORIZED PERSON'S SIGNATURE I authorize the release of any medical or other information necessary to process this claim. I also request payment of government benefits either to myself or to the party who accepts assignment below.

SIGNED Signature on file DATE 4-4-01

13. INSURED'S OR AUTHORIZED PERSON'S SIGNATURE I authorize payment of medical benefits to the undersigned physician or supplier for services described below.

SIGNED Signature on file

14. DATE OF CURRENT: MM DD YY 03 31 01 ◄ ILLNESS (First symptom) OR INJURY (Accident) OR PREGNANCY(LMP)

15. IF PATIENT HAS HAD SAME OR SIMILAR ILLNESS. GIVE FIRST DATE MM DD YY

16. DATES PATIENT UNABLE TO WORK IN CURRENT OCCUPATION
FROM MM DD YY TO MM DD YY

17. NAME OF REFERRING PHYSICIAN OR OTHER SOURCE
Manda Rae Yuricich, DC

17a. I.D. NUMBER OF REFERRING PHYSICIAN

18. HOSPITALIZATION DATES RELATED TO CURRENT SERVICES
FROM MM DD YY TO MM DD YY

19. RESERVED FOR LOCAL USE

20. OUTSIDE LAB? ☐ YES ☐ NO $ CHARGES

21. DIAGNOSIS OR NATURE OF ILLNESS OR INJURY. (RELATE ITEMS 1,2,3 OR 4 TO ITEM 24E BY LINE)
1. 724.2
2. 723.1, 784.0
3. 840.9
4. 728.85

22. MEDICAID RESUBMISSION CODE ORIGINAL REF. NO.

23. PRIOR AUTHORIZATION NUMBER

24. A DATE(S) OF SERVICE From MM DD YY / To MM DD YY	B Place of Service	C Type of Service	D PROCEDURES, SERVICES, OR SUPPLIES (Explain Unusual Circumstances) CPT/HCPCS MODIFIER	E DIAGNOSIS CODE	F $ CHARGES	G DAYS OR UNITS	H EPSDT Family Plan	I EMG	J COB	K RESERVED FOR LOCAL USE
1	4 4 01	3	9	97140	1,2,3,4	25	—	1			
2	4 4 01	3	9	97140	1,2,3,4	25	—	1			
3	4 4 01	3	9	97140	1,2,3,4	25	—	1			
4	4 4 01	3	9	97140	1,2,3,4	25	—	1			
5											
6											

25. FEDERAL TAX I.D. NUMBER SSN EIN
91-1777771 ☐ ☒

26. PATIENT'S ACCOUNT NO.

27. ACCEPT ASSIGNMENT? (For govt. claims, see back)
☐ YES ☐ NO

28. TOTAL CHARGE $ 100 —

29. AMOUNT PAID $ 0

30. BALANCE DUE $ 100

31. SIGNATURE OF PHYSICIAN OR SUPPLIER INCLUDING DEGREES OR CREDENTIALS (I certify that the statements on the reverse apply to this bill and are made a part thereof.)
SIGNED Helena La Luna, CR 4-4-01 DATE

32. NAME AND ADDRESS OF FACILITY WHERE SERVICES WERE RENDERED (If other than home or office)

33. PHYSICIAN'S, SUPPLIER'S BILLING NAME, ADDRESS, ZIP CODE & PHONE #
Helena La Luna, CR
123 Sun Moon and Stars Dr.
Capitol Hill, WA 98119
PIN# (206) 555-4446 GRP#

FORM HCFA-1500 (12-90)
NORTHWEST BUSINESS FORMS (206) 728-8181

PLEASE PRINT OR TYPE

FORM OWCP-1500 FORM RRB-1500 APPROVED OMB-0938-0008
(APPROVED BY AMA COUNCIL ON MEDICAL SERVICE 8/88)

CARRIER

PATIENT AND INSURED INFORMATION

PHYSICIAN OR SUPPLIER INFORMATION

Figure 8-3. HCFA 1500 Billing form.

188

HANDS HEAL:
COMMUNICATION,
DOCUMENTATION,
AND INSURANCE BILLING
FOR MANUAL THERAPISTS

1. Check the box that applies to the type of insurance for the patient. For health insurance, check the Group Health Plan box and write either the patient's social security number or the insurance ID number in the space 1a. For personal injury cases or worker's comp cases, check the Other box and write the claim number in 1a.

2. In Boxes 2 through 7, fill in the patient's name, address, and phone. If the patient is also the insured, record "same" as the insured's name. If the insured is someone other than the patient, fill in the insured's name, address, and phone number. For example, Darnel's nephew was the owner of the car Darnel was riding in when the accident occurred. Therefore, you would fill in the nephew's name, address, and phone number as the primary insured. (See Figure 8-3, **#4** and **#7**.) His insurance is first in line to cover Darnel's medical expenses. A common situation in which the insured is not the patient occurs when the spouse is insured through work and the insurance policy covers the patient. Check the box that signifies the patient's relationship to the insured.

8. Self explanatory

9. Other Insured refers to second party coverage. For example, this may be the patient's car insurance, if the primary coverage is someone else's, or it may be the patient's health insurance, if the car insurance does not provide PIP. For example, Darnel's other insured, or secondary coverage, is his car insurance. If he does not drive and does not carry auto insurance, his health insurance is considered the other insured.

10. Self explanatory

11. Fill in the insured's policy number. This might be the group number or the plan number, whichever identifies the type of plan the insured has. Fill in the date of birth and sex. The employer or school is necessary only if the insurance plan is provided through either. Personal injury cases do not require this information unless the injury occurred while the patient was working. Fill in the plan name, and answer the question regarding secondary insurance coverage.

12. The patient is required to authorize the release of any medical information necessary to process the claim. The patient does not have to sign every billing form if he has signed a release on file in the chart. This release is included on the Billing Information form. Check to make sure the patient signs the release when he fills out the form and note "Signature on File" instead of having the patient sign every bill. The date for this section should reflect the date the patient signed the Insurance Information form.

13. Here, the patient's signature authorizes the insurance company to pay the health care provider directly. Payment will be written and mailed to the provider listed in **#33**. This is also included on the Billing Information form. Again, rather than requiring the patient to sign every bill, "Signature on File" will suffice if the patient's signature is on the intake form.

14. Boxes 14 and 15 are self explanatory.

16. Boxes 16 and 18. This may not apply to adjunctive care and can be left blank.

17. Fill in the referring HCP's name and provider number, if applicable.

19. Boxes 19 and 20. Leave blank.

21. Most insurance carriers require a diagnosis to reimburse for services, regardless of your ability to diagnose. If diagnosing is not within your scope of practice, simply transfer the diagnosis from the prescription to the HCFA 1500. Filling in the diagnosis code on an HCFA 1500 form will not be construed as acting outside your scope of practice, as long as a referring HCP provided the codes for you and the prescription is on file.

22. Boxes 22 and 23. Leave blank.

24A. Dates of Service has two sections: From and To. Record the dates you provided the service in the From section.

24B. Place of Service codes vary among carriers and may be found in the company's billing manual. Some use numbers, such as:

1. Inpatient Hospital
2. Outpatient Hospital
3. Office
4. Residence
5. Emergency Room
6. Other Medical/Surgical Facilities
7. Nursing Home
8. Other Location

Or

11. Office
12. Home
21. In Hospital
22. Outpatient Hospital
24. Ambulatory Surgical Center
25. Birthing Center
33. Custodial Care Facility
34. Hospice

Others use letters:

AC—Ambulatory Surgical Center
ER—Emergency Room
HM—Patient's Home
HS—Hospice
IH—Inpatient Hospital
NH—Nursing Home
OH—Outpatient Hospital
OF—Practitioner's Office

Check with the insurance representative for the preferred codes, or request a billing manual to ensure accurate billing.

24C. Type of Service also varies among insurance carriers. The following is one example of a carrier's code list:

01. Medical Care
02. Surgery
03. Consultation
04. Diagnostic x-ray
05. Diagnostic labs
06. Radiation therapy
07. Anesthesia
08. Surgical assistant
09. Other medical services

Again, check with the insurance carrier for its preferred codes.

24D. The services you bill for must be listed by CPT code unless state regulations dictate otherwise. Refer to the list on the insurance verification form for each patient and

190

HANDS HEAL:
COMMUNICATION,
DOCUMENTATION,
AND INSURANCE BILLING
FOR MANUAL THERAPISTS

use the codes that describe your services, are within your scope of practice, and are reimbursable within the patient's plan.

24E. The diagnosis codes are numbered in section 21. Fill in the number that corresponds to the diagnosis of the conditions that you treated in the session. For example, the patient might have two conditions, low back pain and cervical subluxation, and two diagnosis codes listed for each condition. Last Tuesday, you treated the low back pain only and did not have time to treat the neck condition. For that session, you would fill in the numbers "1, 2." This Monday you were able to address both conditions, and put "1, 2, 3, 4" in this section.

24F. Charges should reflect the total amount for the line item. A common mistake is to give the value of one unit of service instead of the total for all units of service. If you provided 4 units of the service listed, and each unit is billed at $15 per unit, the total charges would be $60.

24G. Units refer to a designated period of time or a single, specified procedure. Each CPT code lists a unit of time in the description. Some are 15-minute units, others are 30-minute units. If no unit of time is provided in the description, the CPT code refers to the procedure as a single unit, independent of the amount of time it takes to perform the procedure. For example, hot and cold packs may be applied as a procedure undefined by time; whereas neuromuscular reeducation is billable in 15-minute units, and an extended new patient office visit is defined as a 45-minute unit. Check the CPT code book for the definition of units to ensure accurate billing for your services.

24H, I, J, K. Leave blank.

25. Self explanatory

26. This is optional. If you organize your office records by assigning your patients numbers, put the patient's number here to assist you in filing the bills.

27. Leave blank.

28. Total all the charges for each line item.

29. Fill in any payments from the patient.

30. Fill in the balance due.

31. Boxes 31 and 32 are self explanatory.

33. Make sure this is legible. The checks will be made payable to the name listed here and sent to the address listed here. Include your phone number. If there are any questions regarding the bill, a bill processor may prefer to call you before denying the bill or sending it back in the mail.

TIMING

Submit the HCFA 1500 billing form immediately after the first session. If there are any problems with the billing procedures, it is best to work out the glitches early in the reimbursement process. The most common delay in billing is a simple lack of information, such as failure to attach a copy of the prescription, or an inappropriate diagnosis code that is easily corrected. Once the complete and accurate information is provided, the billing usually proceeds smoothly.

Bill as often as you are comfortable billing. Many computerized billing programs make it easy to bill after each session. Other practitioners find it easier to designate one day every week or two for office work, and do all of the billing, report writing, and correspondence on that day. Whichever you choose, make sure you bill treatment dates within the same month. It is easier on the other end to organize and track reimbursement if the dates of services all fall within a calendar month. This may be stipulated in your contract under billing procedures.

Bill frequently to avoid reimbursement delays. High dollar amounts often require additional signatures or a higher authority to authorize payment.

Re-bill every 30 days on the balance due. Stamp the HCFA 1500 form with the word "COPY—resubmitted _____" and write the date you are resubmitting the bill. Attach an invoice adding interest charges, if applicable, and state the new balance. If you are a preferred provider under contract with the carrier, check your contract for stipulations regarding interest. Also, check for state regulations regarding interest charges on medical services. For example, Washington State limits interest on medical services to 12% simple interest annually, or one percent per month applied only to the treatment amount (meaning you can't apply interest to interest). Typically, providers will accrue interest 90 days after the billing date. Provide the patient and the insurance company with 30 days' notice before assigning interest, and calculate it according to state regulations.

PAYMENT LOGS

Create a payment log for each patient. (See Figure 8-4) Track the billing dates, reimbursement dates, and payment amounts. File all payment logs in a three-ring binder in alphabetical order. Go through the binder twice monthly to determine whom to re-bill at 30-day intervals.

Enter all payments onto the logs before depositing funds. Verify the dates of service for each reimbursement check. This is critical. Each check will specify the dates of service that the payment applies toward on the **Explanation of Benefits** (EOB). Sometimes the payment for one bill may not follow the previous payment. For example, Helena has sent three billing statements to HealthCo. The first bill was for treatment provided on 4/12/01. The second bill was for treatments on 4/15/01, 4/18/01, and 4/24/01. The third bill was for treatment on 5/01/01. The first payment received was for treatment on 4/12/01. The second payment received was for treatment on 5/01/01. Helena erroneously applies the second payment to the second treatment that appears chronologically on the payment log. Then, after Helena resubmits a modified bill for the second billing statement and a copy of the third bill, HealthCo informs Helena that she has already been paid for services provided on 5/01/01 and refuses to pay the third bill. She receives only partial payment for the second bill because of the modified statement and no payment for the third bill, and cannot contest it successfully until she resolves the misapplied amount.

Strategies for Managing Reimbursement Challenges

Private health insurance companies are required by law to respond to a designated number of claims within a specified amount of time. (This does not include personal injury insurance or workers' comp.) For example, Washington State law requires 95% of clean claims to be paid within 30 days, and 95% of unclean claims to be paid or denied within 60 days.[8] **Clean claims** are bills submitted with complete and accurate information, for covered services that the patient is eligible for and the practitioner is authorized to provide. **Unclean claims** lack information or contain disputable information, such as a procedure that is not authorized for the diagnosis.

Reimbursement for unclean claims can be delayed, denied, or reversed. Most unclean claims are returned to the practitioner for clarification or correction, and must be

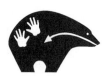

Helena LaLuna, CR
123 Sun Moon and Stars Drive
Capital Hill, WA   98119
TEL   206 555 4446

PAYMENT LOG

Name _Zamora Hostetter_   Date _6-18-01_

Date of Injury _3-31-01_   Insurance ID# _C98-7654321_

Billing Date: _5-18-01_   Total Billed: $ _100_

Patient Paid: $ _0_   Insurance Paid: $ _0_   Total Paid: $ _0_

If Total Paid does NOT equal Total Billed, complete below for each date of service (from lines 1-6, Section 24 of HCFA 1500)

Line 1, Initial Billing
Treatment Date: _5-18-01_ Bill Date: _5-18-01_
Charges: _100_ Adjustments: _0_ Amount Billed: _100_
Due from patient: _0_ Due from Insurance: _100-_
Patient Paid: _0_   Insurance paid: _0_

Line 1, Rebilling
Rebill Date: _6-18-01_ Rebilled to: _Ins._
Outstanding: _100-_ Interest: _0_ Amount Billed: _100-_
Rebill Date: _7-18-01_ Rebilled to: _Ins._
Outstanding: _100-_ Interest: _1%_ Amount Billed: _101-_
Rebill Date: _____ Rebilled to: _____
Outstanding: _____ Interest: _____ Amount Billed: _____

Line 2, Initial Billing
Treatment Date: _____ Bill Date: _____
Charges: ____ Adjustments: ____ Amount Billed: ____
Due from patient: _____ Due from Insurance: _____
Patient Paid: _____ Insurance paid: _____

Line 2, Rebilling
Rebill Date: _____ Rebilled to: _____
Outstanding: _____ Interest: _____ Amount Billed: _____
Rebill Date: _____ Rebilled to: _____
Outstanding: _____ Interest: _____ Amount Billed: _____
Rebill Date: _____ Rebilled to: _____
Outstanding: _____ Interest: _____ Amount Billed: _____

Line 3, Initial Billing
Treatment Date: _____ Bill Date: _____
Charges: ____ Adjustments: ____ Amount Billed: ____
Due from patient: _____ Due from Insurance: _____
Patient Paid: _____ Insurance paid: _____

Line 3, Rebilling
Rebill Date: _____ Rebilled to: _____
Outstanding: _____ Interest: _____ Amount Billed: _____
Rebill Date: _____ Rebilled to: _____
Outstanding: _____ Interest: _____ Amount Billed: _____
Rebill Date: _____ Rebilled to: _____
Outstanding: _____ Interest: _____ Amount Billed: _____

Line 4, Initial Billing
Treatment Date: _____ Bill Date: _____
Charges: ____ Adjustments: ____ Amount Billed: ____
Due from patient: _____ Due from Insurance: _____
Patient Paid: _____ Insurance paid: _____

Line 4, Rebilling
Rebill Date: _____ Rebilled to: _____
Outstanding: _____ Interest: _____ Amount Billed: _____
Rebill Date: _____ Rebilled to: _____
Outstanding: _____ Interest: _____ Amount Billed: _____
Rebill Date: _____ Rebilled to: _____
Outstanding: _____ Interest: _____ Amount Billed: _____

Line 5, Initial Billing
Treatment Date: _____ Bill Date: _____
Charges: ____ Adjustments: ____ Amount Billed: ____
Due from patient: _____ Due from Insurance: _____
Patient Paid: _____ Insurance paid: _____

Line 5, Rebilling
Rebill Date: _____ Rebilled to: _____
Outstanding: _____ Interest: _____ Amount Billed: _____
Rebill Date: _____ Rebilled to: _____
Outstanding: _____ Interest: _____ Amount Billed: _____
Rebill Date: _____ Rebilled to: _____
Outstanding: _____ Interest: _____ Amount Billed: _____

Line 6, Initial Billing
Treatment Date: _____ Bill Date: _____
Charges: ____ Adjustments: ____ Amount Billed: ____
Due from patient: _____ Due from Insurance: _____
Patient Paid: _____ Insurance paid: _____

Line 6, Rebilling
Rebill Date: _____ Rebilled to: _____
Outstanding: _____ Interest: _____ Amount Billed: _____
Rebill Date: _____ Rebilled to: _____
Outstanding: _____ Interest: _____ Amount Billed: _____
Rebill Date: _____ Rebilled to: _____
Outstanding: _____ Interest: _____ Amount Billed: _____

Figure 8-4. Payment Log.

returned clean within a designated time frame to prevent further delay in payment. Other claims require investigation from a **utilization review** board. Peer reviews determine the following:

- Treatment was appropriate
- Treatment was effective
- Cost of care was reasonable

Peer reviewers determine whether claims meet these requirements by studying patient files, looking for answers to the following questions:

- Did the provider deliver the promised services?
- Did the provider deliver the promised services in the agreed upon time?
- Did the intervention deliver the expected outcome?
- Did the provider charge **usual, customary, and regular fees (UCR)** for services?

Claims that are denied result in partial payment, no payment, or a reversal in payment. Partial payment is often the result of:

- Treating outside the diagnosis. For example, Raphael treated a patient diagnosed with an ankle sprain by administering manual therapy to the upper extremities, in addition to the lower extremities. The insurance claims processor determined that the treatment was not consistent with the diagnosis, and awarded a partial payment. Sixty percent of the treatment was designated appropriate treatment and 40% was deemed unnecessary treatment. The partial payment reflected 60% of the total fee for all treatments. Appeals of this type can be successful if you prove the necessity of care.
- Treating outside the time frame authorized for treatments. For example, authorization was obtained for six sessions within 30 days, and the sixth treatment was given on day 32. Be aware of time limitations. Appeals caused by scheduling negligence rarely succeed.
- Treating beyond the standard of care for the condition. For example, 10 sessions are the maximum allowable for low back pain, and 13 were provided. This is easily avoided by verifying the number of sessions authorized before administering the treatment.

Payment denial is common when:

- Billing for treatment outside your scope of practice
- Billing for services not provided for the diagnosis
- Bills for multiple visits of similar modalities are provided on the same day. For example, the patient receives both physical therapy and massage therapy on the same day. The practitioner who submits the claim first will usually be the only one reimbursed.

Reversal of payment occurs when the practitioner is found guilty of fraudulent or abusive billing practices, such as charging for procedures that were not performed, billing for services in addition to those actually performed, charging for medically unnecessary services, submitting claims with misleading diagnostic codes so as to receive benefits for an excluded service, or billing at a higher rate than would be charged in the absence of third-party reimbursement.

194

HANDS HEAL:
COMMUNICATION,
DOCUMENTATION,
AND INSURANCE BILLING
FOR MANUAL THERAPISTS

It is illegal to charge different rates to different people or organizations. It is appropriate, however, to charge different fees for different services, or to offer reasonable discounts for payment on the day of service, as long as the discount is offered to all patients equally. For example, if a patient pays cash but is submitting the bill to the insurance carrier for reimbursement, she must be offered the same discount at the time of service as any other patient. Acceptable discounts range between 5% and 15%, depending on state regulations. Consistent across insurance carriers, billing insurance companies one rate and cash patients another is considered fraudulent and abusive, particularly when the cash patient then seeks reimbursement at the higher rate.

During peer reviews for fraudulent billing, all of the provider's files are seized and reviewed for consistency. If, for example, the massage therapist clearly charges one fee for relaxation massage and one fee for treatment massage, the difference in fees is justified. But if the review board finds that the practitioner's primary techniques—manual lymphatic drainage and neuromuscular reeducation—are performed equally among relaxation patients and insurance patients, the different fee schedules are not justifiable. The practitioner may be required to reimburse insurance payments for as far back as 7 years, depending on the laws of the state.

▼

STORY TELLER 8-1
Usual and Customary Fees

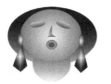

A local physical therapist was found guilty of fraudulent billing practices and was responsible for reimbursing the Department of Labor and Industries (L&I) over $4,800 in back payments plus interest and penalties. She was not a dishonest person but misinterpreted the fee schedule provided by L&I for treating workers' comp cases. The fee schedule stated that the maximum payable for manual therapy was $76 per visit. She assumed that L&I was offering to pay her that amount for her services, regardless of her usual and customary fee. She charged her cash patients and the health insurance plans $65 per visit. The contract she signed with L&I stipulated that she was to charge her usual and customary fee *up to* $76. Her negligence in reading the contract carefully resulted in financial hardship and she was forced to relocate her practice.

Insurance billing can be risky; billing challenges are unavoidable. Staying on top of outstanding bills is imperative. The following sections offer successful strategies for managing insurance reimbursement.

PROVIDE COMPLETE AND ACCURATE INFORMATION

Patient information and insurance information must be complete and accurate to avoid delays in payment. Follow these guidelines to avoid challenges relating to patient documentation:

◆ Take a comprehensive history on each patient.
◆ Keep SOAP charts on every session.
◆ Make sure the treatments noted reflect the procedures billed.
◆ Document subjective and objective data that validate the treatment provided.
◆ Set goals that reflect progress in the patient's everyday activities.
◆ Create a treatment plan to accomplish the patient's functional goals.
◆ Evaluate patient progress regularly.

- Make adjustments to the treatment plan to meet the patient's changing needs.
- Date all forms and SOAP charts.
- Make sure treatment dates correspond accurately with billing dates.
- Write monthly progress reports.
- Make sure the progress reports reflect information in the SOAP charts.
- Write legibly.
- Take notes that are spontaneous and unique to each individual patient.

Follow these guidelines to make sure the insurance information is complete and accurate:

- Have the patient fill out a Billing Information form.
- Go over the completed Billing Information form with the patient to verify content.
- Make sure the patient and insured's information—especially the patient's social security number and insurance policy numbers—is accurately transposed onto the billing form.
- Require a prescription from the patient's primary HCP.
- In case of an incomplete prescription, provide a prescription form for the referring HCP to complete, or gather necessary information over the phone.
- Complete the Insurance Verification form with assistance from the patient's referring HCP, attorney, employer, and insurance representative, as necessary.
- Verify insurance coverage for your services, given your professional scope.
- Verify patient eligibility for the services, given the diagnosis.
- Inform the insurance representative in advance of your fee, unless dictated by contract.
- Double-check the provider information on the billing form to eliminate mistakes such as transposed numbers, inaccurate procedure codes, or incomplete diagnosis.
- Make sure the treatment dates on the billing form correspond with the SOAP notes.
- Know what information should accompany the billing form and send it as required: SOAPs, progress reports, and prescriptions.

STAY WITHIN DESIGNATED TIME LIMITS

Specific requirements must be met by the patient and the practitioner to ensure payment. Many of the requirements revolve around time. Stay within designated time limits when providing treatments, submitting bills, and seeking reimbursement:

- Provide treatment within the time period authorized.
- Make sure prescriptions cover all dates of treatment.
- Submit bills in a timely fashion. Never wait more than 30 days to submit a bill.
- Monitor the time frames for deductibles—when they are satisfied and when they are renewed—and collect appropriate fees at the time of service.
- Record the names, dates, and times of all phone conversations with insurance representatives.
- Resubmit bills after 31 days without payment. Stamp each bill with the rebilling date. Follow up with a phone call.
- Resubmit bills after 61 days without payment. Include the following statement: "This claim is over 60 days past due. If this claim is not paid or denied within 30 days, a writ-

196

HANDS HEAL:
COMMUNICATION,
DOCUMENTATION,
AND INSURANCE BILLING
FOR MANUAL THERAPISTS

ten complaint will be submitted to the Insurance Commissioner." (See Appendix: Contact Information Offices of Insurance Commissioners.) Follow up with a phone call.

◆ Return unclean claims with the requested information as soon as possible.

◆ Appeal denied claims within the time limit specified.

◆ Monitor expiration dates of medical liens and authorizations for release of medical records.

◆ Know the statute of limitations for filing a lawsuit.

PROVE MEDICAL NECESSITY

Practitioners must be able to prove that the treatment provided was medically necessary. Follow these guidelines to avoid dispute over medical necessity:

◆ Make sure prescriptions state the adjunctive care as integral to the treatment plan.

◆ Prove progress specific to the patient's daily activities.

◆ Treat within the diagnosis. For holistic treatments, ensure the prescription requests treatment to structures outside the diagnosis, and if denied, you can confidently justify full-body treatment.

◆ Document active as well as passive care. Educate patients in self-care: self-massage, breathing exercises, application of hot and cold packs, stretching and strengthening exercises, ergonomics and movement mechanics, and increased awareness of aggravating activities.

◆ If a formal appeal is necessary, educate the reviewer on the necessity of treatment and the benefits of manual therapy. Some insurers will see CAM care as experimental treatment and not reimbursable. Be prepared to send research articles and write letters detailing the benefits of manual therapy.

FILE LIENS ON PERSONAL INJURY CASES

Medical or health care liens are used to guarantee payment for treatments provided to people who have sustained a personal injury. The intent is to place a hold on the patient's claim until satisfying the outstanding medical bills. Depending on state law, the health care provider must file the lien in a specified way. For example, in Washington, the lien must be filed with the county auditor before settlement and payment have been made to the injured party.

File medical liens on all personal injury cases where payment has been deferred. Send copies of the lien to the patient, both insurance companies (the patient's and the at-fault party's), and the patient's attorney, if applicable. [6]

MISCELLANEOUS REIMBURSEMENT TIPS

◆ Establish positive, cooperative relationships with insurance representatives. Your attitude may affect the reimbursement results.

◆ Read insurance contracts carefully. Follow the contractual language of the policy.

◆ Correctly apply all payments according to the dates of treatment stated on the EOB.

◆ Be prepared. Know the standard billing practices and procedure codes for your profession for each type of insurance before agreeing to provide billing services.

- Type the information onto the HCFA 1500 form or use computerized billing. Handwritten bills are difficult to read and will result in delays.
- Ask the patient to intervene. If the insurance company is delaying payment, a phone call from the patient can speed up claims processing.
- Ask the attorney to intervene. A letter or a phone call can be very effective in prompting payment.
- If necessary, ask the insurance commissioner's office (OIC) to intervene. A formal complaint to the OIC reflects badly on the insurance company, often results in an investigation, and remains in the insurance carriers' file for several years.
- Require attorney liens or medical liens for all personal injury cases. If the attorney refuses to sign the letter guaranteeing payment from the settlement, stop deferring payment immediately, file a medical lien, and require the patient to make regular payments on the outstanding balance.

State regulatory agencies, such as the Office of the Insurance Commissioner (OIC), may provide additional assistance to manual therapists and patients. Generally, the OIC investigates formal complaints against insurance carriers, and assists with writing, interpreting, and implementing rules that providers and insurers must follow. These regulations offer support and protection for both the health care providers and their patients. Additionally, staff members can be strong advocates for patients and providers, helping patients receive appropriate levels of benefits based on the insurance packages purchased, and supporting providers in receiving fair treatment by insurers, such as prompt payment. Individual provider assistance varies State by State. (See Appendix: Contact Information—Offices of Insurance Commissioners.)

Appealing Claims Denials

Claims can be denied before treatment is provided, during treatment (with the frequent result of discontinued care), or after the services have been provided. There is no financial risk to the practitioner or the patient if the claim is denied before treatment is provided, or if the denial simply prevents ongoing care. If a claim is denied after the service has been delivered, the practitioner has financial motivation to appeal the claim and ease the financial hardship for herself and ultimately for the patient.

Financial hardship is not the only reason to **appeal** a claim. You may have a great deal of emotional investment in getting the patient the needed care. You can be successful in appealing claims if the lack of treatment can result in harm to the patient. The process of appeals becomes an opportunity to educate the insurance representatives on the benefits of manual therapy and the patient's level of need.

The denial may be the result of a simple mistake that can be corrected and the denial reversed, or it may be a valid response to an infraction of policy undeserving of an appeal. However, if a denial is issued when treatment is critical for the health of the patient, and the denial is a result of the insurance carrier's failure to cover the needs of the patient, or of the insurance representative's failure to understand the patient's condition and need for care, an appeal is warranted. Appeals are commonly needed for chronic conditions or conditions poorly understood by health professionals and claims managers alike, such as lymphedema and fibromyalgia. Plans rarely cover chronic conditions because they consider treatment for these conditions to be preventative or palliative (since the symptoms do not subside), even though a lack of treatment may result in a substantial decrease in the

198

HANDS HEAL:
COMMUNICATION,
DOCUMENTATION,
AND INSURANCE BILLING
FOR MANUAL THERAPISTS

patient's ability to function and ultimately leave the patient predisposed to serious acute flare-ups.

Appeals must be written in such a way as to validate treatment based on the patient's specific condition, proving that such care is neither preventative nor palliative, and is necessary for the patient's ability to function in everyday activities. Without the treatment, the quality of the patient's life is diminished.

Appeals must be filed within a specified time frame, or the appeal does not have to be heard. Refer to your provider contract for rules of appeals.

▼

STORY TELLER 8-2

Winning Appeals

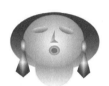

Karin was pregnant. She injured her low back at work and was coming to Lakeside Massage Clinic for manual therapy treatments to ease the pain and muscle spasms in her low back and supporting musculature. Because of the baby, it was difficult to treat the muscles of her anterior lumbar spine and hip flexors. I used foot reflexology to address the structures I could not treat directly with safety. The insurance company paid only for 68% of the amount billed, refusing to pay for foot massage, which they considered palliative. I filed an appeal, did my research, and wrote a letter explaining the patient's condition and the need for indirect treatment in response to the patient's overriding safety concerns. I also defended my decision to treat the opposing flexors as well as the extensors that were directly injured, and provided documentation of the effectiveness of reflexology techniques. I was paid the remaining 32% within 2 weeks of submitting the appeal.

Insurance companies have internal quotas regarding claims denials. It is common knowledge that employees are instructed to deny a minimum percentage of claims to ensure reserve funds for the company and discourage ongoing treatment. Many hope the patient or the practitioner will give up on seeking reimbursement. As a result, it is inevitable that you will be face-to-face with a reimbursement challenge. The best thing to do is stay on top of unpaid claims and limit the financial risk to your patient and yourself. When you find yourself faced with a denied claim for necessary treatment after the service has already been provided, follow these guidelines:

◆ Identify the cause for the denial.
◆ Submit a written request, outlining your objection to the denial.
◆ Write a detailed request for reconsideration, including the patient's situation and the benefits of the treatment provided or proposed.
◆ Cite references from the insurance carrier's policy manual to support your case.
◆ Cite state law if applicable, as in disputes over scope of practice.
◆ Request support from the HCP who referred the patient for treatment. Enclose any supportive statements or reports.
◆ Cite research on the efficacy of the treatment provided or proposed.
◆ Provide photocopies of articles and other documents that will help the claims investigation.
◆ Cite references from the patient's SOAP charts and progress reports to demonstrate the treatment planning and the progress resulting from the treatments provided, if applicable.

Select your appeals wisely. Insurance billing often involves an ethical dilemma: when is it the insurance company's responsibility to pay for treatment and when is care the patient's responsibility? When have we finished treating the condition and begun providing palliative or preventative care?

Once you have identified worthy cases, arm yourself with facts, knowledge, and a desire to educate. Take a positive approach; assume the review board has the patient's best interest in mind and simply did not have the information necessary to come to the appropriate conclusion. Provide the board with more information than necessary to reverse the decision. Be honest and thorough, and communicate respectfully.

SUMMARY

Insurance billing has it benefits and its risks. Limit the risks by familiarizing yourself with the various types of insurance, following the billing strategies presented, and educating yourself on common billing practices specific to your state and profession. Reap the benefits of an increased patient load, a variety of patients offering accelerated learning opportunities, and the satisfaction of influencing the health care community.

Three types of insurance commonly reimburse for manual therapy:

◆ Personal injury insurance
◆ Workers' compensation
◆ Private health insurance

Each plan has its own billing protocols and reimbursement methods, but use a standard billing form and universal procedure codes and diagnostic codes. All plans require alert claims management and tenacious follow-through to ensure payment. Follow these strategies for successful insurance reimbursement:

◆ Provide accurate and complete patient documentation and insurance information.
◆ Stay within designated time limits when providing treatment, billing for services, and appealing claims denials.
◆ Be prepared to prove medical necessity by obtaining prescriptions for services, documenting patient progress, and providing effective treatment.
◆ File attorney liens or medical liens on all personal injury cases.
◆ Maintain accurate payment logs.
◆ Communicate with insurance representatives professionally, respectfully, and cooperatively.

REFERENCES

1. Hands On, The Newsletter of the American Massage Therapy Association, vol. XVI. #4, July/August 2000.
2. Owens C. Managed Care Organizations, Practical Implications for Medical Practices and Other Providers. Los Angeles: PMIC, 1996.
3. Dolan DW. Insurance Reimbursement & Specialty Physician Referrals. Jacksonville: American Health Press, 1998.
4. Foreman SM, Croft AC. Whiplash Injuries The Cervical Acceleration/Deceleration Syndrome. 2nd ed. Baltimore: Williams & Wilkins, 1995.

200

HANDS HEAL:
COMMUNICATION,
DOCUMENTATION,
AND INSURANCE BILLING
FOR MANUAL THERAPISTS

5. Grigsby B, Rosen S. Some Contracts are Not Worth Signing, The Journal A Publication of the American Massage Therapy Association–Washington Chapter, Vol. 16 #1, January 2000.

6. Adler◆Giersch Seminars, Whiplash, Spinal Trauma, and the Chiropractic Personal Injury Case, Adler◆Giersch PS, Seattle, 2000.

7. Alternáre Health Network Seminar, Seattle, 1997.

8. WAC 284-43-321: Provider Contracts—Terms and Conditions of Payment.

CHAPTER 9

Ethics

*A*fter just six additional sessions, Sandee is able to garden, play with her grandson, and clean her house. She even took up bike riding this summer! She has enjoyed all this activity without acute flare-ups of her chronic low back pain. She stretches daily, adding warm-up and cool-down exercises with more strenuous activities, and she stops and rests when her body becomes stiff or achy. She has learned that if she doesn't exercise and rest, the ensuing pain and stiffness will limit her activities for several days.

If you remember from Chapter 4, Sandee had nearly given up on her massage therapist, Holly. After reviewing her SOAP charts, Sandee decided to recommit to Holly's treatment plan—with alterations. Together, they set and accomplished goals and reviewed clinical and functional progress frequently. Sandee's awareness of her body's needs increased, and she learned to identify effective self-care exercises in response to those needs. Sandee's healing curve rose dramatically with her renewed commitment and enhanced communication skills.

Now Sandee is faced with another dilemma. Her insurance company has notified Holly that Sandee has reached maximum benefit and coverage is no longer available. Sandee feels that care is being terminated prematurely. She is not yet pain free and without ongoing care, she and Holly both fear that the symptoms could return.

Sandee's insurance policy defines reasonable and necessary care as care provided to correct the presenting condition, bringing it to maximum improvement. The policy clearly states that maintenance or wellness care is not a covered benefit and is the financial responsibility of the patient. Holly knows that Sandee may never be completely pain free, and she feels that Sandee *is* managing her chronic pain successfully. Should Holly support Sandee in fighting for coverage until she is pain free, or support the insurance company in the decision to discontinue coverage?

Faced with an ethical dilemma, Holly reaches out to her peers for support. She invites three fellow manual therapists over for dessert. All share a passion for chocolate and experience with various insurance companies. Holly explains her patient's situation (respecting patient confidentiality by not mentioning Sandee's name), and the four friends share experiences and opinions. They imagine an ideal world where the patient's health always takes precedence over profits, and they discuss what actions best serve the patient's long-term health in the real world.

In the end, they all agree on one thing. This patient *is* successfully managing her chronic pain, a condition that has plagued her for many years. At this point, it is more important to celebrate the success of the treatments and instill confidence in the patient's ability to manage her health than to prove to the insurance company that she still suffers from chronic pain.

Holly's friends also agree that now is not the time to withdraw all support. Old habits are easy to fall into. Sandee may not be able to afford ongoing care weekly nor does she need that level of care anymore, but monthly treatments for 3 months will maintain progress and monitor any potential flare-ups. It is important for Sandee to realize that preventative care is available and affordable. After 3 months of monthly treatments, Sandee could choose to continue treatments with Holly on a monthly or quarterly basis to maintain her progress or to schedule appointments as needed.

As a result of their discussion, Holly and her friends recognize that they typically treat patients until the prescription runs out or until the insurance benefit is depleted. Preventative health care is the sensible approach; but is it ethical to provide maintenance care when the insurance company clearly states that prevention and maintenance are not covered? Is it ethical to continue care just because the prescription has not been fulfilled or the benefit has not been exhausted? Together they agree to consider the question, "When is treatment finished?" They want to celebrate when patients accomplish their goals ahead of schedule, and educate their patients on the importance of prioritizing regular preventative care in their budgets and on their schedules.

Introduction

Webster's defines ethics as the study of standards of conduct and moral judgment. Ethics comes from the Greek word *ethos*, which means the characteristic and distinguishing attitudes, habits, and beliefs of an individual or a group. By definition, manual therapists are students of right and wrong, striving to be moral and just and to respect and uphold the standards of the profession.

With few written guidelines and a great desire to be of service, we learn how to conduct ourselves professionally by taking risks. Life is our classroom; our pursuit of excellence provides the lessons. Obstacles that challenge our sense of fairness and test our integrity serve to develop our beliefs and shape our character.

As students, we learn by engaging in debates with our peers, questioning our teachers, and consulting our mentors. Through these activities, our visceral and intellectual understanding of right and wrong expands; and our ability to speak honestly, act without fear and greed, and express compassion without prejudice matures. Eventually, we become role models to others, and our learning expands through interactions with those who seek guidance from us.

As health care providers, we care deeply for our patients and strive to nurture and heal their bodies and souls. In our efforts to be successful, we are influenced by fears, needs, desires, and spiritual longings. Ethical dilemmas are unavoidable. It is critical that we take steps to encourage personal and professional growth and protect those we intend to serve by setting standards for our business practices, evaluating them regularly, and discussing ethical beliefs with others. For example:

- Define your ethical standards. Write them down. If your professional organization has a Code of Ethics, frame it and hang it in your office. Read it often.
- Create office policies, distribute them to your patients, and stick to them.
- Join a supervision group. If you cannot find one, form your own.
- Evaluate your business practices and professional relationships monthly.
- Invite others to review your business practices annually.
- Establish a relationship with a mentor.
- Mentor others.

This chapter first presents several current ethical dilemmas for manual therapists, in the areas of documentation and insurance billing, treatment practices, and relationships with other health care professionals. It then recommends steps for building and maintaining an ethical practice: a sample code of ethics, a self-evaluation tool for reviewing your business practices and relationships, and an outline for organizing and participating in supervision groups and mentoring. Be a role model for your peers, patients, and to other health care providers.

Ethical issues involving emotional and physical relationships between the practitioner and the patient, such as dual relationships and patient confidentiality, are not discussed in this chapter because of the scope of this subject matter. Many books are dedicated to such

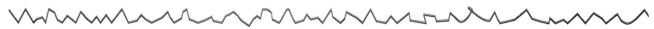

1. Benjamin BE, Sohnen-Moe C. The Ethics of Touch. Tucson, AZ: SMA Inc, 2001.
2. McIntosh N. The Educated Heart: Professional Guidelines for Massage Therapists, Bodyworkers, and Movement Teachers. Memphis, TN: Decatur Bainbridge Press, 1999.
3. Taylor K. The Ethics of Caring: Honoring the Web of Life in our Professional Healing Relationships. 2nd ed. Santa Cruz, CA: Hanford Mead Publishers, 1995.

Figure 9-1. Books on ethics.

topics. A resource list of books on ethical issues in the practitioner-patient relationships is provided. (See Figure 9-1)

Current Ethical Dilemmas: Billing and Documentation Practices

RESPONSIBILITY FOR PAYMENT

The opening story poses an interesting dilemma: when is treatment finished and when does maintenance or wellness care begin? There is a fine line between the two, especially if the condition is chronic. If we can identify guidelines for delineating treatment verses wellness care, we can ethically apply those standards to the insurance issue: who is responsible for paying for care?

The insurance issue is often clouded by our beliefs and experiences, for example, that too often insurance policies or case managers limit access to manual therapy and prevent patients from receiving the number of treatments necessary to recover from their injuries. Therefore, in the seemingly few situations in which authorized treatment exceeds the number of sessions necessary for healing, we often feel we are justified in continuing to provide care. Certainly, the patients are willing to continue: manual therapy feels good and is effective. And it makes sense to continue; after all, an ounce of prevention is worth a pound of cure!

According to standard insurance definitions, treatment is warranted until the condition is corrected or maximum improvement is made. These definitions also state that treatment must provide the patient with appropriate instruction for follow-up, self-care, and prevention of future occurrences. All maintenance and wellness care are the financial responsibility of the patient unless otherwise specified by the insurance plan. Given those parameters, how do we determine when treatment ends and maintenance care begins?

Sometimes it is obvious when the patient has reached maximum healing: the patient is pain free and fully functional. Other times, as with chronic pain, things are not so clear. In such cases, wellness is determined by the patient's ability to manage pain and successfully modify activities. The focus is not on living pain free, but on quality of life: the patient's ability to participate in everyday activities. Use these guidelines to determine when treatments are no longer necessary for resolving the patient's condition:

- The patient is able to function normally, or functional progress has plateaued.
- The patient has no significant symptomology, or clinical progress has plateaued.
- The patient demonstrates self-awareness by identifying situations (activities, emotions, etc.) that exacerbate his condition.

◆ The patient applies self-care techniques to limit exacerbations and to remedy exacerbations when they do occur.

Test your findings by discontinuing care for a predetermined length of time. For example, if after 4 weeks without treatment, Darnel is sufficiently symptom-free and active, care can be reduced to a monthly or maintenance level of care. If Darnel experiences an exacerbation or acceleration of the condition, in spite of performing his self-care routines, ongoing treatment is warranted.

Most patients who reach maximum improvement for their conditions would benefit from wellness care. Encourage the patient to return monthly for wellness care for 3 months after terminating treatment. During that time, provide care as needed, and fine-tune the patient's self-care instructions. If his health deteriorates without regular care, you have a case to reinstate insurance coverage. If he is able to administer appropriate self-care and maintain his health status, celebrate his accomplishments and invite him to continue monthly or quarterly wellness sessions, or refer him to someone who specializes in wellness care.

PREFERRED PROVIDER STATUS

Insurance carriers contract with health care providers in an attempt to limit who provides health care services and how much they reimburse for those services. The carriers either contract with providers directly, or purchase provider contracts through an **insurance network**. The insurance carrier then provides incentives to insureds who seek health care services from preferred providers such as reduced co-pays or waived deductibles.

Insurance networks and insurance carriers can only support a limited number of providers. Set numbers of providers are credentialed for a given area based on the number of insureds or lives that reside in that area. As the number of covered lives changes in a given area, the network or panel may open to new providers until the ratio of lives to providers is considered adequate.

Only the credentialed manual therapists are permitted to bill under the preferred provider contract. It is unethical and often illegal for non-credentialed practitioners to bill for services under the license of the credentialed provider.

▼

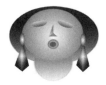

STORY TELLER 9-1

One Preferred Provider in a Clinic of Many

Rosie owns a manual therapy clinic in a bustling urban setting. It's a trendy neighborhood with a reputation for being health-conscious. There is a well-worn walking trail, several juice bars and cafes, a health club, day spas, and wellness centers. Rosie is an excellent practitioner and her services are in high demand. She has added a dozen other manual therapists to her staff over the years to meet the demand. She and her staff receive referrals from the various health care providers in the area, as well as walk-in traffic.

A large insurance network provides manual therapy contracts to most insurance carriers in the area. Rosie was able to get on the preferred provider list several years ago. Because the neighborhood is densely populated with manual therapists, it has become difficult to get new providers credentialed. Rosie is the only practitioner in her clinic with preferred provider status. As a result, she has had to refer her steady cash-paying patients to her staff so that she can accommodate the large number of insurance patients referred to the clinic.

206

HANDS HEAL:
COMMUNICATION,
DOCUMENTATION,
AND INSURANCE BILLING
FOR MANUAL THERAPISTS

Rosie and her regular patients are upset at the turn of events. Rosie wants to be able to see her cash-paying patients, and her regulars miss her care. She decides to have her staff treat the insurance patients and she signs the charts and bills under her name. They are her employees, after all; this must be permissible. She promises to check it out with the insurance network, but never gets around to it.

During a random audit, the insurance company uncovers Rosie's fraudulent billing practices. Her provider status is revoked and her staff is barred from contracting with the company as preferred providers. The company filed a complaint with the state regulatory body requesting disciplinary action against all practitioners involved.

FEE SCHEDULES

Ethical billing practices include charging reasonable and consistent fees for services provided. It is tempting to charge higher fees to insurance companies, because of the time and paperwork required for billing. However, it is unethical and in some cases illegal to charge insurance companies higher rates than patients who do not have insurance coverage for your services. This is commonly referred to as payer discrimination.

Every patient should be charged the same rate for the same service, regardless of who is paying for the service. However, it is more costly to delay payment and bill for services than to accept payment at the time of service. The issue is whether or not you must provide billing services for the patient, not who is being billed. The billing service costs the same whether you send the bills to the patient or to the insurance company. Therefore, it makes sense to offer a cash discount to all patients who pay at the time services are rendered, and to penalize all patients who opt for delaying, regardless of who is responsible for payment. The ethical solution is to offer a modest cash discount as an incentive to patients to pay at the time of service.

What is an ethical discount for payment at the time of service? 5%, 10%, or even 50%? Excessive cash discounts are also considered discriminatory and may provoke an audit by the insurance company. Therefore, it is important to be able to justify the discount by comparing it with the actual expense of billing. Billing agencies generally charge between 7% and 15% of the amount collected. An office providing the service in-house can usually perform the service for less than an outside agency would charge. A discount for payment at the time of service that does not exceed the expense of billing is an ethical discount.

Unethical billing practices also arise when services are chosen because they cost more than other equally appropriate services, or when a practitioner bills for services that pay higher rates than the services actually performed. This course of action is tempting when insurance fee schedules delineate different fees for different manual techniques, as though one technique is better than another. For example, Health R Us published a fee schedule that pays $12 per unit for therapeutic massage, $15 per unit for manual therapy, and $18 per unit for energetic therapeutic touch. It is unethical to bill for four units of energetic therapeutic touch if other techniques were also performed. It is also unethical to use only energetic techniques if other techniques would be equally or more effective.

The key to an ethical fee schedule is in its application. Be consistent and do not discriminate.

- Apply the same fee for the same service to everyone, regardless of the type of payer.
- Provide the service that is most appropriate to the patient, regardless of the reimbursement rate for the service.

TIMELY DOCUMENTATION

Unethical charting practices occur when weeks, months, or years later the chart is filled in because of a request for charts or because payment has been denied and rebilling requires copies of all treatment notes. Charting should be done in a timely fashion. It is difficult to remember a particular session after several other sessions have blurred the details. The best time to chart is during or immediately after the session. Everyone has days, however, when the charts pile up and we don't get to them until the next morning. It is stressful but possible to recreate the session 24 hours later. However, few of us can record a session accurately weeks, months, or years later.

▼

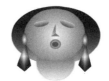

STORY TELLER 9-2

Carbon-Dating?!

An attorney told a story at a billing seminar of a chiropractor whose notes were carbon-dated—a test that establishes the time frame of the record. His patient had been injured in a car accident and the attorney for the at-fault-party suspected tampering with the treatment notes, and therefore ordered the tests. Test results showed that the health care provider had filled in the chart notes 2–3 years after the treatments were provided. The patient's case was adversely affected.

Current Ethical Dilemmas: Treatment Practices
TREATMENT EXPECTATIONS

At times, patients form expectations of us based on hearsay. Patients' healing time and abilities vary in many ways: condition, past history, genetics, emotional complications, daily physical demands, etc. We may or may not be able to live up to the stories our patients have been told by their friends and family. It is critical to represent our abilities honestly and refrain from committing to specific results or time limits for healing.

▼

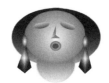

STORY TELLER 9-3

Promises, Promises

Annie experienced what anyone would call a miraculous recovery. She had a long history of head and neck trauma, and after a summer of painting the exterior of her house and working long hours at the computer, she ruptured a disc in her neck. The pain was so intense that she could not lift her head high enough to gaze across the horizon, nor could she hold her head up long enough to eat at the dinner table. The numbness and weakness in her right arm was so great that she could not butter her toast or brush her teeth.

Annie's doctor scheduled an MRI. In the meantime, Annie began seeing her Feldenkrais practitioner, John. The first few visits were house calls, because riding in a car was excruciating for Annie: she had to hold her head in her hands and apply traction so the bumps in the road didn't cause more pain than necessary. By the time the results of the MRI came back and the neurosurgeon met with Annie to discuss treat-

208

HANDS HEAL:
COMMUNICATION,
DOCUMENTATION,
AND INSURANCE BILLING
FOR MANUAL THERAPISTS

ment options, she was pain free, driving to her own appointments, and working part-time. One month from the date of injury, she was working full time and had full mobility in her neck.

John's phone started ringing off the hook. Annie worked in health care and her peers, amazed by Annie's progress, began referring their patients, friends, and family members to John. But not everyone responded to John's care as Annie had, and several were disappointed when they were not symptom-free in 2 weeks.

Annie took care of herself in more ways than John knew or than she told her peers at the clinic. She took naps after every session, limited her activities, and also received acupuncture, Tui Na, Polarity, and lymph drainage. She even had a healing session with a Tibetan Llama. She began her treatment immediately and aggressively after her injury, getting daily care for the first week, and three times a week for the following 3 weeks. She had the resources and knowledge to seek treatment that was effective for her, whether or not it was prescribed by her doctor or covered by her insurance. Annie was willing to do whatever it took to get well, she acted quickly, and she never lost sight of her belief that she could heal instantaneously.

John is a brilliant practitioner. He served all patients equally, to the best of his abilities, given each patient's unique situation. The only thing lacking in his sessions was the conversation about each person's unique healing cycle. Although he made no promises about the results of his treatments, he neglected to address the patient's expectations. He, too, was carried away by his success with Annie. This experience not only increased his skills for working with disc injuries, but also reminded him of the need to communicate clearly with his patients: to hear their expectations and cautiously discuss possible outcomes based on individual circumstances.

Many factors influence healing. As health care providers, we can only try to find the right combination of modalities, communication techniques, and referrals for each patient. Don't take it upon yourself to meet the expectations of everyone who comes to you for help. Instead, talk with each one, find out what her expectations are, tell her what you can honestly predict (which is often nothing more than possibilities), and ask for her help in discovering the best treatment plan for her.

Educate yourself on the state regulations for your profession. Know what claims are legal for your scope. For example, in New York, claims regarding the benefits of massage therapy must be qualified by saying massage therapy "may" reduce inflammation, or "may" improve range of motion. The only concrete claim permissible is that massage therapy increases circulation.

SCOPE OF PRACTICE

Manual therapy encompasses many professions and techniques. Much cross-training occurs, often without knowledge of the licensing laws for each profession in each state. A workshop on a manual technique may be taught by an osteopath, with chiropractors, nurses, physical therapists, dentists, and massage therapists as students. Remember that you may be taught techniques that are outside your scope of practice. Receiving training in a technique does not automatically license you to perform it in your practice.

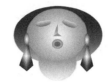
Leisha is a massage therapist in Oregon. To escape the cold winter rains, she travels to Hawaii every January for LomiLomi training in the home of an elder Lomi master. Leisha lives there for 4 weeks each year, and adheres to a rigorous schedule of fasting, taking cleansing herbs, and giving and receiving treatments. She learns to harvest the herbs, make cleansing tonics, perform thrust adjustments on the extremities, and apply vigorous manual techniques to increase the circulation. After 4 years of training, she receives the blessing of the elder to provide this healing ritual to others.

Leisha is confident of her skills but knows that Oregon law does not permit her to perform joint manipulations with a thrusting force. Several months go by without temptation. Then one day Leisha treats a 40-year-old woman with knarled, stiff, and painful toes. Leisha knows that the joint manipulations she learned in her Lomi training would benefit this woman, who is prematurely losing mobility in her toes and feet. What should she do?

If the laws that dictate your profession's scope of practice do not adequately represent the skill and training of those licensed, work to update the laws. Until the laws change, resist the temptation to provide services outside your scope. Create a list of practitioners who can provide those services, and refer out when necessary.

Current Ethical Dilemmas: The Health Care Team
COMMUNICATING WITH REFERRING HEALTH CARE PROVIDERS

As health care is currently structured, a physician or doctor, and possibly a naturopath or chiropractor (depending on the insurance policy and the State regulations), is considered a primary health care provider (HCP). It is the primary HCP's responsibility to diagnose the patient's problem, orchestrate treatment, and refer to adjunctive therapists.

If you are working under the referring HCP's direction but not under his supervision, good communication becomes essential. Provide the referring HCP with clear, complete information so that he can give the patient the best possible treatment.

Occasionally, you may find yourself disagreeing with the referring HCP about a patient's condition or treatment. Do not express this disagreement to the patient. Instead, state your views to the referring HCP—calmly, professionally, tactfully, with all the supporting evidence you can provide. If your input is not considered or if you find that you can't endorse the prescribed treatment, your best choice may be to withdraw from the case. However you choose to handle the situation, remember that the referring HCP is the final authority and that it is unethical for the manual therapist to undermine the relationship between the referring HCP and the patient. If the patient approaches you with complaints about the referring HCP's approach to the treatment plan, support the patient in addressing the issues directly with the referring HCP.

PERMISSION TO CONSULT WITH THE HEALTH CARE TEAM

On the Health Information form is a request for permission to exchange information with the other members of the patient's health care team. In many states, practitioners do not

210

HANDS HEAL:
COMMUNICATION,
DOCUMENTATION,
AND INSURANCE BILLING
FOR MANUAL THERAPISTS

need the patient's consent to speak with referring providers. Regardless, it is a good idea to inform the patient that and with whom information will be shared.

When providing information to other practitioners, respect the patient's confidentiality and limit those conversations to information pertinent to the patient's condition. Omit your personal opinions about the patient and any gossip or details that have no bearing on the case. Refrain from discussing patient cases in public, where others who are not bound by confidentiality can overhear sensitive information.

PAYMENT FOR REFERRALS

As health care providers, we are responsible for serving the patient to the best of our abilities. Accepting payment for referrals can cloud that ability and compromise our ethics. In all cases, this creates a conflict of interest. In many cases it is illegal.

The practice of accepting payment for referrals, or referring to clinics or laboratories in which the provider has a financial interest, is known as **rebating**. Severe penalties can be placed on practitioners who violate laws of this nature.

It is appropriate to refer within a health system network or preferred provider list. It is not appropriate if the referral is based on the prospect of financial gain.

▼

STORY TELLER 9-5

Who is Best for the Patient?

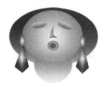

Helena's office is centrally located in town. As a result, several HCPs from around the area refer patients to her. One chiropractor on the north end has expanded his office and needs more patients to meet his expenses. He offers Helena $25 for every patient she refers to him. Typically, Helena provides a list of chiropractors to patients in need of chiropractic services, and highlighted those who are located conveniently for the patient and who specialize in the area of need. After the chiropractor's offer, Helena begins passing out his card to every patient, regardless of which end of town she lives and works in, or what her special needs for care are.

Steps Toward an Ethical Practice
CODE OF ETHICS

Hang your Code of Ethics in your office. This code should be one you strive to abide by, one that reflects your beliefs and professional behavior. Many professional organizations have a Code of Ethics and a disciplinary body to enforce the code. Displaying your ethical standards instills in your patients confidence that the practitioner who cares for them observes a high standard of behavior and is accountable for his actions.

▼

WISE ONE SPEAKS 9-1

Code of Ethics

The following is the Code of Ethics for the American Massage Therapy Association (Reprinted with permission, American Massage Therapy Association, Evanston, 2000, all rights reserved).

This Code of Ethics is a summary statement of the standards by which massage therapists agree to conduct their practice and is a declaration of the general principles of acceptable, ethical, professional behavior.

• Demonstrate commitment to provide the highest quality massage therapy/bodywork to those who seek professional service.

- Acknowledge the inherent worth and individuality of each person by not discriminating or behaving in any prejudicial manner with patients and/or colleagues.
- Demonstrate professional excellence through regular self-assessment of strengths, limitation, and effectiveness by continued education and training.
- Acknowledge the confidential nature of the professional relationship with patients and respect each patient's right to privacy.
- Conduct all business and professional activities within their scope of practice, the law of the land, and project a professional image.
- Accept responsibility to do no harm to the physical, mental, and emotional well-being of the self, patients, and associates.
- Refrain from engaging in any sexual conduct or sexual activities involving their patients.

SELF-EVALUATIONS AND PEER EVALUATIONS

Take time to review your business practices and professional relationships. Regular self-evaluations help identify and resolve difficult situations before they become problems.

When you open a new business, establish office policies and a fee schedule, list your services and office hours, and provide copies to all patients. Setting clear boundaries and business parameters helps you treat all patients fairly and equally, and provides a comfortable working environment for you and your patients. Review those business guidelines monthly and keep them up to date. Patients become confused and frustrated when we distribute policies that no longer apply or are no longer enforced.

As part of your monthly self-evaluation, take 10 minutes to consider the following questions. If your answer highlights a problem situation or call to action, describe the specific situation in writing. Clarify your role in the situation honestly and compassionately. Seek counsel from your peers, if necessary. Identify possible actions and consider the consequences. Determine the timeline for the appropriate action, and follow through.[2]

- Did I conduct myself ethically and legally in all my professional affairs?
- Did I maintain the confidentiality of my patients?
- Did I maintain good boundaries with my patients?
- Was I uncomfortable enforcing any office policies?
- What are my strengths and limitations? What action can I take to improve?
- What steps have I taken to ensure my well-being?
- Are there any issues I should seek counsel on from my peers?

Annually, review your fee schedule, office policies, and business practices with a peer or a mentor. Review your billing and accounting practices with a professional. Implement changes when appropriate.

CONSULTATION GROUPS

Consultation groups, also known as peer supervision or co-vision groups, consist of people with a common interest who meet regularly to share ideas, solve problems, and build a community. The common interest can be as broad as manual therapy or as specific as therapists with AIDS patients.

212

HANDS HEAL:
COMMUNICATION,
DOCUMENTATION,
AND INSURANCE BILLING
FOR MANUAL THERAPISTS

Individuals join consultation groups to get support and information, form professional relationships, and gain skills. Not only do the people who participate in the consultation groups benefit from the results, but so do their patients, the community, and the profession.

Ethics are difficult to learn out of a book. They must be experienced, experimented with, discussed, and hotly debated. By participating in consultation groups, we can study ethical dilemmas from a variety of perspectives and differing levels of experience, sorting out the possible consequences before our patients can be harmed by our actions. The group members hold each other accountable for telling the truth, have compassion and respect for all involved, and offer advice about confusing issues.[2]

Follow these guidelines for establishing a consultation group in your area:

◆ Define goals for establishing a group.
◆ Identify parameters: how many people, how often will you meet, how long will the meetings last, etc.
◆ Create a list of individuals who have similar goals or needs for a group
◆ Check the list for individuals you respect, from whom you can learn. It is important to include people who offer diversity to the group, as well as those who share similar opinions.
◆ Select a date for the first meeting. Explain your vision for the group with those on your list and invite them to join you. If you are lacking in numbers, ask those who are interested in being a part of the group to invite others who may also share the same vision.
◆ Get names and phone numbers of those interested, call back to confirm dates and times, and ask for assistance if necessary.

At the first meeting:

◆ Confirm the dates, locations, and times of the meetings. If it is important to the cohesiveness of the group, get a commitment from everyone to attend four consecutive meetings.
◆ Clarify the goals of the group.
◆ Identify the topics of the first few meetings.
◆ Find out whether a mediator, provocateur, or educator is desired for any of the meetings.
◆ Decide whether you want to rotate responsibilities: host, snacks, facilitator, timekeeper, etc.
◆ Identify guidelines for group interaction, (such as maintaining each other's confidentiality, communicating with respect, speaking honestly), or identify guiding principles that suggest ethical behavior without mandating specific rules. For example, Margaret Wheatly offers guiding principles in her book, *Leadership and the New Science*: take care of yourself, take care of each other, and take care of this place.[3] Kylea Taylor, in *The Ethics of Caring* defines ethical behavior as reverence for life demonstrated by right relationship and offers Buddha's concepts for right relationship: what I do affects you, what you do affects me, and what I do to you ultimately affects me.[4]
◆ At the end of the meeting, evaluate the outcome. Did you meet your goals? Did you have fun? Make adjustments if necessary to ensure the success of future meetings.

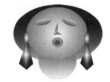

Barb works for a natural foods grocery chain that provides seated massage to customers. There are five stores in her town; each store employs 4–5 manual therapists. Barb discovers that providing massage in front of the check-out lines in a grocery store presents problems that she never had to deal with in her private practice, such as maintaining confidentiality. She can tell her co-workers are also struggling with the same issues but knows it is not appropriate to discuss them at work. She decides to call the practitioners from the stores and try to stir up interest in meeting together and helping each other out with the problems inherent in the work environment.

Barb finds 10 people interested in meeting. She secures a meeting room at the community center and invites one of her teachers from massage school to facilitate the group discussion. She asks a few people to bring snacks and drinks, and someone else to make confirmation calls.

Eight of the 23 massage employees attend the meeting. Barb welcomes everyone and introduces the facilitator. The facilitator leads the group in defining the goals for the meeting and identifying topics for discussion. She suggests some guidelines and creates a safe environment for discussion. The group agrees to communicate respectfully and to use a round robin format to ensure that everyone has the opportunity to speak. The facilitator explains her purpose at the meeting as one to provide organization and keep the discussion moving in a positive direction, not one of offering her opinion. She begins with a story.

MENTORING

One-on-one consultation lacks the diverse perspectives available in consultation groups, but allows for more spontaneous interactions, more personal attention, and a safe environment for those who find it difficult to speak openly in groups.

Mentors influence and shape us by sharing who they are, not just what they know. The study of ethics is about learning how to live and grow and contribute as a human, as well as a professional. Select a mentor who is human, someone who is not afraid of sharing his mistakes as well as his successes, personally and professionally. A role model is not a perfect human being, but someone who is very much like yourself. Marsha Sinetar, in *The Mentor's Spirit* says, "Show me your mentor and I'll show you yourself."[5]

Select a mentor who:

◆ Is available weekly by phone
◆ Is available monthly in person
◆ Has more professional experience than you
◆ Is committed to your growth
◆ Has qualities important to you, such as, compassion, wisdom, ability to confront

SUMMARY

Create an ethical business. Review and revise your business practices regularly. For example:

◆ Set standards for identifying when treatment is complete and wellness care begins, and bill appropriately.

214

HANDS HEAL:
COMMUNICATION,
DOCUMENTATION,
AND INSURANCE BILLING
FOR MANUAL THERAPISTS

◆ Charge reasonable and consistent fees for services.

◆ Provide appropriate treatment and bill for the services provided.

◆ In your charts, do not misrepresent the patient's health or the treatment performed.

◆ Chart patient sessions in a timely fashion.

◆ Represent your services accurately. Discuss treatment outcomes honestly and realistically.

◆ Provide services within your scope of practice. Refer out for services that are outside your scope.

◆ Discuss disagreements about the treatment plan or patient care directly with the referring HCP, never with the patient.

◆ Support the patient in addressing conflicts with other providers directly.

◆ Request permission from the patient to discuss the case with other members of the health care team.

◆ Limit all conversations with the health care team to information pertinent to the patient's condition.

◆ Be an active student of ethics.

◆ Develop your ethical beliefs through discussion with peers and mentors.

◆ Consult your peers and mentors when problems arise in your professional relationships.

◆ Mentor others.

WISE ONE SPEAKS 9-2

Discover What Lies Within

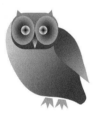

I leave you with the following as an inspiration to be in relationship:

It is during interactions with others that we discover what lies within us. That is the gift of our profession—the gift we offer our patients through our listening and the gift we give ourselves through mentoring.

"We usually look outside ourselves for heroes and teachers. It has not occurred to most people that they may already be the role model they seek. The wholeness they are looking for may be trapped within themselves by beliefs, attitudes, and self-doubt. But our wholeness exists in us now. Trapped though it may be, it can be called upon for guidance, direction, and most fundamentally, comfort. It can be remembered. Eventually we may come to live by it."[6]

REFERENCES

1. Code of Ethics, American Massage Therapy Association, Evanston, 2000.
2. Sohnen-Moe C. Business Mastery: A Guide for Creating a Fulfilling and Thriving Business and Keeping it Successful. 3rd Ed. Tucson: Sohnen-Moe Associates, Inc., 1997.
3. Wheatley M. Leadership and the New Science: Learning about Organization from an Orderly Universe. San Francisco: Berrett-Koehler Publishers, Inc., 1994.
4. Taylor K. The Ethics of Caring: Honoring the Web of Life in Our Professional Healing Relationships. 2nd Ed. Santa Cruz: Hanford Mead Publishers, 1995.
5. Sinetar M. The Mentor's Spirit: Life Lessons on Leadership and the Art of Encouragement. Boulder: Sounds True, 1997.
6. Remen RN. Kitchen Table Wisdom: Stories That Heal. New York: Riverhead Books, 1996.

Appendices

Glossary

active listening: communication tools that demonstrate to the speaker that he/she are being understood and respected. Attending to the speakers' tone, body language, facial expressions, etc.

affinity plan/network: contractual agreement between the provider and the network or carrier to provide a substantial discount directly to the members of the plan.

appeal: request by a party for a higher court or reviewing body to review a lower court's or reviewing body's decision regarding issues of law or policy.

at-fault-party, tort-feasor: person who causes harm to an individual or damages property.

Attorney Lien, Guarantee of Payment: written agreement between a patient and health care provider guaranteeing payment in full to the patient's health care providers upon settlement of a personal injury case. Often, when the patient has an attorney, counsel co-endorses the written agreement.

body language: behavior of a person: facial expressions, postures, gestures, and other actions; a primary system for expressing emotions.

bundling, global fee: type of reimbursement arrangement that combines two or more health care procedures into one procedure code. A flat fee is established to pay for all health care services performed under the single code.

capitation: per-member monthly payment made in advance to a managed care insurer covering contracted services. The insurance provider agrees to provide specified services to eligible members of a plan for this fixed, predetermined payment for a specified length of time, regardless of how many times the member uses the services.

capped fee: predetermined discounted fee allowed for a particular procedure.

clean claims: bills submitted with complete and accurate information, for covered services that the patient is eligible for, and the practitioner is authorized to provide.

co-insurance: provision that the insured and the carrier share losses in agreed proportion. Also known as "percentage participation." In managed care, it refers to the portion of the cost of care for which the individual is responsible, usually determined by a fixed percentage. This often applies after a deductible is met.

co-pay: patient's share of a health care bill, usually a small amount per office visit.

complementary and alternative medicine (CAM): medical/clinical services provided by practitioners not normally taught by conventional medical institutions. Also includes providers whose services are not usually paid by traditional insurance programs.

217

218

HANDS HEAL:
COMMUNICATION,
DOCUMENTATION,
AND INSURANCE BILLING
FOR MANUAL THERAPISTS

complimenting: communication tool used to reinforce behavior. A positive reaction or evaluation by the practitioner in response to the patient, or a question that indirectly implies something positive about the patient.

conversion factors: number of units developed by individual payers (attenuated by market factors, inflation, available resources, geographic variations, etc.) to convert the RVU into a dollar amount for reimbursement purposes.

Current Procedural Terminology (CPT) codes: listing of descriptive terms and identifying codes for reporting health care services and procedures performed by health care providers. The purpose of the terminology is to provide a uniform language that will accurately describe health care services and will thereby provide an effective means for reliable nationwide communication among providers, patients, and third parties. Published by the American Medical Association.

deductible: part of the insured's expenses or loss that must be paid before insurance coverage begins.

deposition: form of discovery whereby the attorney calling for the deposition has the right to ask questions and obtain answers from a party, witness, or expert while that individual is under oath.

disability percentage: overall rating of a physical handicap as determined by scoring the Oswestry or Vernon-Mior Pain and Disability Index.

discharge notes: final summary of the patient's progress, health status, and any subsequent course of action. (SOAP format)

discounted fee: reimbursement arrangement where an insurance carrier contracts with a provider for health care services at a predetermined discounted fee.

door-openers: communication tool used as an invitation to talk. Open-ended questions.

end-of-settlement: personal injury case where the provider must wait until the claim against the at-fault party settles or a judge or jury issues a verdict before receiving payment for services.

Explanation of Benefits (EOB): report from the insurance company to the patient or provider explaining the claims benefit paid, reduced, or denied.

fee-for-service: traditional payment method in US health care, when patients pay doctors, hospitals, and other providers for the services rendered at the time of service, and then seek reimbursement for those costs from their private insurers or the government, if eligible for such a program (e.g. Medicare). The patient is charged according to a fee schedule set for each service or procedure provided.

fee schedule: maximum allowable charge. The amount set by the insurer as the highest amount to be charged for a particular service.

following skills: communication tools—usually open-ended questions—used to discover how a patient views her situation: how the patient feels about something, how she views a situation, who and what is important to the patient.

functional goals: short-term and long-term goals for health based in daily activities the patient is having difficulty performing; goals set by the patient with assistance from the health care provider that address the specific needs of the patient's every day life and lead to an effective treatment plan. Goals must be specific to an activity of daily living, measurable, and achievable in a reasonable amount of time.

functional outcomes: patient's progress toward improved health stated in an increased ability to participate in daily activities; the goals accomplished.

functional outcomes reporting: style of charting which addresses and emphasizes the patient's ability to participate in everyday activities, and setting goals and defining treatments to further participation.

global fee, bundling: type of reimbursement arrangement that combines two or more health care procedures into one procedure code. A flat fee is established to pay for all health care services performed under the single code.

good faith: requirement that the insurer handle insurance matters with its insureds to satisfy provisions of the contract, regulation, or law.

Guarantee of Payment, Attorney Lien: written agreement between a patient and health care provider guaranteeing payment in full to the patient's health care providers upon settlement of a personal injury case. Often, when the patient has an attorney, counsel co-endorses the written agreement.

HCFA: Health Care Financing Administration; the US Department of Health and Human Services agency that administers federal health financing and related regulatory programs, principally Medicare, Medicaid, and Peer Review Organization programs. The contracting agency for HMOs that provide Medicare managed care plans.

HCFA 1500 form: standard billing form approved by federal health and financing agencies.

health care lien: health care provider's legal claim or lien on the patient's personal injury claim to guarantee that the HCP's bills will be paid when the case settles.

Health Maintenance Organizations (HMOs): legal entity that provides health care in a geographic area, and which accepts responsibility to provide directly or by contract an agreed-upon set of health services to a defined, voluntarily-enrolled group of individuals. HMOs are reimbursed through a pre-determined, fixed, periodic prepayment made by or on behalf of each subscriber without regard to the amount of actual services provided. In many states, HMOs are synonymous with managed care. However, in Washington for example, other kinds of health carriers also may employ managed care.

hold harmless: agreements or provisions found in managed care contracts in which the HMO and its providers hold each other not liable for malpractice or corporate malfeasance if either is found liable. This clause is also common for insurance carriers. State law requires this type of clause to prohibit health care providers from billing patients if their managed care company becomes insolvent.

HxTxC charts: History, Treatment, and Comments. A system for documenting wellness sessions with healthy patients.

ICD-10: International Classification of Diseases-10th edition. A statistical classification system that arranges diseases and injuries into groups according to established criteria. Revised approximately every 10 years by the World Health Organization. Published annually by HCFA.

indemnity plan: benefits paid to the insured in a predetermined amount in the event of a covered loss. For example, automobile insurance policies are based on indemnity principles.

independent/insurance medical exam (IME): insurers refer to an IME as an "independent medical exam." Attorneys representing injured people refer to an IME as an "insurance medical exam." An IME is an examination of the patient, her health care records, or both. The insurer selects a doctor of their choice and pays for the examination of the insured. The examination is used in personal injury cases to determine reasonable and necessary care, and to support the insurer's decision to deny, limit, or terminate an insured's health benefits.

initial note: comprehensive notes recording the patient's first visit with a practitioner for a particular condition: exam, findings, treatment, and treatment plan regarding the patient's health and current situation. (SOAP format)

initial report: report following the first visit summarizing the findings and plan for treatment. (Letter format)

insurance companies, insurance carriers, payers: for-profit business primarily engaged in selling indemnification policies to individuals or groups to cover a defined amount of benefits if a loss occurs.

insurance networks: company that contracts with two or more independent group practices or solo practices to provide health services to various insurance carriers' members.

insurance plans, insurance policies: specific benefit package offered by an insurer.

insured, member: party to an insurance agreement to whom, or on behalf of whom, the insurance company agrees to indemnify for losses, provide insurance benefits, or render service. Like "insurer," the term "insured" is functional and unmistakable, and therefore preferred to such terms as "policyholder." In pre-paid hospital service plans, the insured is called the subscriber.

220

HANDS HEAL:
COMMUNICATION,
DOCUMENTATION,
AND INSURANCE BILLING
FOR MANUAL THERAPISTS

IPA: Independent Practice Arrangement/Association. An HMO contract with a physician organization which in turn contracts with individual physicians to provide health services to its members. IPA physicians practice in their own offices and also see fee-for-service patients. The IPA is reimbursed on a capitated basis. The IPA may reimburse its physicians on a capitated or modified fee-for-service basis when physicians charge agree-upon rates to the HMO patients and then bill the IPA.

liability coverage: insurance that pays and renders service on behalf of an insured for loss arising out of his responsibility or negligence, to others imposed by law or assumed by contract.

lives: number of insureds in a given area.

Major Medical: type of health insurance that provides benefits for most types of medical expenses incurred up to a high limit, subject to a large deductible. Such contracts may contain internal limits and a percentage participation clause (sometimes a co-insurance clause). A major medical policy pays expenses both in and out of the hospital.

managed care: philosophy of health care coverage that streamlines health services and creates a health care system that includes both the financing and delivery of services to the consumer. It also takes more responsibility for maintaining subscribers' health, not just curing them once they are sick. It lowers costs by matching the patient with appropriate care as efficiently as possible. Different insurance carriers use different kinds of managed care; often differentiated by reimbursement methods.

manual therapists: health care providers who primarily rely on manual means of providing health care services, such as massage therapists, chiropractors, physical therapists, somatic educators.

maximum benefit, maximum medical recovery: when the injured party has reached a threshold of health improvement.

Medicaid: state program which provides public assistance to persons, regardless of age, whose incomes and resources are insufficient to pay for health care.

medical necessity or medically necessary: covered services required to preserve and maintain the health status of a member or eligible person in accordance with the area's standards of medical practice.

Medical Payments (Med Pay): provision for medical expenses that can be purchased under an automobile insurance policy.

Medicare: federal hospital insurance system and the supplementary medical insurance for the aged created in 1965 by amendment to the Social Security Act.

morning pages: practice of writing 3 pages of "whatever comes to mind" each morning.

narrative report: summary of a patient's injuries, treatment, and progress throughout the entire course of treatment. (Letter format)

network adequacy: basis on which a carrier determines how many providers are necessary to provide services to the lives in each of their plans. The formula used considers a combination of the number of lives within a geographic location, and time and distance traveled to the provider. Requirements are determined by the insurer and available to the Department of Insurance.

no-fault: insurance benefits provided regardless of responsibility or liability of party.

personal injury: bodily injury resulting from the negligence of another person.

Personal Injury Protection (PIP): one component of automobile insurance that provides benefits for medical and hospital services, loss of wages and services, and funeral expenses.

Physician Desk Reference (PDR): resource manual of drugs and medications: generic terms, doses, side effects, etc.

pre-existing conditions: injuries, illnesses, or symptoms that existed prior to the onset of the current injury or condition. The medical-legal-insurance context draws a distinction between asymptomatic or dormant conditions verses symptomatic or active pre-existing conditions. An injury that "lights-up" an asymptomatic or dormant condition requires the responsible party or insurer to cover all reasonable and necessary treatment expenses. However, an injury that "aggravates" a symptomatic or active condition requires the responsible party or insurer to cover only those expenses attributed to the aggravation of the condition.

Preferred Provider Organizations (PPOs): health care arrangement between purchasers of health care such as employers and insurance companies and providers offering benefits at a reasonable cost using incentives, such as lower deductibles and copays to get members to use providers within a network. Use of non-preferred providers would involve a higher cost. Preferred providers must agree to specified fee schedules and are required to comply with certain utilization and review guidelines.

preferred provider status: contracted licensed health care providers who provide specified health care services for a predetermined fee.

prescriptions: formal referrals for adjunctive services. Infers medical necessity. Provides patient information, such as diagnosis (ICD-10 codes), and recommends treatment parameters.

primary care: first care a patient receives. It is often a family physician, although patient may also receive primary care from a nurse, a paramedic, or other types of health care providers, depending on the situation. Managed care systems try to resolve as many health problems as possible at this level.

primary care status: types of health care providers that are allowed to manage a patient's care, as determined by individual health care programs. Often limited to physicians, sometimes includes naturopaths and nurses.

primary insurer: first in line responsible for providing benefits.

private health insurance: insurance against loss by sickness or bodily injury.

problem-oriented medical record (POMR): documentation system introduced by Dr. Lawrence Weed in the 1960's. POMR lists patient problems in the front of the chart, and the practitioner writes a SOAP note to address each problem.

progress notes: comprehensive note recording re-evaluation/re-examination sessions. (SOAP format)

progress reports: summary of patient progress and suggested additions or changes to the treatment plan submitted to the referring provider every 30 days. (Letter format)

Quality Improvement/Assurance programs: internal peer review process used to audit the quality of care provided. Should include an educational mechanism identifying and preventing discrepancies in care.

reasonable and necessary: common insurance or legal term and standard found in automobile and health care insurance policies governing the basis of paying or denying treatment expenses.

rebating: practice of accepting payment for referrals, or referring to clinics or laboratories in which the provider has a financial interest.

referring health care provider: provider who prescribes adjunctive care. Often the primary care provider, or provider with diagnostic scope authorized to manage the patients' health care.

reflecting: communication tool using parroting, paraphrasing, or summarizing the information and feelings the patient has expressed either verbally or nonverbally.

Relative Value Unit (RVU): unit calculated and proposed by the AMA and refined and approved by the HCFA using RBRVS methodology. Individual carriers use a conversion factor as a multiplier to convert the total RVU into a dollar amount for reimbursement purposes.

Resource Based Relative Value Scale (RBRVS): process methodology developed at Harvard University to assess physician work, overhead cost, and malpractice risk for individual CPT codes.

Revised Oswestry Low Back Pain and Disability Index: one type of pain questionnaire used for the low back and lower extremities.

scope of practice: law defining the standards of competence, practice areas, and conduct of a health care provider.

secondary insurer: any coverage that kicks in after primary coverage is exhausted or expires.

222

HANDS HEAL:
COMMUNICATION,
DOCUMENTATION,
AND INSURANCE BILLING
FOR MANUAL THERAPISTS

self-insured, self-insurance: practice of an employer or organization assuming responsibility for the health care losses of its employees. Usually a fund is established against which claims payments are drawn. Claims processing is often handled through an administrative services contract with an independent organization, usually an insurer.

silence: communication tool that allows a patient to sort out her thoughts, take a short breather from the work at hand, or search deeper for answers to the practitioner's questions.

SOAP charting: Subjective, Objective, Assessment, Plan; a standard health care format for charting and documenting treatment sessions. Information is organized into four categories: S: data provided by the patient, O: practitioner findings, A: functional outcomes and diagnoses, and P: treatment recommendations.

Statute of Limitations, statutory time limits: laws enacted by every State which govern the time frame within which a lawsuit must be brought, or otherwise the claim will be barred or dismissed. Statutes of limitations differ from State to State and according to the nature of the claim.

Stipulation for release of medical records: request for medical records which contains the consent of the patient and the patient's attorney to authorize release.

subpoena: written command requiring a person to appear at a certain time and place to give testimony on a certain matter. A subpoena duces tecum is a written command requiring a witness to produce some document or paper that he possesses or controls and is pertinent to the pending issues.

subsequent notes: brief notes addressing the patient's immediate concerns for the day's session. (SOAP format)

Team Therapy Model: paradigm for approaching the interview and information gathering process; a combination of a medical model and intervention-free model of solution building.

third party coverage: liability insurance coverage of the at-fault party or the uninsured/underinsured coverage of the patient.

tort-feasor, at-fault-party: person who causes harm to an individual or damages property.

unclean claims: bills that lack information or contain disputable information.

uninsured motorist coverage: one component of automobile insurance that protects an insured driver from losses that should have been the responsibility of another driver who carried no liability insurance to cover the loss.

upcoding: process of increasing a CPT code from one of a lower value to one of a higher value that results in a higher reimbursement rate.

usual and customary/usual, customary and regular fees (UCR): health insurance plans pay a health care provider's full charge if it is deemed reasonable and does not exceed her usual charges and amount customarily charged by others like health care providers practicing in the area for the service.

Utilization: patterns of use of a service or type of service within a specified time. Usually expressed in rate per unit or population-at-risk for a given period. Utilization experience multiplied by the average cost per unit or service delivered equals capitated costs.

Utilization Management/Review (UM/UR): systematic means to review and control patients' use of medical services and quality of care. Usually involves data collection, review and/or authorization, especially for services such as specialists, emergency room use, and hospitalization.

Vernon-Mior Neck Pain and Disability Index: one type of pain questionnaire used for the neck and upper extremities.

Workers' Compensation: insurance employers are mandated to purchase for all employees. The plans furnish medical and disability benefits for illnesses, injuries, disabilities, and death that result from job-related conditions and activities.

APPENDIX:
Blank Forms

INDEX OF FORMS

224

HANDS HEAL:
COMMUNICATION,
DOCUMENTATION,
AND INSURANCE BILLING
FOR MANUAL THERAPISTS

DESCRIPTION OF FORMS

1. Health Information: Every patient with a health concern completes this two-page form annually, more frequently if the patient's health condition changes rapidly. Healthy patients seeking wellness care may fill out the history section of the HxTxC chart in lieu of this form. This information is useful for designing the treatment plan, and provides contact information.

Attach your logo, name, and contact information to the top of page one. Include your provider number if applicable. Photocopy this form front to back. File completed forms in the patient's chart.

2. Injury Information: Every workers' compensation and personal injury patient completes page one of this form. Every patient whose injury is the result of a motor vehicle accident completes page two of this form. Complete a new form for each incident. This information is useful for designing the treatment plan, and providing proof of significant injury.

Attach your logo, name, and contact information to the top of page one. Include your provider number if applicable. Photocopy this form front to back. Mark a line through page two if not applicable. File completed forms in the patient's chart.

3. Billing Information: If you offer billing services, each patient who requests direct billing to their insurance company fills out this form. Complete a new form for each incident, as billing information can change based on the type of health condition or situation. This information is useful for completing the Insurance Verification form.

Attach your logo, name, and contact information to the top of the page. Include your provider number if applicable. This form stands alone. File completed forms in the patient's chart.

4. Prescription: Send a pad of these forms with your logo, name, and contact information at the top to every potential referring Health Care Provider. HCPs do not have to use your form. If the form they use does not provide the pertinent information, gather the necessary information and attach it to the prescription provided.

Update as needed. If the patient's insurance is paying for care, every session must be medically necessary and accounted for on the prescriptions. File in the patient's chart.

5. Health Report: The patient reports on their current condition. There are multiple uses for this form:
• The patient completes the form before the session every 30 days as a subjective record of ongoing progress.
• The patient completes the form before and after the session every 30 days as a subjective record of immediate treatment results and ongoing progress. This requires a two-sided form, side one is completed before the session, side two is completed after the session.
• The Health Report can be used as a substitute for a SOAP chart. The patient completes side one before the session and side two after the session, as above. The manual therapist records the findings, treatment, and plan in the Comments section.

Attach your logo, name, and contact information to the top of the page. Include your provider number if applicable. Photocopy front to back, when applicable. This form is available in female, male, and non-gender specific versions to use at your discretion. File completed forms in the patient's chart.

6. Pain Questionnaires: Every patient with a complaint of pain resulting in a loss of function completes the applicable form. The Neck Pain Index can be used for the neck as well as any upper extremity pain; the Low Back Pain Index can also be used for any lower extremity pain. If the patient is experiencing mid-back pain, choose the form that best addresses the patient's symptoms. Update the form every 30 days, or until the patient's functional status stabilizes. If the form is used in lieu of a pain diary, the patient completes the form daily or weekly, as recommended by the attorney or HCP.

Attach your logo, name, and contact information to the top of the page. Include your provider number if applicable. The form stands alone, but may be piggybacked with the Health Report and photocopied front to back, when applicable. File completed forms in the patient's chart.

7. Initial Report without Treatment: This is the only acceptable fill-in-the-blank report completed by the practitioner. All other reports should be typed and written in paragraph form. Use this form when you receive a referral or prescription but the patient does not receive a treatment from you.

8. Soap Charts: A SOAP note should be written for each curative treatment session. There are two types of SOAP charts used for recording SOAP notes:

Long version: Use the full page SOAP chart for Initial notes, Progress notes, Discharge notes, or any time additional space is required.

Short version: Use the half page SOAP chart for subsequent notes or health conditions that do not require extensive space for recording information.

Attach your logo, name, and contact information to the top of each page. Include your provider number if applicable. Photocopy the long version as page one and the short version as page two. Also photocopy the short version back to back. This chart is available in female, male, and non-gender specific versions to use at your discretion. File completed forms in the patient's chart.

9. HxTxC Charts: A HxTxC note should be written for each wellness session. There are three types of HxTxC charts provided, any of which can be modified to enhance specific charting needs.

Standard HxTxC: This is useful for table work, as the figures are in a standing position.

Seated HxTxC: This is useful for On-Site sessions, as the figures are in a seated position.

Sports HxTxC: This is useful for sporting events. The intake questions are designed for the needs of treating athletes before and after competition. Treatments are general and rarely require additional notation.

Attach your logo, name, and contact information to the top of each page. Include your provider number if applicable. The Standard and Seated HxTxC charts have a page two for ongoing care. Photocopy page one and page two together, back-to-back. Page two can also be photocopied back-to-back, as the intake form only needs to be completed annually or bi-annually. The Sports HxTxC only has one page, and can be photocopied back-to-back.

Patients receiving ongoing care should have individual files. File charts for events by event and date, rather than by patient's name.

10. Range of Motion: Use this for ease in charting range of motion tests. Space is provided for pre- and post-treatment assessment, for up to three joint assessments. You may use one form for up to three sessions if you are only assessing the motion of one joint by writing the treatment date next to each test. If you photocopy back-to-back, one piece of paper can be used for up to six treatment sessions.

Attach your logo, name, and contact information to the top of the page. Include your provider number if applicable. File completed forms in the patient's chart.

11. Insurance Status—Personal Injury: If the patient has retained an attorney to represent them in a personal injury case, the attorney completes this form. Send this form along with a letter of introduction and request for information, and a self-addressed, stamped envelope. Complete a new form for each incident. This information is useful for completing the Insurance Verification form.

Attach your logo, name, and contact information to the top of the page. Include your provider number if applicable. This form stands alone. File in the patient's chart.

226

HANDS HEAL:
COMMUNICATION,
DOCUMENTATION,
AND INSURANCE BILLING
FOR MANUAL THERAPISTS

12. Guarantee of Payment: If the patient has retained an attorney to represent them in a personal injury case, and there is no PIP, Med Pay, or UIM or the policy limit has been reached, have the patient and their attorney sign and date this form. File in the patient's chart.

13. Insurance Verification and 14. Re-Authorization/Verification: Complete this form using the information provided on the Health Information form, Prescription, Billing Information form, and Insurance Status—Personal Injury form. Gather the remaining information from an insurance representative. Verify coverage and authorize services. Before providing additional services, complete the Reauthorization/Verification section. For multiple reauthorizations, use the Reauthorization/Verification form.

Complete a new form with each incident. This form is useful for assessing the risk involved in billing the patient's insurance company.

Attach your logo, name, and contact information to the top of page one. Include your provider number if applicable. Photocopy front-to-back. File in the patient's chart.

15. Payment Log: Complete this form each time the payment does not match the amount billed. Attach to the corresponding HCFA 1500 form. File in billing binder earmarked for rebilling. Follow through with phone calls and resending bills every 30 days until payment matches the amount billed.

Provider Name _____ **HEALTH INFORMATION**

Patient Name _____ Date _____

Date of Injury_____ Insurance ID# _____

A. Patient Information

Address _____

City_____ State _____ Zip _____

Phone: Home _____

   Work _____ Cell/Pgr_____

Date of Birth_____

Employer _____

Occupation _____

Emergency Contact _____

Phone: Home _____

   Work _____ Cell/Pgr_____

Primary Health Care Provider

Name_____

Address _____

City/State/Zip_____

Phone: _____ Fax _____

I give my manual therapist permission to
consult with my referring health care provider
regarding my health and treatment.

Comments _____

Initials _____ Date _____

B. Current Health Information

List Health/Concerns Check all that apply

Primary _____
☐ mild ☐ moderate ☐ disabling
☐ constant ☐ intermittant
☐ symptoms ↑ w/activity   ☐ ↓ w/activity
☐ getting worse ☐ getting better ☐ no change
treatment received _____

Secondary _____
☐ mild ☐ moderate ☐ disabling
☐ constant ☐ intermittant
☐ symptoms ↑ w/activity   ☐ ↓ w/activity
☐ getting worse ☐ getting better ☐ no change
treatment received _____

Additional _____
☐ mild ☐ moderate ☐ disabling
☐ constant ☐ intermittant
☐ symptoms ↑ w/activity   ☐ ↓ w/activity
☐ getting worse ☐ getting better ☐ no change
treatment received _____

Have you ever received Manual Therapy
before? ☐ Y ☐ N Frequency? _____

List all conditions currently monitored by a
Health Care Provider _____

_____

_____

List the medications you took today
(include pain relievers and herbal remedies)

_____

_____

List all other medications taken in the last
3 months _____

_____

List Daily Activities

Work _____

_____

Home/Family _____

_____

Social/Recreational _____

_____

Circle the activities affected by your condition,
☐ all of the above
Check other activities affected: ☐ sleep
☐ washing ☐ dressing ☐ fitness
How do you reduce stress? _____

_____

Pain? _____

_____

What are your goals for receiving Manual
Therapy?_____

C. Health History

List and Explain. Include dates and treatment
received.

Surgeries _____

_____

Accidents _____

_____

Major Illnesses _____

_____

227

General

current   past   comments
- ☐ ☐ headaches _____
- ☐ ☐ pain _____
- ☐ ☐ sleep disturbances _____
- ☐ ☐ fatigue_____
- ☐ ☐ infectious _____
- ☐ ☐ fever_____
- ☐ ☐ sinus _____
- ☐ ☐ other_____

Skin Conditions

current   past   comments
- ☐ ☐ rashes_____
- ☐ ☐ athlete's foot, warts _____
- ☐ ☐ other_____

Allergies

current   past   comments
- ☐ ☐ scents, oils, lotions _____
- ☐ ☐ detergents _____
- ☐ ☐ other_____

Muscles and Joints

current   past   comments
- ☐ ☐ rheumatoid arthritis _____
- ☐ ☐ osteoarthritis_____
- ☐ ☐ osteoporosis_____
- ☐ ☐ scoliosis _____
- ☐ ☐ broken bones _____
- ☐ ☐ spinal problems _____
- ☐ ☐ disk problems_____
- ☐ ☐ lupus_____
- ☐ ☐ TMJ, jaw pain_____
- ☐ ☐ spasms, cramps
- ☐ ☐ sprains, strains
- ☐ ☐ tendonitis, bursitis
- ☐ ☐ stiff or painful joints _____
- ☐ ☐ weak or sore muscles ____
- ☐ ☐ neck, shoulder, arm pain _____
- ☐ ☐ low back, hip, leg pain _____
- ☐ ☐ other_____

Nervous System

current   past   comments
- ☐ ☐ head injuries, concussions _____
- ☐ ☐ dizziness, ringing in the ears _____
- ☐ ☐ loss of memory, confusion_____
- ☐ ☐ numbness, tingling _____
- ☐ ☐ sciatica, shooting pain _____
- ☐ ☐ chronic pain _____
- ☐ ☐ depression _____
- ☐ ☐ other_____

Respiratory, Cardiovascular

current   past   comments
- ☐ ☐ heart disease _____
- ☐ ☐ blood clots _____
- ☐ ☐ stroke _____
- ☐ ☐ lymphadema_____
- ☐ ☐ high, low blood pressure _____
- ☐ ☐ irregular heart beat_____
- ☐ ☐ poor circulation _____
- ☐ ☐ swollen ankles _____
- ☐ ☐ varicose veins _____
- ☐ ☐ chest pain, shortness of breath _____
- ☐ ☐ asthma _____

Digestive/Elimination System

current   past   comments
- ☐ ☐ bowel dysfunction _____
- ☐ ☐ gas, bloating _____
- ☐ ☐ bladder/kidney dysfunction _____
- ☐ ☐ abdominal pain _____
- ☐ ☐ other _____

Endocrine System

current   past   comments
- ☐ ☐ thyroid dysfunction _____
- ☐ ☐ diabetes _____

Reproductive System

current   past   comments
- ☐ ☐ pregnancy _____
- ☐ ☐ painful, emotional menses _____
- ☐ ☐ fibrotic cysts _____

Cancer/Tumors

current   past   comments
- ☐ ☐ benign _____
- ☐ ☐ malignant _____

Habits

current   past   comments
- ☐ ☐ tobacco _____
- ☐ ☐ alcohol_____
- ☐ ☐ drugs _____
- ☐ ☐ coffee, soda _____

Contract for Care

I promise to participate fully as a member of my health care team. I will make sound choices regarding my treatment plan based on the information provided by my manual therapist and other members of my health care team, and my experience of those suggestions. I agree to participate in the self care program we select. I promise to inform my practitioner any time I feel my well-being is threatened or compromised. I expect my manual therapist to provide safe and effective treatment.

Consent for Care

It is my choice to receive manual therapy, and I give my consent to receive treatment. I have reported all health conditions that I am aware of and will inform my practitioner of any changes in my health.

Signature _____ Date _____

Signature of parent or guardian _____ Date _____
(If patient is a minor)

Provider Name _____   **INJURY INFORMATION**

Patient Name _____ Date _____

Date of Injury_____ Insurance ID# _____

A. General Injury Information

1. How did the accident occur?
   ☐ Auto   ☐ On-the-Job   ☐ Other _____

2. Was a police report filed?   ☐Yes   ☐ No
   Was a work incident report filed?
   ☐Yes   ☐No

3. Describe your injury and how it occurred:
   _____
   _____
   _____
   _____
   _____
   _____

4. Describe how you felt during and
   immediately after the injury:
   _____
   _____

   Later that same day: _____
   _____

   The next day: _____
   _____

   The next week: _____
   _____

   The next month: _____
   _____

   Describe any bruises, cuts, or abrasions
   as a result of the injury:
   _____
   _____

5. Are your symptoms ☐ getting better
   ☐ getting worse   ☐ no change
   What makes them better? _____
   _____
   _____
   _____

   Worse? _____
   _____
   _____

6. Did you return to work on the day of the
   injury? ☐ Yes   ☐ No
   Have you lost time from work since the
   injury? ☐ Yes   ☐ No

7. What are your work responsibilities?
   _____
   _____

   Which work activities are affected by this
   injury? _____
   _____

   Have your work responsibilities changed as
   a result of this injury?   ☐ Yes   ☐ No

   Explain _____
   What other daily activities are affected by
   this injury? _____
   _____

8. Did you go to the emergency room?
   ☐ Yes   ☐ No
   Were you hospitalized?   ☐ Yes   ☐ No
   List the health care providers who have
   treated you for this injury, the type of
   treatment provided, and their diagnosis.
   _____
   _____
   _____
   _____

9. Have you ever had this type of injury
   before?   ☐ Yes   ☐ No
   Explain _____
   _____

   Did you have any physical complaints
   before the injury? ☐ Yes   ☐ No
   Explain _____
   _____

   Do you have any illnesses or previous
   injuries that may have been affected by
   this injury?   ☐ Yes   ☐ No
   Explain _____
   _____

Signature _____ Date _____

229

B. Motor Vehicle Accident Information

1. Did the police arrive at the accident?
☐ Yes ☐ No

2. How was your vehicle hit?
☐ Rear end ☐ Head on ☐ Side swipe
OR Did your vehicle hit another vehicle/object?
☐ Rear end ☐ Head on ☐ Side swipe
If you were hit from behind, was your vehicle pushed forward upon impact?
☐ Yes ☐ No If yes, how much?
_____
Did your vehicle hit anything else after the initial impact? ☐ Yes ☐ No
Explain _____
_____
_____
_____

3. Were you at a stop or moving at the time of impact? ☐ Stopped ☐ Moving
If you were stopped, was your foot on the brake? ☐ Yes ☐ No
If you were moving, were you:
☐ Increasing speed
☐ Decreasing speed
☐ Traveling at a steady speed
Was the other vehicle moving at the time of impact? ☐ Yes ☐ No
If yes, was it: ☐ Increasing speed
☐ Decreasing speed ☐ Traveling at a steady speed

4. Where were you seated in the vehicle?
_____
_____
_____

5. Which way was your head facing upon impact?
_____
_____
_____

6. Were you aware of the approaching vehicle or did the impact catch you by surprise?
☐ Aware ☐ Surprise

7. Did you lose consciousness?
☐ Yes ☐ No

8. Were you wearing a seat belt? ☐ No
☐ Lap belt ☐ Shoulder harness ☐ Both

9. Is your vehicle equipped with an airbag?
☐ Yes ☐ No
Did it activate? ☐ Yes ☐ No

10. Is the top of your head rest:
☐ Above your head ☐ Below your head
Does your head touch the head rest?
☐ Yes ☐ No
If no, how far in front of the head rest is your head?
_____

11. What were the road conditions?
☐ Wet ☐ Dry ☐ Icy ☐ Oily

12. What type of vehicle were you in? (make, model, year)
_____
What type of vehicle hit you? (make, model, year)
_____

13. Did any part of your body come into contact with the vehicle? ☐ Yes ☐ No
Explain _____
_____
_____
_____
Did any parts of the vehicle break?
☐ Yes ☐ No
Explain _____
_____
_____
_____

14. Check all of the following symptoms that you have experienced since the accident:
☐ Loss of memory _____
☐ Loss of balance_____
☐ Visual disturbances _____
☐ Hearing difficulties _____
☐ Difficulty breathing_____
☐ Sleep disturbances_____

15. Anything else you want to tell me about the accident or how you feel?
_____
_____
_____

Patient Signature_____Date _____

Provider Name _____

BILLING INFORMATION

Patient Name _____ Date _____

Date of Injury_____ Insurance ID# _____

A. Patient Information

Address _____
City _____ State _____ Zip _____
Phone: Home _____
        Work _____ Cell/Pgr _____
Date of Birth _____
☐ Male   ☐ Female
Marital Status: ☐ Single ☐ Married ☐ Partnered
Relationship of Patient to Insured:
☐ Self ☐ Spouse ☐ Partner ☐ Child ☐ Other
☐ Employed ☐ Student
Employer's Name or School Name:

_____
Phone _____ Fax _____
Is patient's condition related to:
Employment   ☐ Yes   ☐ No
Auto Accident   ☐ Yes   ☐ No
If Auto Accident, in what state? _____
Other Accident   ☐ Yes   ☐ No
Illness   ☐ Yes   ☐ No

Primary Health Care Provider

Name _____
Address _____
City _____ State _____ Zip _____
Phone _____ Fax _____

Attorney

Has an attorney been consulted? ☐ Yes ☐ No
Retained?   ☐ Yes   ☐ No
Name _____
Address _____
City _____ State _____ Zip _____
Phone _____ Fax _____

B. Insured (if other than patient)

Name _____
Insurance ID# _____
Date of Birth _____
☐ Male   ☐ Female
Address _____
City _____ State _____ Zip _____
Phone: Home _____
        Work _____ Cell/Pgr _____
Employer's Name or School Name:

_____
Phone _____ Fax _____

Signature _____ Date _____

C. Primary Insurance Coverage

Insurance Carrier _____
Contact _____
Group Number _____
Plan # or Name _____
Billing Address _____
City _____ State _____ Zip _____
Phone _____ Fax _____

D. Secondary Insurance Coverage

Insured _____
Insurance ID# _____
Date of Birth _____
☐ Male   ☐ Female
Address _____
City _____ State _____ Zip _____
Phone: Home _____
        Work _____ Cell/Pgr _____
Employer's Name or School Name:

_____
Phone _____ Fax _____
Insurance Carrier _____
Contact _____
Group Number _____
Plan # or Name _____
Billing Address _____
City _____ State _____ Zip _____
Phone _____ Fax _____

E. Assignment of Benefits

My signature below authorizes and directs payment of medical benefits for services billed to my health care provider.

F. Release of Medical Records

My signature below authorizes the release of my medical records including intake forms, chart notes, reports, and billing statements to my attorneys, health care providers, and insurance case managers, for the purpose of processing my claims. (I will inform my practitioner immediately upon signing any exclusive Release of Medical Records with my attorney.)

G. Financial Responsibility

It is my responsibility to pay for all services provided. In the unfortunate event that my insurance company denies payment or makes a partial payment, I am responsible for the balance. If you have contracted with my insurance company at a discount rate and the agreed-upon fee has been satisfied, the balance will be waived.

231

Provider Name _____   **PRESCRIPTION**

Patient Name _____ Date _____

Date of Injury _____ Insurance ID# _____

A. Diagnosis

(Include ICD-10 codes that specifically address Manual Therapy Treatment)

_____

_____

_____

_____

Condition is related to
☐ Auto Accident
☐ Work Injury
☐ Illness
☐ Other:_____

_____

_____

B. Medically Necessary Treatment: Implement Plan as Prescribed Below

Application (Direct & Indirect)
☐ Head _____
☐ Neck _____
☐ Chest _____
☐ Shoulders _____
☐ Abdomen _____
☐ Back _____
☐ Lowback/Hips _____
☐ Upper extremities _____
☐ Lower extremities _____
☐ All of the above _____
☐ Other: _____

Duration & Frequency
☐ 1× wk for _____ wks
☐ 2× wk for _____ wks
☐ 3× wk for _____ wks
☐ 2× month for _____ months
☐ 1× month for _____ months

Specific Instructions:

_____

_____

_____

Treatment Type
☐ Manual Therapy _____
☐ Hydrotherapy _____
☐ Self-Care Education _____
☐ Other _____

Treatment Goals
☐ Decrease Pain
☐ Decrease Inflammation
☐ Decrease Muscle Tension/Spasms
☐ Decrease Compensatory Patterns
☐ Increase Mobility
☐ Increase Strength
☐ Restore Function
☐ Restore Posture
☐ Maintain Associated Structures
☐ All of the Above
☐ Other

C. Referring Health Care Provider (HCP)

Contact Information
HCP Name _____
Provider No. _____
Address _____
City _____ State ____ Zip _____
Phone _____
Fax _____

Reporting
☐ Send Report After Initial Visit
☐ Send Report at End of Prescription
☐ Send Copies of Chart Notes at End of Prescription
☐ Fax Information
☐ Mail Information
☐ Email Information

HCP Signature: _____ Date _____

Revised and reprinted with permission, Adler ◆ Giersch, PS

232

Provider Name _____

Patient Name _____ Date _____

Date of Injury_____ Insurance ID# _____

A. Draw today's symptoms on the figures.

1. Identify CURRENT symptomatic areas in your body by marking letters on the figures below. Use the letters provided in the key to identify the symptoms you are feeling today.
2. Circle the area around each letter, representing the size and shape of each symptom location.

Key
P = pain or tenderness
S = joint or muscle stiffness
N = numbness or tingling

B. Identify the intensity of your symptoms.

1. Pain Scale: Mark a line on the scale to show the amount of pain you are experiencing today.

No Pain |————————————————————————————————| Unbearable Pain

2. Activities Scale: Mark a line on the scale to show the limitations you are experiencing today in your daily activities.

Can Do Anything I Want |————————————————————————————| Cannot Do Anything

C. Comments

_____

_____

_____

_____

Signature _____ Date _____

233

HEALTH REPORT-M

Patient Name _____ Date _____

Date of Injury_____ Insurance ID# _____

A. Draw today's symptoms on the figures.

1. Identify CURRENT symptomatic areas in your body by marking letters on the figures below. Use the letters provided in the key to identify the symptoms you are feeling today.
2. Circle the area around each letter, representing the size and shape of each symptom location.

Key
P = pain or tenderness
S = joint or muscle stiffness
N = numbness or tingling

B. Identify the intensity of your symptoms.

1. Pain Scale: Mark a line on the scale to show the amount of pain you are experiencing today.

No Pain ├───┤ Unbearable Pain

2. Activities Scale: Mark a line on the scale to show the limitations you are experiencing today in your daily activities.

Can Do Anything I Want ├──────────────────────────────────┤ Cannot Do Anything

C. Comments

_____
_____
_____
_____

Signature _____ Date _____

Provider Name _____

Patient Name _____ Date _____

Date of Injury_____ Insurance ID# _____

A. Draw today's symptoms on the figures.

1. Identify CURRENT symptomatic areas in your body by marking letters on the figures below. Use the letters provided in the key to identify the symptoms you are feeling today.
2. Circle the area around each letter, representing the size and shape of each symptom location.

Key
P = pain or tenderness
S = joint or muscle stiffness
N = numbness or tingling

B. Identify the intensity of your symptoms.

1. Pain Scale: Mark a line on the scale to show the amount of pain you are experiencing today.

   No Pain ┠─────────────────────────────────────┨ Unbearable Pain

2. Activities Scale: Mark a line on the scale to show the limitations you are experiencing today in your daily activities.

   Can Do Anything I Want ┠─────────────────────────────┨ Cannot Do Anything

C. Comments

_____

_____

_____

Signature _____ Date _____

Provider Name _____

Patient Name _____ Date _____

Date of Injury_____ Insurance ID# _____

This questionnaire has been designed to give the health care provider information as to how your neck pain has affected your ability to manage everyday life. Please answer every section and mark in each section only the **ONE** box which applies to you. We realize you may consider that two of the statements in any one section relate to you, but please just mark the box which most closely describes your problem today.

Section 1 - Pain Intensity
☐ I have no pain at the moment.
☐ The pain is very mild at the moment.
☐ The pain is moderate at the moment.
☐ The pain is fairly severe at the moment.
☐ The pain is very severe at the moment.
☐ The pain is the worst imaginable at the moment.

Section 2 - Personal Care
(washing, dressing, etc.)
☐ I can look after myself normally without causing pain.
☐ I can look after myself normally but it causes extra pain.
☐ It is painful to look after myself and I am slow and careful.
☐ I need some help but manage most of my personal care.
☐ I need help every day in most aspects of self care.
☐ I do not get dressed, I wash myself with difficulty and I stay in bed.

Section 3 - Lifting
☐ I can lift heavy weights without extra pain.
☐ I can lift heavy weights but it causes extra pain.
☐ Pain prevents me from lifting heavy weights off the floor, but I can manage if they are conveniently positioned, e.g. on a table.
☐ Pain prevents me from lifting heavy weights, but I can manage light to medium weights if they are conveniently positioned.
☐ I can lift very light weights.
☐ I cannot lift or carry anything at all.

Section 4 - Reading
☐ I can read as much as I want to with no pain in my neck.
☐ I can read as much as I want to with slight pain in my neck.
☐ I can read as much as I want to with moderate pain in my neck.
☐ I can't read as much as I want to because of moderate pain in my neck.
☐ I can hardly read at all because of severe pain in my neck.
☐ I cannot read at all.

Section 5 - Headaches
☐ I have no headaches at all.
☐ I have slight headaches which come infrequently.
☐ I have moderate headaches which come infrequently.
☐ I have moderate headaches which come frequently.
☐ I have severe headaches which come frequently.
☐ I have headaches almost all of the time.

Section 6 - Concentration
☐ I can concentrate fully when I want to with no difficulty.
☐ I can concentrate fully when I want to with slight difficulty.
☐ I have a fair degree of difficulty in concentrating when I want to.
☐ I have a lot of difficulty concentrating when I want to.
☐ I have a great deal of difficulty in concentrating when I want to.
☐ I cannot concentrate at all.

Section 7 - Work
☐ I can do as much work as I want to.
☐ I can do my usual work but no more.
☐ I can do most of my usual work but no more.
☐ I cannot do my usual work.
☐ I can hardly do any work at all.
☐ I can't do any work at all.

Section 8 - Driving
☐ I can drive my car without any neck pain.
☐ I can drive my car as long as I want with slight pain in my neck.
☐ I can drive my car as long as I want with moderate pain in my neck.
☐ I can't drive my car as long as I want because of moderate pain in my neck.
☐ I can hardly drive at all because of severe pain in my neck.
☐ I can't drive my car at all.

Section 9 - Sleeping
☐ I have no trouble sleeping.
☐ My sleep is slightly disturbed (less than 1 hour sleepless).
☐ My sleep is mildly disturbed (1–2 hours sleepless).
☐ My sleep is moderately disturbed (2–3 hours sleepless).
☐ My sleep is greatly disturbed (3–5 hours sleepless).
☐ My sleep is completely disturbed (5–7 hours sleepless).

Section 10 - Recreation
☐ I am able to engage in all my recreational activities with no neck pain at all.
☐ I am able to engage in all my recreational activities with some pain in my neck.
☐ I am able to engage in most, but not all of my usual recreational activities because of pain in my neck.
☐ I am able to engage in a few of my usual recreational activities because of pain in my neck.
☐ I can hardly do any recreational activities because of pain in my neck.
☐ I can't do recreational activities at all.

Signature _____ Date _____

LOW BACK PAIN & DISABILITY INDEX

Provider Name _____

Patient Name _____ Date _____

Date of Injury_____ Insurance ID# _____

This questionnaire has been designed to give the health care provider information about how your back pain has affected your ability to manage everyday life. Please answer every section and mark in each section only the **ONE** box which applies to you. We realize you may consider that two statements in any one section relate to you, but please just mark the box which most closely describes your problem today.

Section 1 - Pain Intensity
☐ The pain comes and goes and is mild.
☐ The pain is mild and does not vary much.
☐ The pain comes and goes and is moderate.
☐ The pain is moderate and does not vary much.
☐ The pain comes and goes and is severe.
☐ The pain is severe and does not vary much.

Section 2 - Personal Care
☐ I can look after myself normally without causing pain.
☐ I can look after myself normally but it causes extra pain.
☐ It is painful to look after myself and I am slow and careful.
☐ I need some help but manage most of my personal care.
☐ I need help every day in most aspects of self care.
☐ I do not get dressed, I wash myself with difficulty, and I stay in bed.

Section 3 - Lifting
☐ I can lift heavy weights without extra pain.
☐ I can lift heavy weights but it causes extra pain.
☐ Pain prevents me from lifting heavy weights off the floor, but I can manage if they are conveniently positioned, e.g. on a table.
☐ Pain prevents me from lifting heavy weights, but I can manage light to medium weights if they are conveniently positioned.
☐ I can lift very light weights.
☐ I cannot lift or carry anything at all.

Section 4 - Walking
☐ I have no pain on walking.
☐ I have some pain on walking but it does not increase with distance.
☐ I cannot walk more than 1 mile without increasing pain.
☐ I cannot walk more than 1/2 mile without increasing pain.
☐ I cannot walk more than 1/4 mile without increasing pain.
☐ I cannot walk at all without increasing pain.

Section 5 - Sitting
☐ I can sit in any chair as long as I like.
☐ I can only sit in my favorite chair as long as I like.
☐ Pain prevents me from sitting more than 1 hour.
☐ Pain prevents me from sitting more than 1/2 hour.
☐ Pain prevents me from sitting more than 10 minutes.
☐ I avoid sitting because it increases my pain straight away.

Section 6 - Standing
☐ I can stand as long as I want without pain.
☐ I have some pain on standing but it does not increase with time.
☐ I cannot stand for longer than 1 hour without increasing pain.
☐ I cannot stand for longer than 1/2 hour without increasing pain.
☐ I cannot stand for longer than 10 minutes without increasing pain.
☐ I avoid standing because it increases the pain straight away.

Section 7 - Sleeping
☐ I have no trouble sleeping.
☐ My sleep is slightly disturbed (less than 1 hour sleepless).
☐ My sleep is mildly disturbed (1–2 hours sleepless).
☐ My sleep is moderately disturbed (2–3 hours sleepless).
☐ My sleep is greatly disturbed (3–5 hours sleepless).
☐ My sleep is completely disturbed (5–7 hours sleepless).

Section 8 - Social Life
☐ My social life is normal and gives me no pain.
☐ My social life is normal but increases the degree of pain.
☐ Pain has no significant effect on my social life apart from limiting my more energetic interests, e.g. dancing, etc.
☐ Pain has restricted my social life and I do not go out very often.
☐ Pain has restricted my social life to my home.
☐ I hardly have any social life because of the pain.

Section 9 - Traveling
☐ I get no pain while traveling.
☐ I get some pain while traveling but none of my usual forms of travel make it any worse.
☐ I get extra pain while traveling but it does not compel me to seek alternate forms of travel.
☐ I get extra pain while traveling which compels me to seek alternative forms of travel.
☐ Pain restricts all forms of travel.
☐ Pain prevents all forms of travel except that done lying down.

Section 10 - Changing Degree of Pain
☐ My pain is rapidly getting better.
☐ My pain fluctuates but overall is definitely getting better.
☐ My pain seems to be getting better but improvement is slow at present.
☐ My pain is neither getting better nor getting worse.
☐ My pain is gradually worsening.
☐ My pain is rapidly worsening.

Signature _____ Date _____

Dear _____:

Thank you for referring _____ to my office. Your patient and I were unable to connect for the following reason(s):

_____ The patient did not schedule an appointment.

_____ The patient did not attend the scheduled appointment.

_____ I am not scheduling new patients at this time. I anticipate my schedule to open back up again _____.

_____ I am unable to benefit the patient for the following reason(s):

_____

_____

_____

_____

Thank you for the referral. I hope to work with you again in the future.

Yours in health,

Provider Name _____

Patient Name _____ Date _____

Date of Injury _____ Insurance ID# _____ Current Meds _____

S Focus for Today

    Symptoms: Location/Intensity/Frequency/Duration/Onset

    Activities of Daily Living: Aggravating/Relieving

O Findings: Visual/Palpable/Test Results

    Modalities: Applications/Locations

    Response to Treatment (see Δ)

A Prioritize Functional Limitations

    Goals: Long-term/Short-term

P Future Treatment/Frequency

    Homework/Self-care

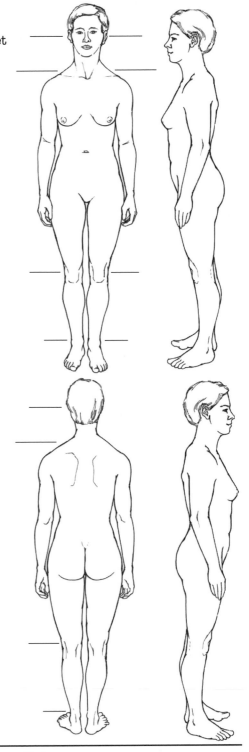

Provider Signature _____ Date _____

Legend:

℮ TP	• TeP	○ Ⓟ	⋇ Infl	≡ HT	≈ SP
✕ Adh	≋ Numb	◯ rot	╱ elev	⊢⊣ Short	⟷ Long

SOAP CHART-M

Patient Name _____ Date _____

Date of Injury_____ Insurance ID# _____ Current Meds _____

S Focus for Today

Symptoms: Location/Intensity/Frequency/Duration/Onset

Activities of Daily Living: Aggravating/Relieving

O Findings: Visual/Palpable/Test Results

Modalities: Applications/Locations

Response to Treatment (see Δ)

A Prioritize Functional Limitations

Goals: Long-term/Short-term

P Future Treatment/Frequency

Homework/Self-care

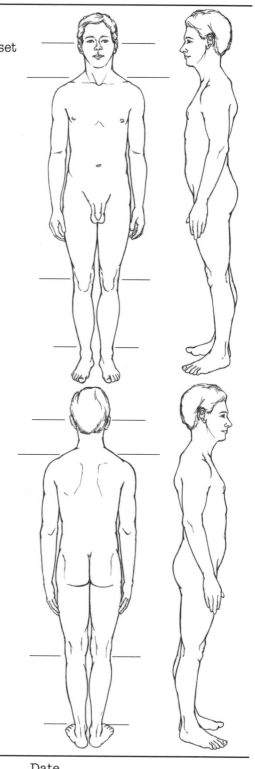

Provider Signature _____ Date _____

Legend:

⊚ TP	• TeP	○ ℗	☀ Infl	≡ HT	≈ SP
✕ Adh	≫ Numb	◯ rot	╱ elev	⊶ Short	⟷ Long

Provider Name _____

SOAP CHART

Patient Name _____ Date _____

Date of Injury_____ Insurance ID# _____ Current Meds _____

S Focus for Today

    Symptoms: Location/Intensity/Frequency/Duration/Onset

    Activities of Daily Living: Aggravating/Relieving

O Findings: Visual/Palpable/Test Results

    Modalities: Applications/Locations

    Response to Treatment (see Δ)

A Prioritize Functional Limitations

    Goals: Long-term/Short-term

P Future Treatment/Frequency

    Homework/Self-care

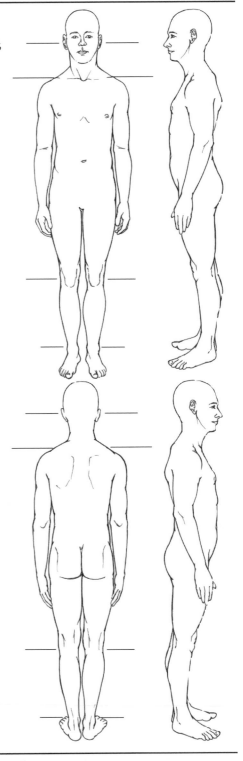

Provider Signature _____ Date _____

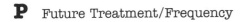

Legend:

ℰ TP	● TeP	○ Ⓟ	✳ Infl	≡ HT	≈ SP
✕ Adh	≫ Numb	⌒ rot	╱ elev	⊢ Short	↔ Long

Provider Name _____

Patient Name _____ Date _____

Date of Injury_____ Insurance ID# _____ Current Meds _____

S

O

A

P

Provider Signature _____ Date _____

S

O

A

P

Provider Signature _____ Date _____

Legend:

ℰ TP	● TeP	○ Ⓟ	⋇ Infl	≡ HT	≈ SP
✕ Adh	≷ Numb	⟲ rot	╱ elev	⤙ Short	↔ Long

Provider Name _____

Patient Name _____ Date _____

Date of Injury_____ Insurance ID# _____ Current Meds _____

S

O

A

P

Provider Signature _____ Date _____

S

O

A

P

Provider Signature _____ Date _____

Legend: ℮ TP   ● TeP   ○ Ⓟ   ✳ Infl   ≡ HT   ≈ SP

        ✕ Adh   ≈ Numb   ⬭ rot   ╱ elev   ⊶ Short   ↔ Long

Provider Name _____   **SOAP CHART**

Patient Name _____   Date _____

Date of Injury_____ Insurance ID# _____ Current Meds _____

S

O

A

P

Provider Signature _____ Date _____

S

O

A

P

Provider Signature _____ Date _____

Legend: ℮ TP   • TeP   ○ Ⓟ   ⸬ Infl   ≡ HT   ≈ SP

✕ Adh   ≫ Numb   ↻ rot   ╱ elev   ⤝ Short   ⟷ Long

244

Provider Name _____ **STANDARD HxTxC Chart-F**

Name _____ Date _____

Phone _____ Address _____

1. What are your goals for health, and how may I assist you in achieving your goals? _____
_____ .

2. Are you currently experiencing any of the following? If yes, please explain.

   pain, tenderness   ☐ No   ☐ Yes: _____   stiffness   ☐ No   ☐ Yes: _____
   numbness or tingling   ☐ No   ☐ Yes: _____   swelling   ☐ No   ☐ Yes: _____
   allergies   ☐ No   ☐ Yes: _____

3. List all illnesses, injuries, and health concerns you have now or have had in the past 3 years. (Examples: arthritis, diabetes, car accident, pregnancy) _____
_____

4. List medications and pain relievers taken today. _____
_____

5. I have provided all my known medical information. I acknowledge that manual therapy is not a substitute for medical diagnosis and treatment. I give my consent to receive treatment.

   Signature _____ Date _____

   Tx: _____
   _____
   C: _____
   _____

initials _____

Name _____ Current Meds _____

Tx: _____   Tx: _____

C: _____   C: _____

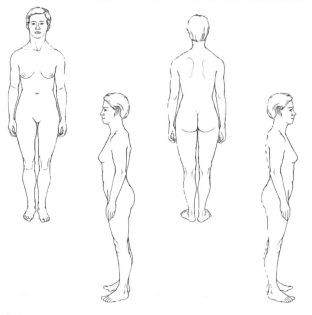

date _____ initials _____

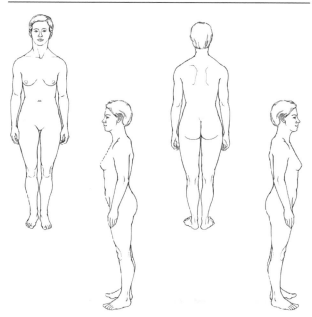

date _____ initials _____

Tx: _____   Tx: _____

C: _____   C: _____

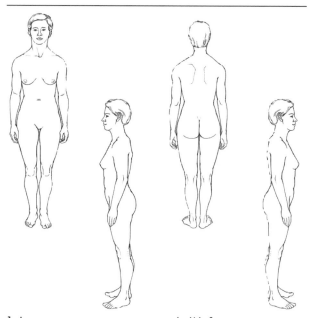

date _____ initials _____

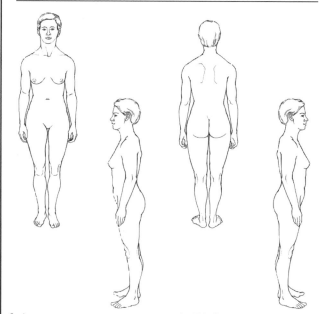

date _____ initials _____

Provider Name _____

STANDARD HxTxC Chart-M

Name _____ Date _____

Phone _____ Address _____

1. What are your goals for health, and how may I assist you in achieving your goals? _____
   _____.

2. Are you currently experiencing any of the following? If yes, please explain.

   pain, tenderness   ☐ No ☐ Yes: _____   stiffness ☐ No ☐ Yes: _____
   numbness or tingling ☐ No ☐ Yes: _____   swelling ☐ No ☐ Yes: _____
   allergies   ☐ No ☐ Yes: _____

3. List all illnesses, injuries, and health concerns you have now or have had in the past 3 years.
   (Examples: arthritis, diabetes, car accident, pregnancy) _____
   _____

4. List medications and pain relievers taken today. _____
   _____

5. I have provided all my known medical information. I acknowledge that manual therapy is not
   a substitute for medical diagnosis and treatment. I give my consent to receive treatment.

   Signature _____ Date _____

   Tx: _____
   _____

   C: _____

initials _____

Name _____   Current Meds _____

Tx: _____

C: _____

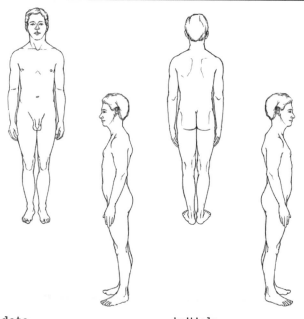

date _____   initials _____

Tx: _____

C: _____

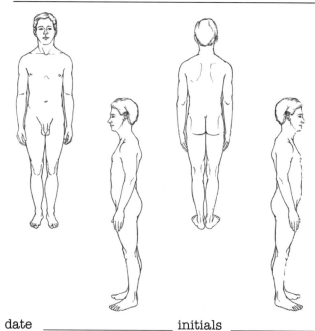

date _____   initials _____

Tx: _____

C: _____

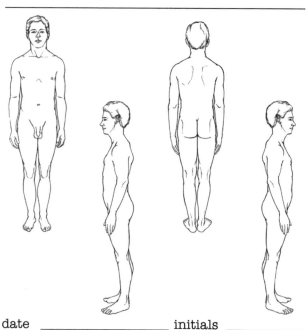

date _____   initials _____

Tx: _____

C: _____

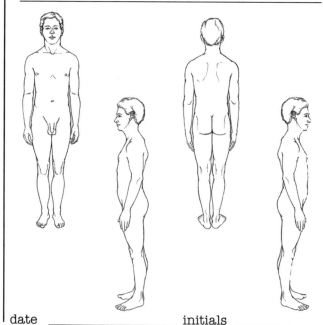

date _____   initials _____

Provider Name _____

STANDARD HxTxC Chart

Name _____ Date _____

Phone _____ Address _____

1. What are your goals for health, and how may I assist you in achieving your goals? _____
_____ .

2. Are you currently experiencing any of the following? If yes, please explain.

   pain, tenderness   ☐ No ☐ Yes: _____   stiffness ☐ No ☐ Yes: _____
   numbness or tingling ☐ No ☐ Yes: _____   swelling ☐ No ☐ Yes: _____
   allergies   ☐ No ☐ Yes: _____

3. List all illnesses, injuries, and health concerns you have now or have had in the past 3 years.
   (Examples: arthritis, diabetes, car accident, pregnancy) _____
   _____

4. List medications and pain relievers taken today. _____
   _____

5. I have provided all my known medical information. I acknowledge that manual therapy is not
   a substitute for medical diagnosis and treatment. I give my consent to receive treatment.

   Signature _____ Date _____

Tx: _____

_____

C: _____

_____

initials _____

STANDARD HxTxC   page 2

Name _____ Current Meds _____

Tx: _____   Tx: _____
_____   _____

C: _____   C: _____
_____   _____

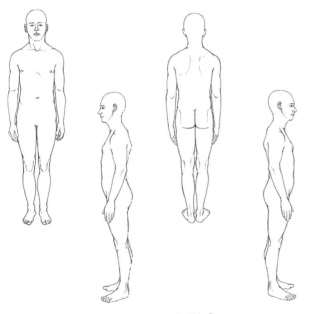

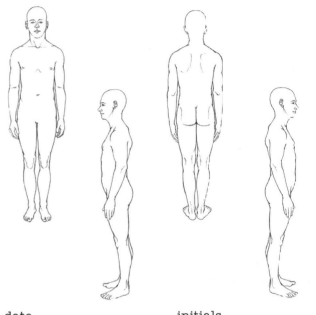

date _____ initials _____   date _____ initials _____

Tx: _____   Tx: _____
_____   _____

C: _____   C: _____
_____   _____

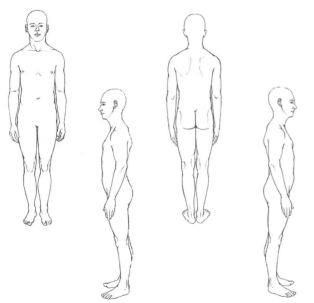

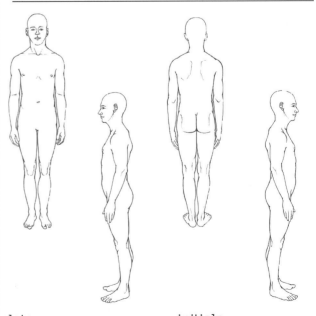

date _____ initials _____   date _____ initials _____

250

Provider Name _____   **SEATED HxTxC Chart**

Name _____   Date _____

Phone _____   Location _____

1. Are you currently experiencing any of the following? If yes, please explain.

   pain, tenderness   ☐ No ☐ Yes: _____   stiffness ☐ No ☐ Yes: _____
   numbness or tingling ☐ No ☐ Yes: _____   swelling   ☐ No ☐ Yes: _____
   allergies   ☐ No ☐ Yes: _____

2. List all illnesses, injuries, and health concerns you have now or have had in the past 3 years.
   (Examples: arthritis, diabetes, car accident, pregnancy) _____
   _____

3. List medications and pain relievers taken today. _____
   _____

4. I have provided all my known medical information. I acknowledge that manual therapy is not
   a substitute for medical diagnosis and treatment. I give my consent to receive treatment.

   Signature _____   Date _____

   Tx: _____

   _____

   C: _____

   _____

initials _____

251

Name _____ Current Meds _____

Tx: _____

C: _____

date _____ initials _____

Tx: _____

C: _____

date _____ initials _____

Tx: _____

C: _____

date _____ initials _____

Tx: _____

C: _____

date _____ initials _____

SPORTS HxTxC CHART

Provider Name _____ Date _____

Event or Race _____ Location _____

Ask each athlete the following: (Note individual responses below—concerns only.)

1. Are you currently experiencing any of the following?
   - pain, tenderness, stiffness
   - swelling
   - numbness, tingling
   - dizziness
   - cold, clammy skin
   - shaking

2. How soon do you compete? / When did you finish competing?

3. Have you warmed up? / Cooled down?

4. Have you consumed water since the event?

Athlete's Name _____

Hx: (note concerns) _____

Tx: (check all that apply) _____ Pre-event _____ Post-event _____ Refer-first aid/med

C: _____

_____ Initials: _____

Athlete's Name _____

Hx: (note concerns) _____

Tx: (check all that apply) _____ Pre-event _____ Post-event _____ Refer-first aid/med

C: _____

_____ Initials: _____

Athlete's Name _____

Hx: (note concerns) _____

Tx: (check all that apply) _____ Pre-event _____ Post-event _____ Refer-first aid/med

C: _____

_____ Initials: _____

Athlete's Name _____

Hx: (note concerns) _____

Tx: (check all that apply) _____ Pre-event _____ Post-event _____ Refer-first aid/med

C: _____

_____ Initials: _____

Provider Name _____ **RANGE OF MOTION**

Patient Name _____ Date _____

Date of Injury_____ Insurance ID# _____

PRE-TEST 1 (circle test parameters)

Position of patient: prone, sidelying, sitting, standing, supine, other: _____

Type of test: active, active assisted, passive, resistive, other: _____

Joint: C-spine, T-spine, L-spine, hip, knee, ankle, shoulder, elbow, wrist, other: _____

Action	Range+Int		Pain+Int		Ltd+Int		Mvmt+Int	
	Ⓡ	Ⓛ	Ⓡ	Ⓛ	Ⓡ	Ⓛ	Ⓡ	Ⓛ

POST-TEST 1 (circle test parameters)

Position of patient: prone, sidelying, sitting, standing, supine, other: _____

Type of test: active, active assisted, passive, resistive, other: _____

Joint: C-spine, T-spine, L-spine, hip, knee, ankle, shoulder, elbow, wrist, other: _____

Action	Range+Int		Pain+Int		Ltd+Int		Mvmt+Int	
	Ⓡ	Ⓛ	Ⓡ	Ⓛ	Ⓡ	Ⓛ	Ⓡ	Ⓛ

PRE-TEST 2 (circle test parameters)

Position of patient: prone, sidelying, sitting, standing, supine, other: _____

Type of test: active, active assisted, passive, resistive, other: _____

Joint: C-spine, T-spine, L-spine, hip, knee, ankle, shoulder, elbow, wrist, other: _____

Action	Range+Int		Pain+Int		Ltd+Int		Mvmt+Int	
	Ⓡ	Ⓛ	Ⓡ	Ⓛ	Ⓡ	Ⓛ	Ⓡ	Ⓛ

POST-TEST 2 (circle test parameters)

Position of patient: prone, sidelying, sitting, standing, supine, other: _____

Type of test: active, active assisted, passive, resistive, other: _____

Joint: C-spine, T-spine, L-spine, hip, knee, ankle, shoulder, elbow, wrist, other: _____

Action	Range+Int		Pain+Int		Ltd+Int		Mvmt+Int	
	Ⓡ	Ⓛ	Ⓡ	Ⓛ	Ⓡ	Ⓛ	Ⓡ	Ⓛ

PRE-TEST 3 (circle test parameters)

Position of patient: prone, sidelying, sitting, standing, supine, other: _____

Type of test: active, active assisted, passive, resistive, other: _____

Joint: C-spine, T-spine, L-spine, hip, knee, ankle, shoulder, elbow, wrist, other: _____

Action	Range+Int		Pain+Int		Ltd+Int		Mvmt+Int	
	Ⓡ	Ⓛ	Ⓡ	Ⓛ	Ⓡ	Ⓛ	Ⓡ	Ⓛ

POST-TEST 3 (circle test parameters)

Position of patient: prone, sidelying, sitting, standing, supine, other: _____

Type of test: active, active assisted, passive, resistive, other: _____

Joint: C-spine, T-spine, L-spine, hip, knee, ankle, shoulder, elbow, wrist, other: _____

Action	Range+Int		Pain+Int		Ltd+Int		Mvmt+Int	
	Ⓡ	Ⓛ	Ⓡ	Ⓛ	Ⓡ	Ⓛ	Ⓡ	Ⓛ

Directions for charting Range of Motion Results: For each test, fill in the form blanks as follows:
ACTION - Identify the action tested: abd, add, DF, ever, ext, ext rot, flex, int rot, inv, lat flex, PF, pro, SB, and Sup
RANGE - Identify the deviation from normal: ↓ (hypomobility), ↑ (hypermobility)
INTENSITY (INT) - Rate the intensity of each finding. L, M, S; 0–5, 0–10; N, G, F, P (normal, good, fair, poor)
PAIN - Identify if pain is present with movement: √ (present), Ø (absent)
LIMITATIONS (LTD) - Identify the cause of the limitation. For example: Adh, ed, HT, LB, Ⓟ, Sp, TP, etc.
MOVEMENT (MVMT) - Identify the quality of the movement: sm, seg, Sp, rig, (smooth, segmented, spastic, rigid)

INSURANCE STATUS—PERSONAL INJURY

Patient Name _____ Date _____

Date of Injury _____ Insurance ID# _____

A. Reporting to Attorney

Which information would you like to receive monthly and how do you prefer to receive information:

☐ copies of billing   ☐ fax
☐ monthly statements   ☐ mail
☐ SOAP charts   ☐ email
☐ Progress reports   ☐ upon request

B. Primary Insurance Coverage

Please provide the following information regarding your client's/my patient's insurance status:

Insured _____
Insurance ID# _____
Insurance Carrier _____
Billing Address _____
City _____ State _____ Zip _____
Adjuster _____
Phone _____ Fax _____
PIP policy amount $ _____
Dates of coverage _____
PIP available $ _____
Med Pay policy amount $ _____
Dates of coverage _____
Med Pay available $ _____

C. Secondary Insurance Coverage

Insured _____
Insurance ID# _____
Insurance Carrier _____
Billing Address _____
City _____ State _____ Zip _____
Adjuster _____
Phone _____ Fax _____
PIP policy amount $ _____
Dates of coverage _____
PIP available $ _____
Med Pay policy amount $ _____
Dates of coverage _____
Med Pay available $ _____

If secondary coverage is through the patients' private health insurance, is manual therapy a covered benefit: ☐ Yes   ☐ No   ☐ Don't Know

D. Third Party Insurance Coverage

Insured _____
Insurance ID# _____
Insurance Carrier _____
Billing Address _____
City _____ State _____ Zip _____
Adjuster _____
Phone _____ Fax _____
Liability policy amount $ _____
Dates of coverage _____
Liability available $ _____
Uninsured/underinsured Motorist (UIM)$ _____
Policy Amount $ _____
UIM available $ _____

CONTRACTUAL GUARANTEE OF PAYMENT FOR MEDICAL SERVICES

I hereby authorize and direct you, my attorney, to pay directly to my health care provider(s), _____, the total dollar amount owing for health care services, including applicable interest charges, provided for injuries arising from the motor vehicle accident on _____. I hereby authorize my attorney and the involved insurance companies to withhold sums from any settlement, judgment, or verdict as may be necessary to adequately protect my health care provider(s) and their office. I hereby further consent to a lien being filed on my case by said health care provider(s) and their office against any and all proceeds of my settlement, judgment, or verdict which may be paid to you, my attorney, or myself as the result of the injuries for which I have been treated.

I agree never to rescind this document and that any attempt at recession will not be honored by my attorney. I hereby instruct that in the event another attorney is substituted in this matter, the new attorney shall honor this Contractual Guarantee of Payment for Health Care Services as inherent in the settlement and enforceable upon the case as if it were executed by him/her.

I fully understand that I am directly and fully responsible to said health care provider(s) or their office for all health care bills submitted by them for services rendered to me. Further, this agreement is made solely for said health care providers' additional protection and in consideration of their forbearance on payment. I also understand that such payment is not contingent on any settlement, judgment, or verdict by which I may eventually recover damages.

I specifically request my attorney to acknowledge this letter by signing below and returning it to the office of said health care provider(s). I have been advised that if my attorney does not wish to cooperate in protecting the health care providers' interest, the health care provider(s) will not await payment, but will require me to make payments on a current basis.

Date _____ Patient's Signature _____

Patient's Social Security Number or Driver's License Number _____

The undersigned, being attorney of record for the above patient, does hereby agree to observe all the terms of the above, and agrees to withhold such sums from any settlement, judgment, or verdict as may be necessary to adequately protect said health care provider(s) named above.

Date _____ Attorney's Signature _____

Please date, sign, and return one original to _____

_____

_____

_____

_____

THANK YOU.

Revised and reprinted with permission, Adler ◆ Giersch, PS

INSURANCE VERIFICATION

Provider Name _____

Name _____ Date _____

Date of Injury _____ Insurance ID# _____

A. Patient Information

Employment

Employer _____

Phone _____ Fax _____

Currently Employed? ☐ Y ☐ N

Effective date of benefits _____

Expiration date of benefits _____

Contact name _____

Date/Time verified _____

Attorney

Name _____

Phone _____ Fax _____

Guarantee of Payment filed? ☐ Y ☐ N

Medical Lien filed? ☐ Y ☐ N

   Date _____ Expires _____

   Renewed _____ Expires _____

Copies of patient file requests

   Date requested _____ Date sent _____

   Date requested _____ Date sent _____

Primary Health Care Provider

Name _____

Phone _____ Fax _____

Attending provider for this injury/illness? ☐ Y ☐ N

Referring provider for manual therapy services? ☐ Y ☐ N

Prescription received? ☐ Y ☐ N

Prescription date _____ # of Tx _____

   Tx duration/frequency_____

   Diagnosis (ICD-10 codes) _____

   _____

First Renewal date _____ # of Tx _____

   Tx duration/frequency_____

Second Renewal date _____ # of Tx _____

   Tx duration/frequency_____

B. Insurance Information

Workers Compensation Insurance

Contact _____

Phone _____ Fax _____

Date/Time verified _____

   Is claim open? ☐ Y ☐ N

   Date Opened _____ Date Closed _____

   Date Reopened _____

Private Health Insurance

Insurer_____

Contact _____

Phone _____ Fax _____

Date/Time verified _____

Personal Injury Insurance

Primary Insurer_____

  Adjuster _____

  Phone _____ Fax _____

  Date/Time verified _____

    PIP policy amount $ _____

    Dates of coverage _____

    PIP available $ _____

    Med Pay policy amount $ _____

    Dates of coverage _____

    Med Pay available $ _____

Secondary Insurer _____

  Adjuster _____

  Phone _____ Fax _____

  Date/Time verified _____

    PIP policy amount $ _____

    Dates of coverage _____

    PIP available $ _____

    Med Pay policy amount $ _____

    Dates of coverage _____

    Med Pay available $ _____

C. Verify Benefits/Authorize Services

Ask the insurance representative the following questions regarding the patient's coverage:

1. Is manual therapy a covered benefit? ☐ Y ☐ N
2. Is the patient eligible for the manual therapy benefit for this condition (supply diagnosis/ICD-10 codes)? ☐ Y ☐ N
3. Am I eligible to provide manual therapy services (supply professional license/certification)? ☐ Y ☐ N

If the answer to any one of these questions is No, bill the patient for manual therapy services.

If the answer to all three questions is Yes, continue verification on page two, and bill the insurance company for manual therapy services.

C. Verify Benefits/Authorize Services, cont.

Record the answers you get to questions 4, 5, and 6 in this table. In the first column list the services you provide. In the second column, record the corresponding CPT code. Complete the table with the answers you get to questions 4, 5, and 6.

4. Which manual therapy services are authorized? (Go through each one listed below.)
5. Are there any restrictions or limitations to each authorized service?
6. What is the maximum allowable reimbursement rate for each authorized service?

Service Item	CPT code	4. Authorized?	5. Restrictions?	6. Max Rate?
1. _____	_____	☐Y ☐N	_____	_____
2. _____	_____	☐Y ☐N	_____	_____
3. _____	_____	☐Y ☐N	_____	_____
4. _____	_____	☐Y ☐N	_____	_____
5. _____	_____	☐Y ☐N	_____	_____
6. _____	_____	☐Y ☐N	_____	_____
7. _____	_____	☐Y ☐N	_____	_____
8. _____	_____	☐Y ☐N	_____	_____
9. _____	_____	☐Y ☐N	_____	_____
10. _____	_____	☐Y ☐N	_____	_____

Complete 7-17 as applicable

7. Does a deductible apply? ☐Y ☐N Amount $ _____

Paid to date $ _____

Policy year dates _____

8. Does a Co-Pay apply? ☐Y ☐N Amount $ _____

9. Does a co-insurance apply? ☐Y ☐N Amount % _____

10. Is there a limit on the # of sessions per policy year?

☐Y ☐N Total per year _____

Number available to date _____

11. Is there a limit on the total $ spent on these services or similar services per policy year? ☐Y ☐N Amount $ _____

Amount available to date _____

12. Treatment dates authorized _____

13. Number of sessions authorized _____

14. Preferred billing method/form:

☐HCFA 1500 ☐Electronic ☐Other _____

15. Send with each bill:

☐Prescription ☐SOAP notes ☐Progress Reports

☐License/Certification ☐Other _____

16. What is the expected turnaround time on claim reimbursement? _____

17. Are you able to authorize payment? ☐Y ☐N

If Yes, authorization # _____

If No, can you connect me with someone who is able to authorize payment? ☐Y ☐N

Name _____

Phone _____ Fax _____

Send a copy of this form to the insurance representative with a letter confirming the information gathered.

Date sent _____

Re-Authorization/Verification

Contact _____

Phone _____ Fax _____

Date/Time verified _____

Treatment dates authorized _____

Number of sessions authorized _____

Is payment authorized? ☐Y ☐N

Authorization # _____

Confirmation sent? ☐Y ☐N Date sent _____

Verify remainder of policy year, if applicable:

1. Deductible paid to date $ _____

2. Total # of sessions to date _____

3. Total $ spent to date $ _____

Re-Authorization/Verification

Contact _____

Phone _____ Fax _____

Date/Time verified _____

Treatment dates authorized _____

Number of sessions authorized _____

Is payment authorized? ☐Y ☐N

Authorization # _____

Confirmation sent? ☐Y ☐N Date sent _____

Verify remainder of policy year, if applicable:

1. Deductible paid to date $ _____

2. Total # of sessions to date _____

3. Total $ spent to date $ _____

Provider Name _____ **RE-AUTHORIZATION / VERIFICATION**

Patient Name _____ Date _____

Date of Injury_____ Insurance ID# _____

Re-Authorization/Verification

Contact _____
Phone_____ Fax _____
Date/Time verified _____
Treatment dates authorized _____
Number of sessions authorized _____
Is payment authorized? ☐Y ☐N
  Authorization # _____
Confirmation sent? ☐Y ☐N Date sent _____
Verify remainder of policy year, if applicable:
1. Deductible paid to date $ _____
2. Total # of sessions to date _____
3. Total $ spent to date $ _____

Re-Authorization/Verification

Contact _____
Phone_____ Fax _____
Date/Time verified _____
Treatment dates authorized _____
Number of sessions authorized _____
Is payment authorized? ☐Y ☐N
  Authorization # _____
Confirmation sent? ☐Y ☐N Date sent _____
Verify remainder of policy year, if applicable:
1. Deductible paid to date $ _____
2. Total # of sessions to date _____
3. Total $ spent to date $ _____

Re-Authorization/Verification

Contact _____
Phone_____ Fax _____
Date/Time verified _____
Treatment dates authorized _____
Number of sessions authorized _____
Is payment authorized? ☐Y ☐N
  Authorization # _____
Confirmation sent? ☐Y ☐N Date sent _____
Verify remainder of policy year, if applicable:
1. Deductible paid to date $ _____
2. Total # of sessions to date _____
3. Total $ spent to date $ _____

Re-Authorization/Verification

Contact _____
Phone_____ Fax _____
Date/Time verified _____
Treatment dates authorized _____
Number of sessions authorized _____
Is payment authorized? ☐Y ☐N
  Authorization # _____
Confirmation sent? ☐Y ☐N Date sent _____
Verify remainder of policy year, if applicable:
1. Deductible paid to date $ _____
2. Total # of sessions to date _____
3. Total $ spent to date $ _____

Re-Authorization/Verification

Contact _____
Phone_____ Fax _____
Date/Time verified _____
Treatment dates authorized _____
Number of sessions authorized _____
Is payment authorized? ☐Y ☐N
  Authorization # _____
Confirmation sent? ☐Y ☐N Date sent _____
Verify remainder of policy year, if applicable:
1. Deductible paid to date $ _____
2. Total # of sessions to date _____
3. Total $ spent to date $ _____

Re-Authorization/Verification

Contact _____
Phone_____ Fax _____
Date/Time verified _____
Treatment dates authorized _____
Number of sessions authorized _____
Is payment authorized? ☐Y ☐N
  Authorization # _____
Confirmation sent? ☐Y ☐N Date sent _____
Verify remainder of policy year, if applicable:
1. Deductible paid to date $ _____
2. Total # of sessions to date _____
3. Total $ spent to date $ _____

259

PAYMENT LOG

Name _____ Date _____

Date of Injury_____ Insurance ID# _____

Billing Date: _____ Total Billed: $ _____

Patient Paid: $ _____ Insurance Paid: $ _____ Total Paid: $ _____

If Total Paid does NOT equal Total Billed, complete below for each date of service (from lines 1-6, Section 24 of HCFA 1500)

Line 1, Initial Billing

Treatment Date: _____ Bill Date: _____

Charges: _____ Adjustments: _____ Amount Billed: _____

Due from patient: _____ Due from Insurance: _____

Patient Paid: _____ Insurance paid: _____

Line 1, Rebilling

Rebill Date: _____ Rebilled to: _____

Outstanding: _____ Interest: _____ Amount Billed: _____

Rebill Date: _____ Rebilled to: _____

Outstanding: _____ Interest: _____ Amount Billed: _____

Rebill Date: _____ Rebilled to: _____

Outstanding: _____ Interest: _____ Amount Billed: _____

Line 2, Initial Billing

Treatment Date: _____ Bill Date: _____

Charges: _____ Adjustments: _____ Amount Billed: _____

Due from patient: _____ Due from Insurance: _____

Patient Paid: _____ Insurance paid: _____

Line 2, Rebilling

Rebill Date: _____ Rebilled to: _____

Outstanding: _____ Interest: _____ Amount Billed: _____

Rebill Date: _____ Rebilled to: _____

Outstanding: _____ Interest: _____ Amount Billed: _____

Rebill Date: _____ Rebilled to: _____

Outstanding: _____ Interest: _____ Amount Billed: _____

Line 3, Initial Billing

Treatment Date: _____ Bill Date: _____

Charges: _____ Adjustments: _____ Amount Billed: _____

Due from patient: _____ Due from Insurance: _____

Patient Paid: _____ Insurance paid: _____

Line 3, Rebilling

Rebill Date: _____ Rebilled to: _____

Outstanding: _____ Interest: _____ Amount Billed: _____

Rebill Date: _____ Rebilled to: _____

Outstanding: _____ Interest: _____ Amount Billed: _____

Rebill Date: _____ Rebilled to: _____

Outstanding: _____ Interest: _____ Amount Billed: _____

Line 4, Initial Billing

Treatment Date: _____ Bill Date: _____

Charges: _____ Adjustments: _____ Amount Billed: _____

Due from patient: _____ Due from Insurance: _____

Patient Paid: _____ Insurance paid: _____

Line 4, Rebilling

Rebill Date: _____ Rebilled to: _____

Outstanding: _____ Interest: _____ Amount Billed: _____

Rebill Date: _____ Rebilled to: _____

Outstanding: _____ Interest: _____ Amount Billed: _____

Rebill Date: _____ Rebilled to: _____

Outstanding: _____ Interest: _____ Amount Billed: _____

Line 5, Initial Billing

Treatment Date: _____ Bill Date: _____

Charges: _____ Adjustments: _____ Amount Billed: _____

Due from patient: _____ Due from Insurance: _____

Patient Paid: _____ Insurance paid: _____

Line 5, Rebilling

Rebill Date: _____ Rebilled to: _____

Outstanding: _____ Interest: _____ Amount Billed: _____

Rebill Date: _____ Rebilled to: _____

Outstanding: _____ Interest: _____ Amount Billed: _____

Rebill Date: _____ Rebilled to: _____

Outstanding: _____ Interest: _____ Amount Billed: _____

Line 6, Initial Billing

Treatment Date: _____ Bill Date: _____

Charges: _____ Adjustments: _____ Amount Billed: _____

Due from patient: _____ Due from Insurance: _____

Patient Paid: _____ Insurance paid: _____

Line 6, Rebilling

Rebill Date: _____ Rebilled to: _____

Outstanding: _____ Interest: _____ Amount Billed: _____

Rebill Date: _____ Rebilled to: _____

Outstanding: _____ Interest: _____ Amount Billed: _____

Rebill Date: _____ Rebilled to: _____

Outstanding: _____ Interest: _____ Amount Billed: _____

Case Studies

Personal Injury

Flow Charts: Use of Intake Forms, Progress Summaries, Treatment Notes, and Billing Forms as needed for Personal Injury Cases, Workers' Compensation, and Wellness Care.

This flow chart demonstrates which forms are recommended for use with patients involved in personal injury cases: who completes the form, how often the form is used, and any additional comments for using the form.

Personal Injury INTAKE FORMS	Who	Frequency	Comments
Fees and Policies	Patient	initial visit	update as needed
Health Information	Patient	initial visit	update annually
History section of HxTxC	—		
Injury Information, part 1	Patient	initial visit	per incident
Injury Information, part 2	Patient	initial visit	per incident
Billing Information	Patient	initial visit	if you provide billing services
Prescription	HCP	as needed	a progress report should precede each renewal

PROGRESS SUMMARIES			
Health Report	Patient	monthly	patient reports current status
Pain Questionnaires	Patient	monthly	daily or weekly, if used as a pain journal
Initial Report w/o Tx	MT	as needed	if patient does not receive tx
Initial Report w/ Tx	MT	initial visit	summarizes tx and proposes tx plan
Progress Report	MT	monthly	practitioner reports to HCP
Narrative Report	MT	1x	if requested by patient's attorney

TREATMENT NOTES			
Initial SOAP	MT	initial visit	summarizes all findings; sets goals, plan
Subsequent SOAP	MT	each visit	(excluding initial, progress, and discharge sessions) brief, focused
Progress SOAP	MT	monthly	summarizes all findings; updates goals, plan
Discharge SOAP	MT	final visit	summarizes all findings; ongoing care plan
HxTxC	—		
Range of Motion	MT	as needed	

BILLING FORMS			
Insurance Status–Personal Injury	Attny	as needed	if patient has an attorney
Guarantee of Payment	MT, patient, Attny		if end-of-settlement case
Insurance Verification	MT	as needed	with renewal of prescribed services
HCFA 1500 billing form	MT	each visit	may bill for multiple sessions per HCFA form after initial billing if total amount is under $250
Payment Log	MT	as needed	if payments do not match bills

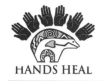

John Olson, LMP, GCFP
345 Moon River Rd. Ste. 6
Minnehaha, MN   55987
Tel   612 555 9889

FEES AND POLICIES

A. Fee Schedule

Fees for services are as follows:

- CranioSacral/Lymph Drainage $80 per hour
  (97140)   ($20 per 15 minute units)
- Feldenkrais $80 per hour
  (97112)   ($20 per 15 minute unit)
- Hot and Cold Packs $15 per session
  (97101)   ($15 per session)
- Therapeutic Massage $60 Per Hour
  (97124)   ($15 per 15 minute unit)

B. Payment Policies

Cash or Check

- A 10% discount is available when payment is made at the time services are provided.
- Pre-payment discounts: 6 sessions for the price of 5.

Billing

I will bill your insurance company directly under the following conditions:

Private Health: verbal verification of coverage
Worker's Compensation: verbal verification of coverage

Auto Accident

- PIP: verbal verification of coverage
- Second Party Coverage: written verification of coverage
- Third Party Coverage: health care lien will be filed and/or letter of guarantee signed by the patient's attorney

All insurance accounts not paid in full within 90 days from date of service will be charged interest. Interest rates are 12% annually and are charged at 1% monthly. Interest is calculated on the principal amount; interest is not compounded.

C. Office Policies

Cancellations

Cancellations must be made 24 hours in advance of the scheduled appointment time. If cancellations are not made within 24 hours, payment in full is required. This charge will be waived if a replacement can be found for your appointment time. Your insurance company will not be charged for your missed appointment; you will be responsible for payment out-of-pocket.

Right of Refusal

I reserve the right to refuse service to anyone. This includes but is not limited to anyone who requests treatment or services that are outside my scope of practice. I will exercise this right if anyone arrives for treatment under the influence of alcohol or recreational drugs; I reserve the right to charge for the session time, whether or not services were rendered, if I so choose.

Patient Agreement

I have read the policies stated above and agree to abide by them.

Signature ___Darnel G. Washington_____   Date ___2-6-01___

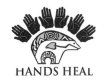

HANDS HEAL

John Olson, LMP, GCFP

345 Moon River Rd. Ste. 6
Minnehaha, MN   55987
Tel   612 555 9889

HEALTH INFORMATION

Patient Name   Darnel G. Washington   Date 2-6-01

Date of Injury   1-6-01   Insurance ID#   123-45-6789

A. Patient Information

Address   1209 Lake Winnetonka Dr.

City Minnehaha   State MN Zip 55987

Phone: Home   (612) 555-1515

  Work   N/A   Cell/Pgr   555-5511

Date of Birth   4-22-37

Employer   IBM

Occupation   retired

Emergency Contact   Shalonda-wife

Phone: Home   same

  Work N/A   Cell/Pgr   555-5511

Primary Health Care Provider

Name Sage Redtree, MD

Address   87 Old Trail Pkwy

City/State/Zip   Minnehaha MN 55987

Phone: 555-0009   Fax 555-9000

I give my manual therapist permission to consult with my referring health care provider regarding my health and treatment.

Comments

Initials DGW   Date 2-6-02

B. Current Health Information

List Health/Concerns Check all that apply

Primary   back pain

☐ mild ☒ moderate ☐ disabling

☒ constant ☐ intermittant

☐ symptoms ↑ w/activity   ☐ ↓ w/activity

☒ getting worse ☐ getting better ☐ no change

treatment received   pain pills, back brace

Secondary   headaches

☐ mild ☒ moderate ☐ disabling

☐ constant ☒ intermittant

☐ symptoms ↑ w/activity   ☐ ↓ w/activity

☒ getting worse ☐ getting better ☐ no change

treatment received   pain pills

Additional   neck stiff

☒ mild ☐ moderate ☐ disabling

☒ constant ☐ intermittant

☐ symptoms ↑ w/activity   ☐ ↓ w/activity

☐ getting worse ☒ getting better ☐ no change

treatment received   stretching

Have you ever received Manual Therapy before? ☐ Y ☒ N Frequency? _____

List all conditions currently monitored by a Health Care Provider   scoliosis

List the medications you took today (include pain relievers and herbal remedies) hydrocodone

List all other medications taken in the last 3 months   flu vaccination

List Daily Activities

Work   N/A

Home/Family   gardening, vacuuming

Social/Recreational play w/ grandchildren, dancing, bowling, bridge group

Circle the activities affected by your condition, ☒ all of the above

Check other activities affected: ☒ sleep

☐ washing ☐ dressing ☒ fitness

How do you reduce stress? watch sports, garden

Pain?   heat, back brace, meds

What are your goals for receiving Manual Therapy? get around easier, less pain

C. Health History

List and Explain. Include dates and treatment received.

Surgeries   appendicitis 1949 removed, torn meniseus ⓇT knee 1980 arthoscopy

Accidents   bowling injury ⓇT knee 1979 no treatment until surgery 1980

Major Illnesses   scoliosis 1949 Milwaukee brace, exercise, pain meds

General

current	past		comments
☒	☐	headaches	
☒	☒	pain	*scoliosis*
☒	☐	sleep disturbances	*can't get comfortable*
☐	☒	fatigue	*scoliosis*
☐	☐	infectious	
☐	☐	fever	
☐	☐	sinus	
☐	☐	other	

Skin Conditions

current	past		comments
☐	☐	rashes	
☐	☐	athlete's foot, warts	
☐	☐	other	

Allergies

current	past		comments
☐	☐	scents, oils, lotions	
☐	☐	detergents	
☐	☐	other	

Muscles and Joints

current	past		comments
☐	☐	rheumatoid arthritis	
☒	☐	osteoarthritis	
☐	☐	osteoporosis	
☒	☒	scoliosis	
☐	☐	broken bones	
☐	☐	spinal problems	
☐	☐	disk problems	
☐	☐	lupus	
☐	☐	TMJ, jaw pain	
☐	☐	spasms, cramps	
☐	☐	sprains, strains	
☐	☐	tendonitis, bursitis	
☐	☐	stiff or painful joints	
☐	☒	weak or sore muscles	*scoliosis*
☐	☐	neck, shoulder, arm pain	
☒	☒	low back, hip, leg pain	*MVA, scoliosis*
☐	☐	other	

Nervous System

current	past		comments
☐	☐	head injuries, concussions	
☐	☐	dizziness, ringing in the ears	
☐	☐	loss of memory, confusion	
☐	☐	numbness, tingling	
☐	☐	sciatica, shooting pain	
☐	☐	chronic pain	
☐	☐	depression	
☐	☐	other	

Respiratory, Cardiovascular

current	past		comments
☐	☐	heart disease	
☐	☐	blood clots	
☐	☐	stroke	
☐	☐	lymphadema	
☐	☐	high, low blood pressure	
☐	☐	irregular heart beat	
☐	☐	poor circulation	
☐	☐	swollen ankles	
☐	☐	varicose veins	
☐	☐	chest pain, shortness of breath	
☐	☐	asthma	

Digestive/Elimination System

current	past		comments
☐	☐	bowel dysfunction	
☐	☐	gas, bloating	
☐	☐	bladder/kidney dysfunction	
☐	☐	abdominal pain	
☐	☐	other	

Endocrine System

current	past		comments
☐	☐	thyroid dysfunction	
☐	☐	diabetes	

Reproductive System

current	past		comments
☐	☐	pregnancy	
☐	☐	painful, emotional menses	
☐	☐	fibrotic cysts	

Cancer/Tumors

current	past		comments
☐	☐	benign	
☐	☐	malignant	

Habits

current	past		comments
☐	☒	tobacco	*quit chew 30 yrs ago*
☐	☐	alcohol	
☐	☐	drugs	
☒	☐	coffee, soda	*1-2 cups/day*

Contract for Care

I promise to participate fully as a member of my health care team. I will make sound choices regarding my treatment plan based on the information provided by my manual therapist and other members of my health care team, and my experience of those suggestions. I agree to participate in the self care program we select. I promise to inform my practitioner any time I feel my well-being is threatened or compromised. I expect my manual therapist to provide safe and effective treatment.

Consent for Care

It is my choice to receive manual therapy, and I give my consent to receive treatment. I have reported all health conditions that I am aware of and will inform my practitioner of any changes in my health.

Signature   *Darnel G. Washington*   Date   *2-6-01*

Signature of parent or guardian _____   Date _____
(If patient is a minor)

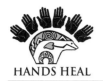

HANDS HEAL

John Olson, LMP, GCFP
345 Moon River Rd. Ste. 6
Minnehaha, MN   55987
TEL   612 555 9889

INJURY INFORMATION

Patient Name   _Darnel G. Washington_   Date _2-6-01_

Date of Injury _1-6-01_   Insurance ID# _123-45-6789_

A. General Injury Information

1. How did the accident occur?
   ☒ Auto   ☐ On-the-Job   ☐ Other _____

2. Was a police report filed?   ☒ Yes   ☐ No
   Was a work incident report filed?
   ☐ Yes   ☒ No

3. Describe your injury and how it occurred:
   My nephew was driving. We were slowing
   down for a yellow light and a truck hit us
   from behind

4. Describe how you felt during and
   immediately after the injury:
   fine

   Later that same day: _soreness and stiff neck_
   and back after sitting at hockey game, headache
   The next day: _headache - pounding, stiff and_
   sore neck and back

   The next week: _headache worse, neck_
   stiffness better but back pain worse
   The next month: _headache and back pain_

   Describe any bruises, cuts, or abrasions
   as a result of the injury:
   _0_

5. Are your symptoms ☐ getting better
   ☒ getting worse   ☐ no change
   What makes them better? _____
   nothing yet

   Worse? _sitting, lifting grandkids,_
   pushing them in swing, bending over in
   garden

6. Did you return to work on the day of the
   injury? ☐ Yes   ☐ No
   Have you lost time from work since the
   injury? ☐ Yes   ☐ No

7. What are your work responsibilities?

   _N/A_

   Which work activities are affected by this
   injury? _____

   Have your work responsibilities changed as
   a result of this injury? ☐ Yes   ☐ No
   Explain _____
   What other daily activities are affected by
   this injury? _____

8. Did you go to the emergency room?
   ☐ Yes   ☒ No
   Were you hospitalized?   ☐ Yes   ☒ No
   List the health care providers who have
   treated you for this injury, the type of
   treatment provided, and their diagnosis.
   Dr. Redtree—pain pills, back support,
   stretching exercises, says I have mild
   whiplash and a reoccurance of scolios

9. Have you ever had this type of injury
   before? ☒ Yes   ☐ No
   Explain _I've had scoliosis most of my life._

   Did you have any physical complaints
   before the injury? ☐ Yes   ☒ No
   Explain _My scoliosis wasn't bothering_
   me at all

   Do you have any illnesses or previous
   injuries that may have been affected by
   this injury? ☒ Yes   ☐ No
   Explain _just the scoliosis_

Signature   _Darnel G. Washington_   Date _2-6-01_

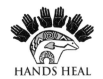

HANDS HEAL

John Olson, LMP, GCFP
345 Moon River Rd. Ste. 6
Minnehaha, MN   55987
Tᴇʟ   612 555 9889

B. Motor Vehicle Accident Information

1. Did the police arrive at the accident?
   ☒ Yes   ☐ No

2. How was your vehicle hit?
   ☒ Rear end   ☐ Head on   ☐ Side swipe
   OR Did your vehicle hit another vehicle/object?
   ☐ Rear end   ☐ Head on   ☐ Side swipe
   If you were hit from behind, was your vehicle pushed forward upon impact?
   ☒ Yes   ☐ No   If yes, how much?
   about 50 feet
   Did your vehicle hit anything else after the initial impact?   ☐ Yes   ☐ No
   Explain _____
   _____
   _____
   _____

3. Were you at a stop or moving at the time of impact?   ☐ Stopped   ☒ Moving
   If you were stopped, was your foot on the brake?   ☐ Yes   ☐ No
   If you were moving, were you:
   ☐ Increasing speed
   ☒ Decreasing speed
   ☐ Traveling at a steady speed
   Was the other vehicle moving at the time of impact?   ☒ Yes   ☐ No
   If yes, was it: ☒ Increasing speed
   ☐ Decreasing speed   ☐ Traveling at a steady speed

4. Where were you seated in the vehicle?
   passenger side-front seat
   _____
   _____

5. Which way was your head facing upon impact?
   facing nephew-driver, we were talking
   _____
   _____

6. Were you aware of the approaching vehicle or did the impact catch you by surprise?
   ☐ Aware   ☒ Surprise

7. Did you lose consciousness?
   ☐ Yes   ☒ No

8. Were you wearing a seat belt?   ☐ No
   ☐ Lap belt   ☐ Shoulder harness   ☒ Both

9. Is your vehicle equipped with an airbag?
   ☐ Yes ☒ No
   Did it activate?   ☐ Yes   ☐ No

10. Is the top of your head rest:
    ☐ Above your head   ☒ Below your head
    Does your head touch the head rest?
    ☐ Yes   ☒ No
    If no, how far in front of the head rest is your head?
    a few inches

11. What were the road conditions?
    ☐ Wet   ☐ Dry   ☒ Icy   ☐ Oily

12. What type of vehicle were you in? (make, model, year)
    '82 Honda Accord
    What type of vehicle hit you? (make, model, year)
    '91 Ford F250 Truck

13. Did any part of your body come into contact with the vehicle?   ☐ Yes   ☒ No
    Explain _____
    _____
    _____
    Did any parts of the vehicle break?
    ☒ Yes   ☐ No
    Explain _fender damage_
    _____
    _____

14. Check all of the following symptoms that you have experienced since the accident:
    ☐ Loss of memory _____
    ☐ Loss of balance _____
    ☒ Visual disturbances _eye strain_
    ☐ Hearing difficulties _____
    ☒ Difficulty breathing _tight & painful_
    ☒ Sleep disturbances _pain keeps me up_

15. Anything else you want to tell me about the accident or how you feel?
    _____
    _____
    _____

Patient Signature _Darnel G. Washington_   Date _2-6-01_

268

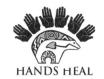

HANDS HEAL

John Olson, LMP, GCFP
345 Moon River Rd. Ste. 6
Minnehaha, MN   55987
TEL   612 555 9889

BILLING INFORMATION

Patient Name **Darnel G. Washington**   Date _____   updated
                                                                    3-15-01
Date of Injury **1-6-01**   Insurance ID# **123-45-6789**   **JO**

A. Patient Information
Address **1209 Lake Winnetonka Dr.**
City **Minnehaha**   State **MN** Zip **55987**
Phone: Home **(612)555-1515**
            Work **N/A**   Cell/Pgr **555-1155**
Date of Birth **4-22-37**
☒ Male   ☐ Female
Marital Status: ☐ Single ☒ Married ☐ Partnered
Relationship of Patient to Insured:
☐ Self ☐ Spouse ☐ Partner ☐ Child ☒ Other
☐ Employed ☐ Student
Employer's Name or School Name:

Phone _____ Fax _____
Is patient's condition related to:
Employment   ☐ Yes   ☒ No
Auto Accident   ☒ Yes   ☐ No
If Auto Accident, in what state? **MN**
Other Accident   ☐ Yes   ☒ No
Illness   ☐ Yes   ☒ No

Primary Health Care Provider
Name **Sage Redtree, MD**
Address **87 Old Trail Pkwy**
City **Minnehaha**   State **MN** Zip **55987**
Phone **(612)555-0009** Fax **555-9000**

Attorney   updated 3-15-01 JO
Has an attorney been consulted? ☒ Yes ☐ No
Retained?   ☒ Yes   ☐ No
Name **B. Charma Storro, JD**
Address **5 Hive Lane**
City **Minnehaha**   State **MN** Zip **55987**
Phone **(612)555-0009** Fax **555-9000**

B. Insured (if other than patient)
Name **James Washington**
Insurance ID# **989-76-6789**
Date of Birth **5-31-60**
☒ Male   ☐ Female
Address **32 W. Holden Court**
City **Minnehaha**   State **MN** Zip **55987**
Phone: Home **(612) 555-7654**
            Work **555-4567** Cell/Pgr **555-6574**
Employer's Name or School Name:
Maad Printing and Design
Phone **555-4567**   Fax **555-7676**

Signature **Darnel G. Washington**

C. Primary Insurance Coverage 3-15-01 JO
Insurance Carrier **Farmington States**
Contact **Clifford Glens**
Group Number **N/A**
Plan # or Name **N/A**
Billing Address **PO Box 3778**
City **O'Claire**   State **MN** Zip **55978**
Phone **(612)555-7887** Fax **555-8778**

D. Secondary Insurance Coverage 3-15-01 JO
Insured **Darnel G. Washington**
Insurance ID# **see patient info**
Date of Birth _____
☐ Male   ☐ Female
Address _____
City _____ State ____ Zip ____
Phone: Home _____
            Work _____ Cell/Pgr _____
Employer's Name or School Name:

Phone _____ Fax _____
Insurance Carrier **Allied**
Contact **Jarma Jones**
Group Number **G 4321**
Plan # or Name **P56789-0**
Billing Address **PO Box 2988**
City **Omaha**   State **NE** Zip **68144**
Phone **(402)555-1991** Fax **555-9119**

E. Assignment of Benefits
My signature below authorizes and directs payment of medical benefits for services billed to my health care provider.

F. Release of Medical Records
My signature below authorizes the release of my medical records including intake forms, chart notes, reports, and billing statements to my attorneys, health care providers, and insurance case managers, for the purpose of processing my claims. (I will inform my practitioner immediately upon signing any exclusive Release of Medical Records with my attorney.)

G. Financial Responsibility
It is my responsibility to pay for all services provided. In the unfortunate event that my insurance company denies payment or makes a partial payment, I am responsible for the balance. If you have contracted with my insurance company at a discount rate and the agreed-upon fee has been satisfied, the balance will be waived.

Date **2-6-01**

HANDS HEAL

John Olson, LMP, GCFP
345 Moon River Rd. Ste. 6
Minnehaha, MN   55987
TEL   612 555 9889

PRESCRIPTION

Patient Name Darnel G. Washington   Date 2-01-02

Date of Injury 1-6-02   Insurance ID# 123-45-6789

A. Diagnosis

(Include ICD-10 codes that specifically
address Manual Therapy Treatment)

Neck Pain   723.1

Spasm   728.85

Thoracic Pain   724.1

Headache   784.0

Condition is related to
- ☒ Auto Accident
- ☐ Work Injury
- ☐ Illness
- ☒ Other: _____

B. Medically Necessary Treatment: Implement Plan as Prescribed Below

Application (Direct & Indirect)
- ☒ Head 1°
- ☒ Neck 1°
- ☒ Chest 1°
- ☒ Shoulders 2°
- ☒ Abdomen 2°
- ☒ Back 1°
- ☒ Lowback/Hips 2°
- ☒ Upper extremities 2°
- ☒ Lower extremities 2°
- ☐ All of the above
- ☐ Other: _____

Duration & Frequency
- ☐ 1× wk for _____ wks
- ☒ 2× wk for 3 wks
- ☐ 3× wk for _____ wks
- ☐ 2× month for _____ months
- ☐ 1× month for _____ months

Specific Instructions:
as needed

Treatment Type
- ☒ Manual Therapy _____
- ☒ Hydrotherapy _____
- ☒ Self-Care Education _____
- ☐ Other _____

Treatment Goals
- ☐ Decrease Pain
- ☐ Decrease Inflammation
- ☐ Decrease Muscle Tension/Spasms
- ☐ Decrease Compensatory Patterns
- ☐ Increase Mobility
- ☐ Increase Strength
- ☐ Restore Function
- ☐ Restore Posture
- ☐ Maintain Associated Structures
- ☒ All of the Above
- ☐ Other _____

C. Referring Health Care Provider (HCP)

Contact Information
HCP Name Sage Redtree MD
Provider No. _____
Address 87 Old Trail PKWY
City Minnehaha   State MN Zip 55987
Phone (612) 555-0009
Fax 555-9000

Reporting
- ☒ Send Report After Initial Visit
- ☒ Send Report at End of Prescription
- ☒ Send Copies of Chart Notes at End of Prescription
- ☒ Fax Information
- ☐ Mail Information
- ☐ Email Information

HCP Signature: Sage Redtree MD   Date 2-01-02

Revised and reprinted with permission, Adler ◆ Giersch, PS

270

John Olson, LMP, GCFP

345 Moon River Rd. Ste. 6
Minnehaha, MN   55987
TEL   612 555 9889

HANDS HEAL

HEALTH REPORT

Patient Name   _Darnel G. Washington_   Date _2-6-01_

Date of Injury _1-6-01_   Insurance ID# _123-45-6789_

A. Draw today's symptoms on the figures.

1. Identify CURRENT symptomatic areas in your body by marking letters on the figures below.
   Use the letters provided in the key to identify the symptoms you are feeling today.
2. Circle the area around each letter, representing the size and shape of each symptom location.

Key
P = pain or tenderness
S = joint or muscle stiffness
N = numbness or tingling

B. Identify the intensity of your symptoms.

1. Pain Scale: Mark a line on the scale to show the amount of pain you are experiencing today.

   No Pain ├──────────────┼──────────────┤ Unbearable Pain   (5.5)

2. Activities Scale: Mark a line on the scale to show the limitations you are experiencing today
   in your daily activities.   (5.5)

   Can Do Anything I Want ├──────────────┼──────────────┤ Cannot Do Anything

C. Comments

_____

_____

_____

_____

Signature _Darnel G. Washington_   Date _2-6-01_

Provider Name _John Olson LMT GCFP_

(revised Oswestry)
LOW BACK PAIN & DISABILITY INDEX

Patient Name _Darnel G. Washington_   Date _2-6-01_

Date of Injury _1-6-01_   Insurance ID# _123-45-6789_

This questionnaire has been designed to give the health care provider information about how your back pain has affected your ability to manage everyday life. Please answer every section and mark in each section only the **ONE** box which applies to you. We realize you may consider that two statements in any one section relate to you, but please just mark the box which most closely describes your problem today.

Section 1 - Pain Intensity
- ☐ The pain comes and goes and is mild.
- ☐ The pain is mild and does not vary much.
- ☐ The pain comes and goes and is moderate.
- ☒ The pain is moderate and does not vary much.   *3*
- ☐ The pain comes and goes and is severe.
- ☐ The pain is severe and does not vary much.

Section 2 - Personal Care
- ☐ I can look after myself normally without causing pain.
- ☐ I can look after myself normally but it causes extra pain.
- ☒ It is painful to look after myself and I am slow and careful.   *2*
- ☐ I need some help but manage most of my personal care.
- ☐ I need help every day in most aspects of self care.
- ☐ I do not get dressed, I wash myself with difficulty, and I stay in bed.

Section 3 - Lifting
- ☐ I can lift heavy weights without extra pain.
- ☐ I can lift heavy weights but it causes extra pain.
- ☐ Pain prevents me from lifting heavy weights off the floor, but I can manage if they are conveniently positioned, e.g. on a table.
- ☒ Pain prevents me from lifting heavy weights, but I can manage light to medium weights if they are conveniently positioned.   *3*
- ☐ I can lift very light weights.
- ☐ I cannot lift or carry anything at all.

Section 4 - Walking
- ☐ I have no pain on walking.
- ☐ I have some pain on walking but it does not increase with distance.
- ☒ I cannot walk more than 1 mile without increasing pain.   *2*
- ☐ I cannot walk more than 1/2 mile without increasing pain.
- ☐ I cannot walk more than 1/4 mile without increasing pain.
- ☐ I cannot walk at all without increasing pain.

Section 5 - Sitting
- ☐ I can sit in any chair as long as I like.
- ☐ I can only sit in my favorite chair as long as I like.
- ☐ Pain prevents me from sitting more than 1 hour.
- ☒ Pain prevents me from sitting more than 1/2 hour.   *3*
- ☐ Pain prevents me from sitting more than 10 minutes.
- ☐ I avoid sitting because it increases my pain straight away.

Section 6 - Standing
- ☐ I can stand as long as I want without pain.
- ☐ I have some pain on standing but it does not increase with time.
- ☒ I cannot stand for longer than 1 hour without increasing pain.   *2*
- ☐ I cannot stand for longer than 1/2 hour without increasing pain.
- ☐ I cannot stand for longer than 10 minutes without increasing pain.
- ☐ I avoid standing because it increases the pain straight away.

Section 7 - Sleeping
- ☐ I have no trouble sleeping.
- ☐ My sleep is slightly disturbed (less than 1 hour sleepless).
- ☐ My sleep is mildly disturbed (1–2 hours sleepless).
- ☒ My sleep is moderately disturbed (2–3 hours sleepless).   *3*
- ☐ My sleep is greatly disturbed (3–5 hours sleepless).
- ☐ My sleep is completely disturbed (5–7 hours sleepless).

Section 8 - Social Life
- ☐ My social life is normal and gives me no pain.
- ☐ My social life is normal but increases the degree of pain.
- ☒ Pain has no significant effect on my social life apart from limiting my more energetic interests, e.g. dancing, etc.   *2*
- ☐ Pain has restricted my social life and I do not go out very often.
- ☐ Pain has restricted my social life to my home.
- ☐ I hardly have any social life because of the pain.

Section 9 - Traveling
- ☐ I get no pain while traveling.
- ☐ I get some pain while traveling but none of my usual forms of travel make it any worse.
- ☒ I get extra pain while traveling but it does not compel me to seek alternate forms of travel.   *2*
- ☐ I get extra pain while traveling which compels me to seek alternative forms of travel.
- ☐ Pain restricts all forms of travel.
- ☐ Pain prevents all forms of travel except that done lying down.

Section 10 - Changing Degree of Pain
- ☐ My pain is rapidly getting better.
- ☐ My pain fluctuates but overall is definitely getting better.
- ☐ My pain seems to be getting better but improvement is slow at present.   *4*
- ☐ My pain is neither getting better nor getting worse.
- ☒ My pain is gradually worsening.
- ☐ My pain is rapidly worsening.

26
x2
52%

Signature _Darnel G. Washington_   Date _2-6-01_

John Olson, LMP, GCFP

345 Moon River Rd. Ste. 6
Minnehaha, MN   55987
TEL   612 555 9889

January 20, 2002

Patient: Darnel G. Washington
DOI: 1-6-01
Claim Number: 123-45-6789
Date of Exam: 1-20-02

Mr. Washington was first seen in my office on 2-6-01 for manual therapy treatment to injuries sustained in a motor vehicle accident on 1-6-01. He was referred by Dr. Sage Redtree, MD, with an initial diagnosis of spinal sprain-strain in the neck, mid-back and low back areas, and headaches. Within 2 months of the accident, Dr. Redtree diagnosed Mr. Washington with a flare-up of scoliosis with accelerated spinal degeneration.

Mr. Washington stated: he was a passenger in a Honda Accord and was rear-ended by a Ford F250 pick-up truck. The Honda was stopping for a yellow light, and the Ford was speeding up to go through the intersection. It was a cold and snowy January afternoon and the roads were slick. The car was pushed across the intersection but did not come in contact with any other vehicles or objects. Mr. Washington was turned to his left in his seat to chat with the driver at the time of impact. His head was thrown from side to side.

Initial Subjective Data:

On 2-6-01, Mr. Washington complained of mild neck pain and stiffness, moderate mid-back pain and stiffness, mild low back stiffness, and a moderate headache. The symptoms were constant since the evening of the accident, and increased in severity when he attempted to lift his granddaughter, garden with his wife, or sit for over 30 minutes playing bridge with the club he presides over.

Initial Objective Findings:

I palpated moderate muscle spasms in the right sternocleidomastoid and scalene muscles, left trapezius and rhomboids, and right quadratus lumborum. Trigger points were elicited with light digital pressure in the paraspinal muscles, intercostals, and diaphragm. Muscle tension was mild to moderate throughout the spinal postural muscles. Cervical range of motion was moderately limited with active flexion and extension, and passive lateral flexion bilateraly. Inflammation was palpable in the cervical and thoracic regions: redness, heat, swelling, and loss of function; pain and inflammation seemed to be preventing full range of motion. Mr. Washington's posture showed a moderate left shoulder elevation with internal rotation, mild right hip elevation, mild "hump" or kyphosis in the mid-back, mild curvature of the thoracic spine, and a mild forward head position. He was weight-bearing moderately more on the right, his leg swing mildly closed on the right and arm swing moderately closed on the left when I observed his gait.

Initial Functional Goals:

Mr. Washington is the primary caregiver for his granddaughter during the day. Because of her age, he needed to pick her up to put her into the high chair at meals, and into the car seat, and to put her to bed at nap time. At the beginning of treatment, he was unable to lift or carry her because of pain and stiffness. His initial goal was to be able to lift her 10 times a day with mild pain and fatigue.

After the scoliosis flared up, his activity level dropped considerably. Simple activities such as getting dressed and driving a car became too painful without assistance or frequent rest periods. His goal was to wash himself, dress himself, and walk around the block every day.

A year later, he was able to accomplish his initial goal.

Current Subjective Data:

Mr. Washington has infrequent and mild episodes of pain and stiffness with mild activity, which increase to moderate episodes of pain and stiffness lasting for several hours if he exceeds the following: 5 minutes of carrying his granddaughter, 1 hour of gardening, and 2 hours of sitting.

Current Objective Data:

Mr. Washington's kyphosis and spinal curvature are more pronounced than they were initially. The muscles around the scoliosis are constantly and moderately tight. His muscles in the mid-back area spasm only with activities in excess of the limitations described above, the rest of the spasms have resolved. The trigger points have resolved except around the scoliosis, the headaches are gone, and his cervical range of motion is normal. His gait is excellent and his posture is compromised only by the scoliosis.

Treatment:

Initially, I used full body lymphatic drainage techniques to reduce the swelling and pain, increase mobility, and strengthen the immune system. Soon I began incorporating movement re-education techniques to find ways that allowed Mr. Washington to move and perform daily activities, such as sitting, standing, and lifting, with more comfort and ease.

Progress Summary:

Within 6 sessions, the neck pain and stiffness, headaches, and low back stiffness were infrequent and mild. Unfortunately, the mid-back pain and stiffness worsened for several months and were debilitating. After several months, the treatments slowly and steadily diminished the pain and increased Mr. Washington's ability to return to a modified level of activity, but it was over a year before Mr. Washington's scoliosis stabilized and he could return to his normal activities.

Mr. Washington is able to lift his granddaughter as needed, but can carry her for only 5 minutes at a time. He is able to garden for up to 1 hour, and can sit at a bridge table for 2 hours, after which time the pain kicks in.

Patient Status:

Mr. Washington participates in a daily stretching and strengthening routine, and comes in monthly for group movement classes to maintain his daily activity level. We have attempted to discontinue his treatments and rely solely on his self-care routine; however, after 45–50 days without treatment, his ability to function is compromised and his pain increases to moderate and frequent.

In summary, Mr. Washington responded positively to treatments and adapted to a higher level of self-care responsibilities. Please call if you have questions.

Yours in health,
John Olson, LMP, GCFP

HANDS HEAL

John Olson, LMP, GCFP
345 Moon River Rd. Ste. 6
Minnehaha, MN   55987
TEL   612 555 9889

SOAP CHART-M

Patient Name   _Darnel G. Washington_   Date _2-6-0_

Date of Injury _1-6-01_   Insurance ID# _123-45-6789_   Current Meds _hydrocodone_

S   Focus for Today   ↓ ⑰ hd, C, T, L

Symptoms: Location/Intensity/Frequency/Duration/Onset

C, T, L ⑰ M Con post MVA   Δ L

HA ⑰ M interm/da post MVA   Δ ⑰

Activities of Daily Living: Aggravating/Relieving

A: sitting (playing bridge), lifting (GD), bowling, dancing, gardening

R: rest, heat

O   Findings: Visual/Palpable/Test Results

V: 1° WB rising and standing – Ⓡ leg & Ft Δ L ↓ bal

  sits Ⓡ pelvis, bends mid – T Δ̸

  BR M shallow RR Δ L & even

  L–M seg mvm't Ⓛ ribs c̄ deep inh Δ smooth

P: M Ⓡ frontal tor Δ L

  M⁺ ⒝⒧ sph decomp Δ M

  L⁺ Adh tent Δ̸

  CSR M weak Ⓡ L Ⓛ
          Δ L   Δ N

Modalities: Applications/Locations

97140   LDT trunk   FI eyes & ft
60 min.   CST hd

Response to Treatment (see Δ)

A   Prioritize Functional Limitations

1. lift GD 2° nec = carseat, highchair, crib

2. gardening 2° pref = veg & flowers, time c̄ wife

Goals: Long-term/Short-term

LTG: Lift GD 10x/da from floor to carry

10 min 5 da/wk c̄ L ⑰ & fatigue–60 da

STG: Lift light weight toys from floor 10x/da

3 da/wk c̄ L ⑰ –2 wks

P   Future Treatment/Frequency

2x/wk for 3 wks, 60 min/tx

LDT, CST, FI-ribs, diap., ↑ mob ↓ Adh

Homework/Self-care

con't heat T, ice only C, L

Deep BR ex

Provider Signature   _JO, LMP, GCFP_   Date _2-6-01_

John Olson, LMP, GCFP
345 Moon River Rd. Ste. 6
Minnehaha, MN   55987
Tel   612 555 9889

HANDS HEAL

SOAP CHART-M

Patient Name _Darnel G. Washington_   Date _2-8-01_

Date of Injury _1-6-01_   Insurance ID# _123-45-6789_   Current Meds _hydrocodone_

S   Focus- ↓Ⓟ hd, C
   M C Ⓟ   Δ L
   M HA Ⓟ   Δ L
   M Stiff C c̄ heat

O   97140 LDT hd, C
   60 min
   all P-Rom C L ↓ c̄ L⁺ Ⓟ e
   end range 2° ↓ Δ L⁻ c̄ L Ⓟ

A   lifting lightweight toys from shelves c̄ M Ⓟ

P   reg. ice
   reg. BR ex

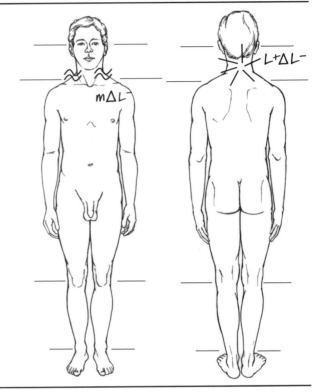

Provider Signature _JO LMP GCFP_   Date

S   Focus - ↓Ⓟ hd, C
   L⁺ C Ⓟ   Δ L⁻
   L⁺ HA Ⓟ   Δ L⁻
   L⁺ stiff C c̄ heat   Δ L⁻

O   97140 LDT C, hd, ch, arms
   60 min
   all P-Rom C L ↓ c̄ L Ⓟ℮
   end range 2° ↓ Δ N c̄ L⁻ Ⓟ

A   con't

P   con't

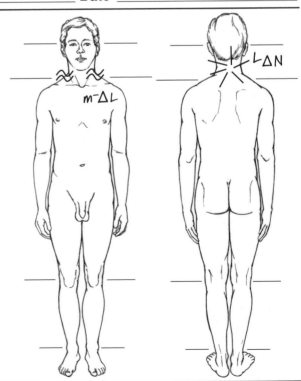

Provider Signature _JO LMP GCFP_   Date _2-11-01_

Legend:	℮ TP	● TeP	○ Ⓟ	✳ Infl	≡ HT	≈ SP
276	✕ Adh	≋ Numb	⌵ rot	╱ elev	⤢ Short	↔ Long

John Olson, LMP, GCFP
345 Moon River Rd. Ste. 6
Minnehaha, MN   55987
TEL   612 555 9889

HANDS HEAL

Patient Name _Darnel G. Washington_   Date _2-11-02_

Date of Injury _1-6-01_   Insurance ID# _123-45-6789_   Current Meds _∅_

S   Focus for Today   ↓ stiff back

Symptoms: Location/Intensity/Frequency/Duration/Onset
Stiff T L cons, 4 da-bridge marathon 2-7-02
Δ WNL

Activities of Daily Living: Aggravating/Relieving
A: carrying GD ↑ 10 min, sit or garden ↑ 2 hrs
R: ex, stretch, rest

O   Findings: Visual/Palpable/Test Results
M weak c̄ sit Δ L
mvm't T vs hip
rib mob M ↓   BR L ↓ Δ N
        Δ L

Modalities: Applications/Locations
97140   Fl ribs T
60 min   CST — C, T, L trac c̄ unwinding
Response to Treatment (see Δ)

A   Prioritize Functional Limitations
has not regained prior functional status since
MVA 1-6-01 (see ADLS)

Goals: Long-term/Short-term
all goals have been reached within the limits of
current health condition

P   Future Treatment/Frequency
con't ATM classes 1x/mth, ↑ prn
released from care, ref. to P HCP

Homework/Self-care
BR ex ribroll ex c̄ ↑ sit
rest + ex ā stiff

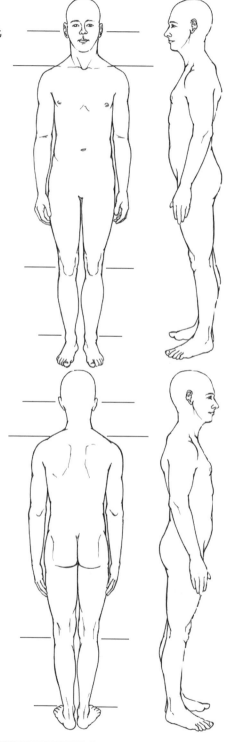

Provider Signature   _JO LMP, GCFP_   Date _____

Legend:
℮ TP	● TeP	○ Ⓟ	✳ Infl	≡ HT	≈ SP
✕ Adh	≋ Numb	◯ rot	╱ elev	⊶ Short	↔ Long

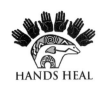

HANDS HEAL

John Olson, LMP, GCFP
345 Moon River Rd. Ste. 6
Minnehaha, MN 55987
TEL 612 555 9889

INSURANCE STATUS—PERSONAL INJURY

Patient Name Darnel G. Washington   Date 2-15-01

Date of Injury 1-6-01   Insurance ID# 123-45-6789

A. Reporting
Which information would you like to receive monthly and how do you prefer to receive information:

☐ copies of billing   ☐ fax
☒ monthly statements   ☒ mail
☒ SOAP charts   ☐ email
☒ Progress reports   ☒ upon request

B. Primary Insurance Coverage
Please provide the following information regarding your client's/my patient's insurance status:
Insured James Washington
Insurance ID# 989-76-6789
Insurance Carrier Farmington States
Billing Address PO Box 3778
City O'Claire   State MN   Zip 55978
Adjuster Clifford Glens
Phone (612) 555-7887   Fax (612) 555-8778
PIP policy amount $ 30,000
Dates of coverage 1-6-01 → 1-6-04
PIP available $ 28,000
Med Pay policy amount $ 10,000
Dates of coverage 1-6-01 → 1-6-02
Med Pay available $ 10,000

C. Secondary Insurance Coverage
Insured Darnel G. Washington
Insurance ID# 123-45-6789
Insurance Carrier Allied
Billing Address PO Box 2988
City Omaha   State NE   Zip 68144
Adjuster Jarma Jones
Phone (402) 555-1991   Fax 555-9119
PIP policy amount $ N/A   Private Health Plan
Dates of coverage
PIP available $
Med Pay policy amount $
Dates of coverage
Med Pay available $
If secondary coverage is through the patients' private health insurance, is manual therapy a
covered benefit: ☐ Yes   ☐ No   ☒ Don't Know

D. Third Party Insurance Coverage
Insured Peter O'Malley
Insurance ID# 987-63-4321
Insurance Carrier Safe Hands
Billing Address PO Box 4321
City St Petersburg   State MD   Zip 10111
Adjuster David Davies
Phone (512) 555-7733   Fax (512) 555-7337
Liability policy amount $ 100,000
Dates of coverage 1-6-01 → 1-6-04
Liability available $ 100,000
Uninsured/underinsured Motorist (UIM)$
Policy Amount $
UIM available $

278

CONTRACTUAL GUARANTEE OF PAYMENT FOR MEDICAL SERVICES

I hereby authorize and direct you, my attorney, to pay directly to my health care provider(s), _John Olson_, the total dollar amount owing for health care services, including applicable interest charges, provided for injuries arising from the motor vehicle accident on _1-6-01_. I hereby authorize my attorney and the involved insurance companies to withhold sums from any settlement, judgment, or verdict as may be necessary to adequately protect my health care provider(s) and their office. I hereby further consent to a lien being filed on my case by said health care provider(s) and their office against any and all proceeds of my settlement, judgment, or verdict which may be paid to you, my attorney, or myself as the result of the injuries for which I have been treated.

I agree never to rescind this document and that any attempt at recession will not be honored by my attorney. I hereby instruct that in the event another attorney is substituted in this matter, the new attorney shall honor this Contractual Guarantee of Payment for Health Care Services as inherent in the settlement and enforceable upon the case as if it were executed by him/her.

I fully understand that I am directly and fully responsible to said health care provider(s) or their office for all health care bills submitted by them for services rendered to me. Further, this agreement is made solely for said health care providers' additional protection and in consideration of their forbearance on payment. I also understand that such payment is not contingent on any settlement, judgment, or verdict by which I may eventually recover damages.

I specifically request my attorney to acknowledge this letter by signing below and returning it to the office of said health care provider(s). I have been advised that if my attorney does not wish to cooperate in protecting the health care providers' interest, the health care provider(s) will not await payment, but will require me to make payments on a current basis.

Date _1-3-02_ Patient's Signature _Darnel G. Washington_

Patient's Social Security Number or Driver's License Number _123-45-6789_

The undersigned, being attorney of record for the above patient, does hereby agree to observe all the terms of the above, and agrees to withhold such sums from any settlement, judgment, or verdict as may be necessary to adequately protect said health care provider(s) named above.

Date _1-6-02_ Attorney's Signature _B. Charma Storro, JD_

Please date, sign, and return one original to

John Olson, LMP, GCFP

345 Moon River Rd. Ste. 6

Minnehaha, MN 55987

_(612) 555-9889_

fax (612) 555-8998

THANK YOU.

Revised and reprinted with permission, Adler ♦ Giersch, PS

Provider Name John Olson, LMP, GCFP

INSURANCE VERIFICATION

Name Darnel G. Washington   Date 3-2-02

Date of Injury 1-6-02   Insurance ID# 123-45-6789

A. Patient Information

Employment

Employer N/A

Phone _____ Fax _____

Currently Employed? ☐Y ☐N

Effective date of benefits _____

Expiration date of benefits _____

Contact name _____

Date/Time verified _____

Attorney

Name B. Charma Storro JD

Phone (612) 555-2337 Fax 555-7332

Guarantee of Payment filed? ☐Y ☒N

Medical Lien filed? ☐Y ☒N

  Date _____ Expires _____

  Renewed _____ Expires _____

Copies of patient file requests

  Date requested _____ Date sent _____

  Date requested _____ Date sent _____

Primary Health Care Provider

Name Sage Redtree MD

Phone 555-0009   Fax 565-9000

Attending provider for this injury/illness? ☒Y ☐N

Referring provider for manual therapy services? ☒Y ☐N

Prescription received? ☒Y ☐N

Prescription date   2-1-02   # of Tx   6

  Tx duration/frequency   2x wk-3 wks

  Diagnosis (ICD-10 codes) 754.2, 723.1,

728.85, 724.1, 784.0

First Renewal date   2-25-02   # of Tx   6

  Tx duration/frequency 1x wk-6 wks

Second Renewal date _____ # of Tx _____

  Tx duration/frequency _____

B. Insurance Information

Workers Compensation Insurance

Contact _____

Phone _____ Fax _____

Date/Time verified _____

  Is claim open? ☐Y ☐N

  Date Opened _____ Date Closed _____

  Date Reopened _____

Private Health Insurance

Insurer _____

Contact _____

Phone _____ Fax _____

Date/Time verified _____

Personal Injury Insurance

Primary Insurer Farmington States

  Adjuster Clifford Glens

  Phone (612)555-7887 Fax 555-8778

  Date/Time verified 3-2-02 per attny request

    PIP policy amount $ 30,000

    Dates of coverage 3 years post DOI

    PIP available $ 28,000

    Med Pay policy amount $ 10,000

    Dates of coverage 1 year post DOI

    Med Pay available $ 10,000

Secondary Insurer Allied

  Adjuster Jarma Jones

  Phone (612)555-1991 Fax 555-9119

  Date/Time verified 3-2-02 per attny request

    PIP policy amount $ 10,000

    Dates of coverage 1 year post DOI

    PIP available $ 10,000

    Med Pay policy amount $ 7,000

    Dates of coverage 1 year post DOI

    Med Pay available $ 7,000

C. Verify Benefits/Authorize Services

Ask the insurance representative the following questions regarding the patient's coverage:

1. Is manual therapy a covered benefit? ☒Y ☐N
2. Is the patient eligible for the manual therapy benefit for this condition (supply diagnosis/ICD-10 codes)? ☒Y ☐N
3. Am I eligible to provide manual therapy services (supply professional license/certification)? ☒Y ☐N

If the answer to any one of these questions is No, bill the patient for manual therapy services.

If the answer to all three questions is Yes, continue verification on page two, and bill the insurance company for manual therapy services.

C. Verify Benefits/Authorize Services, cont.

Record the answers you get to questions 4, 5, and 6 in this table. In the first column list the services you provide. In the second column, record the corresponding CPT code. Complete the table with the answers you get to questions 4, 5, and 6.

4. Which manual therapy services are authorized? (Go through each one listed below.)
5. Are there any restrictions or limitations to each authorized service?
6. What is the maximum allowable reimbursement rate for each authorized service?

Service Item	CPT code	4. Authorized?	5. Restrictions?	6. Max Rate?
1. CST	97140	☒Y ☐N	Reasonable and	UCR
2. Feldy	97112	☒Y ☐N	Necessary only	UCR
3. H/C Pack	97010	☒Y ☐N	" "	UCR
4. Ⓜ	97124	☒Y ☐N	" "	UCR
5.		☐Y ☐N		
6.		☐Y ☐N		
7.		☐Y ☐N		
8.		☐Y ☐N		
9.		☐Y ☐N		
10.		☐Y ☐N		

Complete 7-17 as applicable

7. Does a deductible apply? ☐Y ☒N Amount $_____
Paid to date $_____
Policy year dates _____
8. Does a Co-Pay apply? ☐Y ☒N Amount $_____
9. Does a co-insurance apply? ☐Y ☒N Amount %_____
10. Is there a limit on the # of sessions per policy year? ☐Y ☒N Total per year _____
Number available to date _____
11. Is there a limit on the total $ spent on these services or similar services per policy year? ☐Y ☒N Amount $_____
Amount available to date _____
12. Treatment dates authorized _per MD 'script_
13. Number of sessions authorized _per MD 'script_
14. Preferred billing method/form: ☒HCFA 1500 ☐Electronic ☐Other _____
15. Send with each bill: ☒Prescription ☐SOAP notes ☐Progress Reports ☒License/Certification ☐Other _____
16. What is the expected turnaround time on claim reimbursement? _30 days_
17. Are you able to authorize payment? ☐Y ☒N
If Yes, authorization # _____
If No, can you connect me with someone who is able to authorize payment? ☐Y ☒N
Name _____
Phone_____ Fax_____

Send a copy of this form to the insurance representative with a letter confirming the information gathered.
Date sent _3-2-01_

Re-Authorization/Verification
Contact _____
Phone_____ Fax_____
Date/Time verified _____
Treatment dates authorized _____
Number of sessions authorized _____
Is payment authorized? ☐Y ☐N
Authorization # _____
Confirmation sent? ☐Y ☐N Date sent _____
Verify remainder of policy year, if applicable:
1. Deductible paid to date $_____
2. Total # of sessions to date _____
3. Total $ spent to date $_____

Re-Authorization/Verification
Contact _____
Phone_____ Fax_____
Date/Time verified _____
Treatment dates authorized _____
Number of sessions authorized _____
Is payment authorized? ☐Y ☐N
Authorization # _____
Confirmation sent? ☐Y ☐N Date sent _____
Verify remainder of policy year, if applicable:
1. Deductible paid to date $_____
2. Total # of sessions to date _____
3. Total $ spent to date $_____

PLEASE
DO NOT
STAPLE
IN THIS
AREA

← CARRIER →

HEALTH INSURANCE CLAIM FORM

PICA ☐☐☐   PICA ☐☐☐

| 1. MEDICARE ☐ (Medicare #)   MEDICAID ☐ (Medicaid #)   CHAMPUS ☐ (Sponsor's SSN)   CHAMPVA ☐ (VA File #)   GROUP HEALTH PLAN ☐ (SSN or ID)   FECA BLK LUNG ☐ (SSN)   OTHER ☐ (ID) | 1a. INSURED'S I.D. NUMBER (FOR PROGRAM IN ITEM 1) |

2. PATIENT'S NAME (Last Name, First Name, Middle Initial)
Washington Darnel G.

3. PATIENT'S BIRTH DATE MM 04 DD 22 YY 37   SEX M ☒ F ☐

4. INSURED'S NAME (Last Name, First Name, Middle Initial)
Washington James

5. PATIENT'S ADDRESS (No., Street)
1209 Lake Minnetonka Dr

6. PATIENT RELATIONSHIP TO INSURED
Self ☐ Spouse ☐ Child ☐ Other ☒

7. INSURED'S ADDRESS (No., Street)
32 W. Holden Court

CITY Minnehaha **STATE** MN

8. PATIENT STATUS
Single ☐ Married ☒ Other ☐

CITY Minnehaha **STATE** MN

ZIP CODE 55987 **TELEPHONE (Include Area Code)** (612) 555-1515

Employed ☐ Full-Time Student ☐ Part-Time Student ☐

ZIP CODE 55987 **TELEPHONE (INCLUDE AREA CODE)** (612)555-1515

9. OTHER INSURED'S NAME (Last Name, First Name, Middle Initial)
Washington Darnel G.

10. IS PATIENT'S CONDITION RELATED TO:

11. INSURED'S POLICY GROUP OR FECA NUMBER

a. OTHER INSURED'S POLICY OR GROUP NUMBER
Allied

a. EMPLOYMENT? (CURRENT OR PREVIOUS)
YES ☐ NO ☒

a. INSURED'S DATE OF BIRTH MM 05 DD 31 YY 60   SEX M ☒ F ☐

b. OTHER INSURED'S DATE OF BIRTH MM DD YY   SEX M ☐ F ☐

b. AUTO ACCIDENT? YES ☒ NO ☐ **PLACE (State)** MN

b. EMPLOYER'S NAME OR SCHOOL NAME
Maad Printing & Design

c. EMPLOYER'S NAME OR SCHOOL NAME

c. OTHER ACCIDENT? YES ☐ NO ☒

c. INSURANCE PLAN NAME OR PROGRAM NAME
Farmington States

d. INSURANCE PLAN NAME OR PROGRAM NAME
P56789-0

10d. RESERVED FOR LOCAL USE

d. IS THERE ANOTHER HEALTH BENEFIT PLAN?
YES ☒ NO ☐ If yes, return to and complete item 9 a-d.

READ BACK OF FORM BEFORE COMPLETING & SIGNING THIS FORM.

12. PATIENT'S OR AUTHORIZED PERSON'S SIGNATURE I authorize the release of any medical or other information necessary to process this claim. I also request payment of government benefits either to myself or to the party who accepts assignment below.

SIGNED signature on file DATE 2-6-01

13. INSURED'S OR AUTHORIZED PERSON'S SIGNATURE I authorize payment of medical benefits to the undersigned physician or supplier for services described below.

SIGNED signature on file

14. DATE OF CURRENT: ILLNESS (First symptom) OR INJURY (Accident) OR PREGNANCY(LMP) MM 01 DD 06 YY 01

15. IF PATIENT HAS HAD SAME OR SIMILAR ILLNESS. GIVE FIRST DATE MM DD YY

16. DATES PATIENT UNABLE TO WORK IN CURRENT OCCUPATION FROM MM DD YY TO MM DD YY

17. NAME OF REFERRING PHYSICIAN OR OTHER SOURCE
Sage Redtree, MD

17a. I.D. NUMBER OF REFERRING PHYSICIAN

18. HOSPITALIZATION DATES RELATED TO CURRENT SERVICES FROM MM DD YY TO MM DD YY

19. RESERVED FOR LOCAL USE

20. OUTSIDE LAB? YES ☐ NO ☐ $ CHARGES

21. DIAGNOSIS OR NATURE OF ILLNESS OR INJURY. (RELATE ITEMS 1,2,3 OR 4 TO ITEM 24E BY LINE)

1. 728.85
2. 723.1
3. 724.1
4. 784.0

22. MEDICAID RESUBMISSION CODE ORIGINAL REF. NO.

23. PRIOR AUTHORIZATION NUMBER

24. A. DATE(S) OF SERVICE						B. Place of Service	C. Type of Service	D. PROCEDURES, SERVICES, OR SUPPLIES (Explain Unusual Circumstances) CPT/HCPCS MODIFIER	E. DIAGNOSIS CODE	F. $ CHARGES		G. DAYS OR UNITS	H. EPSDT Family Plan	I. EMG	J. COB	K. RESERVED FOR LOCAL USE
From MM	DD	YY	To MM	DD	YY											
02	06	01				3	9	97140	1,2,3,4	$80	00	4				
02	06	01				3	9	97140	1,2,3,4	$80	00	4				

25. FEDERAL TAX I.D. NUMBER 567-89-1234 SSN ☐ EIN ☒

26. PATIENT'S ACCOUNT NO.

27. ACCEPT ASSIGNMENT? (For govt. claims, see back) YES ☐ NO ☐

28. TOTAL CHARGE $ 160 00

29. AMOUNT PAID $ 0

30. BALANCE DUE $ 160 00

31. SIGNATURE OF PHYSICIAN OR SUPPLIER INCLUDING DEGREES OR CREDENTIALS (I certify that the statements on the reverse apply to this bill and are made a part thereof.)
John Olson LMP, GCFP 2-8-01
SIGNED DATE

32. NAME AND ADDRESS OF FACILITY WHERE SERVICES WERE RENDERED (If other than home or office)

33. PHYSICIAN'S, SUPPLIER'S BILLING NAME, ADDRESS, ZIP CODE & PHONE #
John Olson, LMP, GCFP
345 Moon River Rd. Ste. 6
Minnehaha, MN 55987
PIN# (612) 555-9889 GRP#

FORM HCFA-1500 (12-90)
NORTHWEST BUSINESS FORMS (206) 728-8181

PLEASE PRINT OR TYPE

FORM OWCP-1500   FORM RRB-1500   APPROVED OMB-0938-0008
(APPROVED BY AMA COUNCIL ON MEDICAL SERVICE 8/88)

PATIENT AND INSURED INFORMATION

PHYSICIAN OR SUPPLIER INFORMATION

Workers' Compensation

This flow chart demonstrates which forms are recommended for use with patients involved in workers' compensation cases: who completes the form, how often the form is used, and any additional comments for using the form.

Workers' Compensation	Who	Frequency	Comments
INTAKE FORMS			
Fees and Policies	Patient	initial visit	update as needed
Health Information	Patient	initial visit	update annually
History section of HxTxC	—		
Injury Information, part 1	Patient	initial visit	per incident
Injury Information, part 2	—		
Billing Information	Patient	initial visit	if you provide billing services
Prescription	HCP	as needed	a progress report should precede each renewal
PROGRESS SUMMARIES			
Health Report	Patient	monthly	patient reports current status
Pain Questionnaires	Patient	monthly	daily or weekly, if used as a pain journal
Initial Report w/o Tx	MT	as needed	if patient does not receive tx
Initial Report w/ Tx	MT	initial visit	summarizes tx and proposes tx plan
Progress Report	MT	monthly	practitioner reports to HCP
Narrative Report	—		
TREATMENT NOTES			
Initial SOAP	MT	initial visit	summarizes all findings; sets goals, plan
Subsequent SOAP	MT	each visit	(excluding initial, progress, and discharge sessions) brief, focused
Progress SOAP	MT	monthly	summarizes all findings; updates goals, plan
Discharge SOAP	MT	final visit	summarizes all findings; ongoing care plan
HxTxC	—		
Range of Motion	MT	as needed	minimal ROM assessment necessary each subsequent note, extensive ROM for initial and progress notes
BILLING FORMS			
Insurance Status–Personal Injury	—		
Guarantee of Payment	—		
Insurance Verification	MT	as needed	with renewal of prescribed services
HCFA 1500 billing form	MT	each visit	may bill for multiple sessions per HCFA form after initial billing if total amount is under $250
Payment Log	MT	as needed	if payments do not match bills

Helena LaLuna, CR

123 Sun Moon and Stars Drive
Capital Hill, WA   98119
TEL   206 555 4446

A. My Fees For Services Are As Follows:

Structural Integration	$100 per hour
(CTP code #97140)	($25 per 15 minute Unit)

B. Payment for services are as follows:

Cash, Check, or Credit Card (Mastercard, Visa, or American Express):

- A 15% discount when payment is made at the time of service.
- Monthly accounts may be pre-arranged, payment in full required monthly.

I will bill your insurance company directly under the following conditions:

- Private Health Insurance: No
- Worker's Compensation: Yes—verbal authorization OK, active claims only, HCP prescription required
- Auto Accident:
  - PIP: Yes—written authorization required or Insurance Status–Personal Injury from Attorney verifying insurance status, HCP prescription required
  - Second Party Coverage: Yes—if PIP, see above
  - Third Party Coverage: Yes—Guarantee of Payment contract required, helath care lien required, HCP perscription required

All insurance accounts not paid in full within 90 days from date of service will be charged interest. Interest rates are 12% annually and are charged at 1% monthly. Interest is calculated on the principal amount; interest is not compounded.

C. Office Policies

Cancellations

Cancellations must be made 24 hours in advance of the scheduled appointment time. If cancellations are not made within 24 hours, payment in full is required. This charge will be waived if a replacement can be found for your appointment time. Your insurance company will not be charged for your missed appointment; you will be responsible for payment out-of-pocket.

Right of Refusal

I reserve the right to refuse service to anyone. This includes but is not limited to anyone who requests treatment or services that are outside my scope of practice. I will exercise this right if anyone arrives for treatment under the influence of alcohol or recreational drugs; I reserve the right to charge for the session time, whether or not services were rendered, if I so choose.

Patient Agreement

I have read the policies stated above and agree to abide by them.

Signature   *Zamora Hostetter*   Date   *4-4-01*

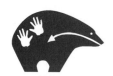

Helena LaLuna, CR
123 Sun Moon and Stars Drive
Capital Hill, WA   98119
TEL   206 555 4446

Patient Name _Zamora Hostetter_   Date _4-4-01_

Date of Injury _3-31-01_   Insurance ID# _C98-7654321_

A. Patient Information

Address _63 18th Ave. W_

City _Capitol Hill_   State _WA_ Zip _98119_

Phone: Home _(206) 555-1221_

   Work _555-2112_ Cell/Pgr _555-1122_

Date of Birth _5-22-80_

Employer _Howling Moon Cafe_

Occupation _Chef_

Emergency Contact _Mary Lou Hostetter_

Phone: Home _(206) 555-0909_

   Work _555-9090_ Cell/Pgr _555-9900_

Primary Health Care Provider

Name _Manda Rae Yuricich, DC_

Address _4041 Bell Town Wy, Ste. 200_

City/State/Zip _Capitol Hill WA 98119_

Phone: _555-3535_   Fax _555-4646_

I give my manual therapist permission to consult with my referring health care provider regarding my health and treatment. _& P.T._

Comments _re: work injury only_

Initials _ZH_   Date _4-4-01_

B. Current Health Information

List Health/Concerns Check all that apply

Primary _shoulder pain_

☐ mild ☐ moderate ☒ disabling

☒ constant ☐ intermittant

☒ symptoms ↑ w/activity   ☐ ↓ w/activity

☐ getting worse ☐ getting better ☒ no change

treatment received _ER-x-rays, sling_

Secondary _back pain_

☐ mild ☒ moderate ☐ disabling

☒ constant ☐ intermittant

☒ symptoms ↑ w/activity   ☐ ↓ w/activity

☐ getting worse ☒ getting better ☐ no change

treatment received _ER, DC-adjust._

Additional _neck pain & headaches_

☒ mild ☐ moderate ☐ disabling

☐ constant ☒ intermittant

☒ symptoms ↑ w/activity   ☐ ↓ w/activity

☐ getting worse ☒ getting better ☐ no change

treatment received _ER, DC_

Have you ever received Manual Therapy before? ☐ Y ☒ N Frequency? _____

List all conditions currently monitored by a Health Care Provider _none_

List the medications you took today (include pain relievers and herbal remedies) _arnica, calcium, vitamins_

List all other medications taken in the last 3 months _none_

List Daily Activities

Work _standing, lifting, cooking, chopping_

Home/Family _cooking, cleaning, yardwork_

Social/Recreational _biking, roller hockey, dancing_

Circle the activities affected by your condition, ☒ all of the above

Check other activities affected: ☒ sleep ☐ washing ☐ dressing ☒ fitness

How do you reduce stress? _sports, being outdoors_

Pain? _arnica, ice packs, visualization_

What are your goals for receiving Manual Therapy? _get back to work & sports_

C. Health History

List and Explain. Include dates and treatment received.

Surgeries _none_

Accidents _Broken arm ℞ fell out of tree house in 1987, cast for 8 wks_

Major Illnesses _none_

General

current	past		comments
☒	☐	headaches	_____
☒	☐	pain _sh, back, neck_	
☒	☐	sleep disturbances	
		pain wakes me up	
☐	☐	fatigue _____	
☐	☐	infectious _____	
☐	☐	fever _____	
☐	☐	sinus _____	
☐	☐	other _____	

Skin Conditions

current	past		comments
☐	☐	rashes _____	
☐	☐	athlete's foot, warts_____	
☐	☐	other _____	

Allergies

current	past		comments
☐	☐	scents, oils, lotions _____	
☐	☐	detergents _____	
☐	☐	other _____	

Muscles and Joints

current	past		comments
☐	☐	rheumatoid arthritis_____	
☐	☐	osteoarthritis _____	
☐	☐	osteoporosis _____	
☐	☐	scoliosis _____	
☐	☒	broken bones _Ⓡ arm_	
☒	☐	spinal problems_____	
		neck & back	
☐	☐	disk problems _____	
☐	☐	lupus _____	
☐	☐	TMJ, jaw pain _____	
☐	☐	spasms, cramps	
☐	☐	sprains, strains	
☐	☐	tendonitis, bursitis	
☒	☐	stiff or painful joints _sh Ⓡ back, neck_	
☐	☐	weak or sore muscles_____	
☒	☐	neck, shoulder, arm pain_____	
☒	☐	low back, hip, leg pain_____	
☐	☐	other _____	

Nervous System

current	past		comments
☐	☐	head injuries, concussions _____	
☐	☐	dizziness, ringing in the ears _____	
☐	☐	loss of memory, confusion _____	
☐	☐	numbness, tingling _____	
☐	☐	sciatica, shooting pain _____	
☐	☐	chronic pain _____	
☐	☐	depression _____	
☐	☐	other _____	

Respiratory, Cardiovascular

current	past		comments
☐	☐	heart disease _____	
☐	☐	blood clots _____	
☐	☐	stroke _____	
☐	☐	lymphadema _____	
☐	☐	high, low blood pressure_____	
☐	☐	irregular heart beat _____	
☐	☐	poor circulation_____	
☐	☐	swollen ankles _____	
☐	☐	varicose veins_____	
☐	☐	chest pain, shortness of breath _____	
☐	☐	asthma_____	

Digestive/Elimination System

current	past		comments
☐	☐	bowel dysfunction _____	
☐	☐	gas, bloating _____	
☐	☐	bladder/kidney dysfunction _____	
☐	☐	abdominal pain _____	
☐	☐	other _____	

Endocrine System

current	past		comments
☐	☐	thyroid dysfunction _____	
☐	☐	diabetes _____	

Reproductive System

current	past		comments
☐	☐	pregnancy _____	
☐	☐	painful, emotional menses _____	
☐	☐	fibrotic cysts _____	

Cancer/Tumors

current	past		comments
☐	☐	benign _____	
☐	☐	malignant_____	

Habits

current	past		comments
☐	☒	tobacco _quit 1998_	
☒	☐	alcohol _mild use_	
☐	☐	drugs _____	
☐	☐	coffee, soda_____	

Contract for Care

I promise to participate fully as a member of my health care team. I will make sound choices regarding my treatment plan based on the information provided by my manual therapist and other members of my health care team, and my experience of those suggestions. I agree to participate in the self care program we select. I promise to inform my practitioner any time I feel my well-being is threatened or compromised. I expect my manual therapist to provide safe and effective treatment.

Consent for Care

It is my choice to receive manual therapy, and I give my consent to receive treatment. I have reported all health conditions that I am aware of and will inform my practitioner of any changes in my health.

Signature _Zamora Hostetter_ _____ Date _4-4-01_

Signature of parent or guardian _____ Date _____
(If patient is a minor)

287

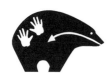

Helena LaLuna, CR

123 Sun Moon and Stars Drive
Capital Hill, WA 98119
TEL 206 555 4446

INJURY INFORMATION

Patient Name _Zamora Hostetter_   Date _4-4-01_

Date of Injury _3-31-01_   Insurance ID# _C98-7654321_

A. General Injury Information

1. How did the accident occur?
   ☐ Auto   ☒ On-the-Job   ☐ Other _____

2. Was a police report filed?   ☐ Yes   ☒ No
   Was a work incident report filed?
   ☒ Yes   ☐ No

3. Describe your injury and how it occurred:
   slipped on banana peel, carrying 25 lb. bag
   of rice over left shoulder, fell backwards
   onto right arm, then right hip, head
   bounced on tile floor, rice landed on top of
   _me._

4. Describe how you felt during and
   immediately after the injury:
   shoulder "popped"-immediate pain, head
   throbbing
   Later that same day: _backache_

   The next day: _neck stiff, back stiff, can't_
   use Right arm at all

   The next week: _N/A_

   The next month: _N/A_

   Describe any bruises, cuts, or abrasions
   as a result of the injury:
   bruise on right hip

5. Are your symptoms ☒ getting better
   ☐ getting worse   ☒ no change _-shoulder_
   What makes them better? _only_
   ice, arnica, visualization ex., chiropractor

   Worse? _everything using my arm, sleep_

6. Did you return to work on the day of the
   injury? ☐ Yes ☒ No
   Have you lost time from work since the
   injury? ☒ Yes ☐ No

7. What are your work responsibilities?
   cooking, prep, stocking supplies

   Which work activities are affected by this
   injury? _everything_

   Have your work responsibilities changed as
   a result of this injury? ☒ Yes ☐ No
   Explain _____
   What other daily activities are affected by
   this injury? _everything using my right arm_

8. Did you go to the emergency room?
   ☒ Yes ☐ No
   Were you hospitalized? ☐ Yes ☒ No
   List the health care providers who have
   treated you for this injury, the type of
   treatment provided, and their diagnosis.
   ER-separated shoulder-sling
   DC-whiplash, spinal subluxations, muscle
   spasms-adjust, ice

9. Have you ever had this type of injury
   before? ☐ Yes ☒ No
   Explain _____

   Did you have any physical complaints
   before the injury? ☐ Yes ☒ No
   Explain _____

   Do you have any illnesses or previous
   injuries that may have been affected by
   this injury? ☐ Yes ☒ No
   Explain _____

Signature _Zamora Hostetter_   Date _4-4-01_

288

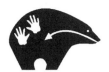

Helena LaLuna, CR
123 Sun Moon and Stars Drive
Capital Hill, WA   98119
TEL   206 555 4446

BILLING INFORMATION

Patient Name _Zamora Hostetter_   Date _4-4-01_

Date of Injury _3-31-01_   Insurance ID# _C98-7654321_

A. Patient Information

Address _63 18th Ave W_

City _Capitol Hill_   State _WA_ Zip _98119_

Phone: Home _(206) 555-1221_
         Work _555-2112_ Cell/Pgr _555-1122_

Date of Birth _5-22-80_

☐ Male   ☒ Female

Marital Status: ☒ Single ☐ Married ☐ Partnered

Relationship of Patient to Insured:

☒ Self ☐ Spouse ☐ Partner ☐ Child ☐ Other

☒ Employed ☐ Student

Employer's Name or School Name:

Howling Moon Cafe

Phone _555-2112_   Fax _555-2211_

Is patient's condition related to:

Employment   ☒ Yes   ☐ No

Auto Accident   ☐ Yes   ☒ No

If Auto Accident, in what state? _____

Other Accident   ☐ Yes   ☒ No

Illness   ☐ Yes   ☒ No

Primary Health Care Provider

Name _Manda Rae Yuricich, OC_

Address _4041 Bell Town Wy Ste. 200_

City _Capitol Hill_   State _WA_ Zip _98119_

Phone _555-3535_   Fax _555-4646_

Attorney

Has an attorney been consulted? ☐ Yes ☒ No

Retained?   ☐ Yes   ☐ No

Name _____

Address _____

City _____ State _____ Zip _____

Phone _____ Fax _____

B. Insured (if other than patient)

Name _____

Insurance ID# _____

Date of Birth _____

☐ Male   ☐ Female

Address _____

City _____ State _____ Zip _____

Phone: Home _____
        Work _____ Cell/Pgr _____

Employer's Name or School Name:

_____

Phone _____ Fax _____

Signature _Zamora Hostetter_

C. Primary Insurance Coverage

Insurance Carrier _WA Dept. L & I_

Contact _claims division_

Group Number _N/A_

Plan # or Name _PO Box 323_

Billing Address _____

City _Olympia_   State _WA_ Zip _98055_

Phone _(360)555-6655_ Fax _555-5566_

D. Secondary Insurance Coverage

Insured _N/A_

Insurance ID# _____

Date of Birth _____

☐ Male   ☐ Female

Address _____

City _____ State _____ Zip _____

Phone: Home _____
        Work _____ Cell/Pgr _____

Employer's Name or School Name:

_____

Phone _____ Fax _____

Insurance Carrier _____

Contact _____

Group Number _____

Plan # or Name _____

Billing Address _____

City _____ State _____ Zip _____

Phone _____ Fax _____

E. Assignment of Benefits

My signature below authorizes and directs payment of medical benefits for services billed to my health care provider.

F. Release of Medical Records

My signature below authorizes the release of my medical records including intake forms, chart notes, reports, and billing statements to my attorneys, health care providers, and insurance case managers, for the purpose of processing my claims. (I will inform my practitioner immediately upon signing any exclusive Release of Medical Records with my attorney.)

G. Financial Responsibility

It is my responsibility to pay for all services provided. In the unfortunate event that my insurance company denies payment or makes a partial payment, I am responsible for the balance. If you have contracted with my insurance company at a discount rate and the agreed-upon fee has been satisfied, the balance will be waived.

Date _4-4-01_

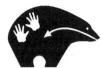

Helena LaLuna, CR
123 Sun Moon and Stars Drive
Capital Hill, WA   98119
Tel   206 555 4446

PRESCRIPTION

Patient Name _Zamora Hostetter_   Date _4-1-01_

Date of Injury _3-31-01_   Insurance ID# _C98-7654321_

A. Diagnosis

(Include ICD-10 codes that specifically
address Manual Therapy Treatment)

Lowback ℗ 724.2

Neck ℗ 723.1

Shoulder sp/st 840.9

Headache 784.0

Spasm 728.85

Condition is related to
- ☐ Auto Accident
- ☒ Work Injury
- ☐ Illness
- ☐ Other:_____

B. Medically Necessary Treatment: Implement Plan as Prescribed Below

Application (Direct & Indirect)
- ☐ Head _____
- ☐ Neck _____
- ☐ Chest _____
- ☐ Shoulders _separated ℝ SH_
- ☐ Abdomen _____
- ☐ Back _____
- ☐ Lowback/Hips _____
- ☐ Upper extremities _as related to sh injury_
- ☐ Lower extremities _a related to LB injury_
- ☒ All of the above _____
- ☐ Other: _____

Treatment Type
- ☒ Manual Therapy _____
- ☒ Hydrotherapy _____
- ☒ Self-Care Education _____
- ☐ Other _____

Treatment Goals
- ☐ Decrease Pain
- ☐ Decrease Inflammation
- ☐ Decrease Muscle Tension/Spasms
- ☐ Decrease Compensatory Patterns
- ☐ Increase Mobility
- ☐ Increase Strength
- ☐ Restore Function
- ☐ Restore Posture
- ☐ Maintain Associated Structures
- ☒ All of the Above
- ☐ Other

Duration & Frequency
- ☐ 1× wk for _____ wks
- ☒ 2× wk for _5_ wks
- ☐ 3× wk for _____ wks
- ☐ 2× month for _____ months
- ☐ 1× month for _____ months

Specific Instructions:
Techniques at your discretion
No strengthening for first 3 wks

C. Referring Health Care Provider (HCP)

Contact Information
HCP Name _Manda Rae Yuricich DC_
Provider No. _22-23-242_
Address _4041 Bell Town Wy Ste 200_
City _Capitol Hill_ State _WA_ Zip _98119_
Phone _206) 555-3535_
Fax _(206) 555-4646_

Reporting
- ☒ Send Report After Initial Visit
- ☒ Send Report at End of Prescription
- ☐ Send Copies of Chart Notes at End of Prescription
- ☒ Fax Information
- ☐ Mail Information
- ☐ Email Information

HCP Signature: _Manda Rae Yuricich, DC_   Date _4-1-01_

Revised and reprinted with permission, Adler ♦ Giersch, PS

Helena LaLuna, CR
123 Sun Moon and Stars Drive
Capital Hill, WA   98119
TEL   206 555 4446

HEALTH REPORT

Patient Name _Zamora Hostetter_   Date _4-4-01_

Date of Injury _3-31-01_   Insurance ID# _C98-7654321_

A. Draw today's symptoms on the figures.

1. Identify CURRENT symptomatic areas in your body by marking letters on the figures below.
   Use the letters provided in the key to identify the symptoms you are feeling today.
2. Circle the area around each letter, representing the size and shape of each symptom location.

Key
P = pain or tenderness
S = joint or muscle stiffness
N = numbness or tingling

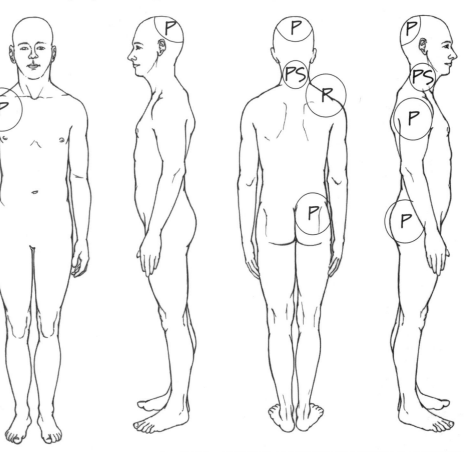

B. Identify the intensity of your symptoms.

1. Pain Scale: Mark a line on the scale to show the amount of pain you are experiencing today.

   No Pain ┠─────────────────┼─────────────────┨ Unbearable Pain   (6.5)

2. Activities Scale: Mark a line on the scale to show the limitations you are experiencing today   (8.75)
   in your daily activities.

   Can Do Anything I Want ┠─────────────────────────┼────────┨ Cannot Do Anything

C. Comments

_____

_____

_____

_____

Signature _Zamora Hostetter_   Date _4-4-01_

Helena LaLuna, CR
123 Sun Moon and Stars Drive
Capital Hill, WA   98119
TEL   206 555 4446

® shoulder   (revised Vernon-Mior)
NECK PAIN & DISABILITY INDEX

Patient Name __Zamora Hostetter__   Date __4-4-01__

Date of Injury __3-31-01__   Insurance ID# __C98-7654321__

This questionnaire has been designed to give the health care provider information as to how your neck pain has affected your ability to manage everyday life. Please answer every section and mark in each section only the **ONE** box which applies to you. We realize you may consider that two of the statements in any one section relate to you, but please just mark the box which most closely describes your problem today.

3 **Section 1 - Pain Intensity**
- ☐ I have no pain at the moment.
- ☐ The pain is very mild at the moment.
- ☐ The pain is moderate at the moment.
- ☒ The pain is fairly severe at the moment.
- ☐ The pain is very severe at the moment.
- ☐ The pain is the worst imaginable at the moment.

3 **Section 2 - Personal Care**
(washing, dressing, etc.)
- ☐ I can look after myself normally without causing pain.
- ☐ I can look after myself normally but it causes extra pain.
- ☐ It is painful to look after myself and I am slow and careful.
- ☒ I need some help but manage most of my personal care.
- ☐ I need help every day in most aspects of self care.
- ☐ I do not get dressed, I wash myself with difficulty and I stay in bed.

5 **Section 3 - Lifting**
- ☐ I can lift heavy weights without extra pain.
- ☐ I can lift heavy weights but it causes extra pain.
- ☐ Pain prevents me from lifting heavy weights off the floor, but I can manage if they are conveniently positioned, e.g. on a table.
- ☐ Pain prevents me from lifting heavy weights, but I can manage light to medium weights if they are conveniently positioned.
- ☐ I can lift very light weights.
- ☒ I cannot lift or carry anything at all.

1 **Section 4 - Reading**
- ☐ I can read as much as I want to with no pain in my neck.
- ☒ I can read as much as I want to with slight pain in my neck.
- ☐ I can read as much as I want to with moderate pain in my neck.
- ☐ I can't read as much as I want to because of moderate pain in my neck.
- ☐ I can hardly read at all because of severe pain in my neck.
- ☐ I cannot read at all.

3 **Section 5 - Headaches**
- ☐ I have no headaches at all.
- ☐ I have slight headaches which come infrequently.
- ☐ I have moderate headaches which come infrequently.
- ☒ I have moderate headaches which come frequently.
- ☐ I have severe headaches which come frequently.
- ☐ I have headaches almost all of the time.

1 **Section 6 - Concentration**
- ☐ I can concentrate fully when I want to with no difficulty.
- ☒ I can concentrate fully when I want to with slight difficulty.
- ☐ I have a fair degree of difficulty in concentrating when I want to.
- ☐ I have a lot of difficulty concentrating when I want to.
- ☐ I have a great deal of difficulty in concentrating when I want to.
- ☐ I cannot concentrate at all.

5 **Section 7 - Work**
- ☐ I can do as much work as I want to.
- ☐ I can do my usual work but no more.
- ☐ I can do most of my usual work but no more.
- ☐ I cannot do my usual work.
- ☐ I can hardly do any work at all.
- ☒ I can't do any work at all.

1 **Section 8 - Driving**
- ☐ I can drive my car without any neck pain.
- ☒ I can drive my car as long as I want with slight pain in my neck.
- ☐ I can drive my car as long as I want with moderate pain in my neck.
- ☐ I can't drive my car as long as I want because of moderate pain in my neck.
- ☐ I can hardly drive at all because of severe pain in my neck.
- ☐ I can't drive my car at all.

4 **Section 9 - Sleeping**
- ☐ I have no trouble sleeping.
- ☐ My sleep is slightly disturbed (less than 1 hour sleepless).
- ☐ My sleep is mildly disturbed (1–2 hours sleepless).
- ☐ My sleep is moderately disturbed (2–3 hours sleepless).
- ☒ My sleep is greatly disturbed (3–5 hours sleepless).
- ☐ My sleep is completely disturbed (5–7 hours sleepless).

30 x 2 = 60%

4 **Section 10 - Recreation**
- ☐ I am able to engage in all my recreational activities with no neck pain at all.
- ☐ I am able to engage in all my recreational activities with some pain in my neck.
- ☐ I am able to engage in most, but not all of my usual recreational activities because of pain in my neck.
- ☐ I am able to engage in a few of my usual recreation activities because of pain in my neck.
- ☒ I can hardly do any recreational activities because of pain in my neck.
- ☐ I can't do recreational activities at all.

Signature __Zamora Hostetter__   Date __4-4-01__

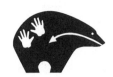

Helena LaLuna, CR
123 Sun Moon and Stars Drive
Capital Hill, WA   98119
TEL   206 555 4446   •   FAX   206 555 4447   •   EMAIL   laluna@email.com

Manda Rae Yuricich, DC
4041 Bell Town Way, Ste. 200
Capitol Hill, WA 98119

Thank you, Dr. Yuricich, for referring Ms. Hostetter to my office. Our first appointment was on April 4, 2001. The results of the sessions are as follows:

Functional goals: Ms. Hostetter would like to return to work as a chef as soon as possible. To facilitate that, our initial goal is to have her cooking for 30 minutes per day, 3 days per week, with moderate pain and fatigue.

Together, we will resolve those findings and accomplish those goals with the following treatment plan: myofascial release for 10 sessions, addressing her shoulder, neck, back and sacral soft tissue injuries, hydrotherapy to reduce the inflammation; and homework exercises to facilitate self-care.

I will report back to you by May 5th. Please contact me if you have questions, comments, or feedback.

Yours in health,

Helena LaLuna, CR

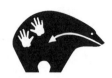

Helena LaLuna, CR

123 Sun Moon and Stars Drive
Capital Hill, WA   98119

TEL   206 555 4446   •   FAX   206 555 4447   •   EMAIL   laluna@email.com

Manda Rae Yuricich, DC
4041 Bell Town Way, Ste. 200
Capitol Hill, WA 98119

Patient: Zamora Hostetter
DOI: 3-31-01
claim #: C98-7654321

Dear Dr. Yuricich:

Thank you for referring Ms. Hostetter to my office for manual therapy. After 10 sessions of myofascial release, Ms. Hostetter has achieved her initial goal. She is able to stand and cook for 30 minutes, while repeatedly lifting and extending up to 25 pounds over a stove and tossing food, 3 days a week, with moderate pain and fatigue.

To facilitate Ms. Hostetter's to return to work, ongoing care is requested. We must extend her cooking time to 90 minutes, 3 days a week, and include 3 hours of additional time at work preparing food. However, Ms. Hostetter is able to sit down at work and take frequent breaks during her preparation time. With 3 additional sessions of myofascial release, we should be able to reach the new goal of cooking for 90 minutes, while repeatedly lifting and extending up to 25 pounds over a stove and tossing food, 3 days a week, with mild pain and moderate fatigue. Ms. Hostetter will attend session weekly for three weeks, receive additional self-care instructions, and participate in home exercises and hydrotherapy during this time.

Please inform me of your decision to continue Ms. Hostetter's manual therapy. I look forward to working with you in the future.

Yours in health,

Helena LaLuna, CR

Helena LaLuna, CR
123 Sun Moon and Stars Drive
Capital Hill, WA   98119
TEL   206 555 4446

Patient Name   Zamora Hostetter   Date   4-4-01

Date of Injury   3-31-01   Insurance ID#   C98-7654321   Current Meds   Arnica

S   Focus for Today   ↓ Ⓟ ↑ Rom SH, neck, LB
Dx: separated shoulder, Sljt subluxation, mild whiplash
Symptoms: Location/Intensity/Frequency/Duration/Onset
SH / Ⓟ / S⁻ / cons / fall – 3-31-01 ΔM
LB / Ⓟ / M / cons / fall – 3-31-01
Δm⁻
Activities of Daily Living: Aggravating/Relieving
Agg: work-lifting, bending, standing, tossing food in pans,
chopping food
Rel: ice, arnica, visualization

O   Findings: Visual/Palpable/Test Results
See chart for spasms, myofascial restrictions and
postural changes

Modalities: Applications/Locations
97140 MFR FB
60 min
Response to Treatment (see Δ)

A   Prioritize Functional Limitations
1. Standing at store, prep counter
2. lifting & tossing food in heavy pans
3. exercise – hockey, biking, hiking

Goals: Long-term/Short-term
2 mths-LTG: stand for 5 hrs cooking-lifting & extending up to
          25 lbs, 5 da/wk c̄ Ⓟ or fatigue
2 wks-STG: Stand for 20 min. slicing Kiwis and decorating a
          cake c̄ M Ⓟ & M fatigue

P   Future Treatment/Frequency
2x/wk for 5 wks
10 session rolfing protocol
focus on Ⓡ SH and Ⓡ Sl jt
Homework/Self-care
ice Ⓡ SH Ⓡ hip 8–10 min prn
SH ex – wall climb ASAP 3–5x/da

Provider Signature   HLL, RC   around bone

Legend:

℮ TP	● TeP	○ Ⓟ	✳ Infl	☰ HT	∿ ≈ SP	
✕ Adh	≋ Numb	⟲ rot	╱ elev	⤙ Short	↔ Long	deep

295

Helena LaLuna, CR
123 Sun Moon and Stars Drive
Capital Hill, WA   98119
TEL   206 555 4446

SOAP CHART-F

Patient Name _Zamora Hostetter_   Date _4-13-01_

Date of Injury _3-31-01_   Insurance ID# _C98-7654321_ Current Meds _Arnica_

S SH Ⓟ Mt cons   Ⱥ
  N&H Ⓟ L interm   Δ Ⓟ
  ADL's Ⱥ

O 97140 MFR FB

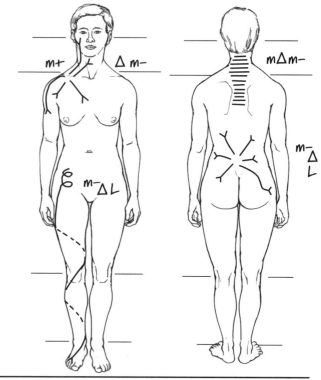

A STG: Brush teeth c̄ Ⓡ arm
  30 sec   1x/da   c̄ L ↑ Ⓟ

P See initial note

Provider Signature   _HLL, CR_   Date   _4-13-01_

S LB Ⓟ M - cons Δ L+
  ADL's - M SH Ⓟ c̄ dressing, washing,
  brushing teeth post tx   4-13-01

O 97140 MFR FB

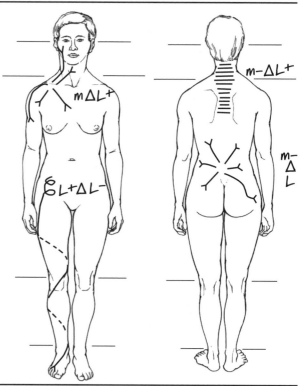

A STG: Stand for 10 min. slicing
  soft fruit, alternating Ⓡ & Ⓛ hands
  c̄ L ↑ Ⓟ & L+ fatigue

P See initial note

Provider Signature   _HLL, CR_   Date   _4-23_

Legend: ℮ TP   • TeP   ○ Ⓟ   ✳ Infl   ≡ HT   ≈ SP
296   ✕ Adh   ≋ Numb   ◯ rot   / elev   ✕ Short   ↔ Long

Patient Name _Zamora Hostetter_   Date _4-4-01_

Date of Injury _3-31-01_   Insurance ID# _C98-7654321_

PRE-TEST 1 (circle test parameters)

Position of patient: prone, sidelying, (sitting,) standing, supine, other: _____

Type of test: (active,) active assisted, passive, resistive, other: _____

Joint: C-spine, T-spine, L-spine, hip, knee, ankle, (shoulder,) elbow, wrist, other _____

Action	Range+Int		Pain+Int		Ltd+Int		Mvmt+Int	
	(R)	(L)	(R)	(L)	(R)	(L)	(R)	(L)
flex	S↓	N	S	O	S(P)	Ø	/	N
ext	S↓	N	S	O	S(P)	Ø	/	N
Abd	S↓	N	S	O	S(P)	Ø	/	N
Add	S↓	N	S	O	S(P)	Ø	/	N

PRE-TEST 2 (circle test parameters)

Position of patient: prone, sidelying, (sitting,) standing, supine, other: _____

Type of test: active, active assisted, (passive,) resistive, other: _____

Joint: C-spine, T-spine, L-spine, hip, knee, ankle, (shoulder,) elbow, wrist, other _____

Action	Range+Int		Pain+Int		Ltd+Int		Mvmt+Int	
	(R)	(L)	(R)	(L)	(R)	(L)	(R)	(L)
flex	S↓	N	S	O	S(P)	Ø	Mseg	N
ext	M↓	N	M	O	M(P)	Ø	Mseg	N
Abd	S↓	N	S	O	S(P)	Ø	Mseg	N
Add	M↓	N	M	O	M(P)	Ø	Mseg	N

PRE-TEST 3 (circle test parameters)

Position of patient: prone, sidelying, sitting, standing, supine, other: _____

Type of test: active, active assisted, passive, resistive, other: _____

Joint: C-spine, T-spine, L-spine, hip, knee, ankle, shoulder, elbow, wrist, other _____

Action	Range+Int		Pain+Int		Ltd+Int		Mvmt+Int	
	(R)	(L)	(R)	(L)	(R)	(L)	(R)	(L)

POST-TEST 1 (circle test parameters)

Position of patient: prone, sidelying, (sitting,) standing, supine, other: _____

Type of test: (active,) active assisted, passive, resistive, other: _____

Joint: C-spine, T-spine, L-spine, hip, knee, ankle, (shoulder,) elbow, wrist, other _____

Action	Range+Int		Pain+Int		Ltd+Int		Mvmt+Int	
	(R)	(L)	(R)	(L)	(R)	(L)	(R)	(L)
flex								
ext								
Abd								
Add								

POST-TEST 2 (circle test parameters)

Position of patient: prone, sidelying, (sitting,) standing, supine, other: _____

Type of test: (active,) active assisted, passive, resistive, other: _____

Joint: C-spine, T-spine, L-spine, hip, knee, ankle, (shoulder,) elbow, wrist, other _____

Action	Range+Int		Pain+Int		Ltd+Int		Mvmt+Int	
	(R)	(L)	(R)	(L)	(R)	(L)	(R)	(L)
flex								
ext								
Abd								
Add								

POST-TEST 3 (circle test parameters)

Position of patient: prone, sidelying, sitting, standing, supine, other: _____

Type of test: active, active assisted, passive, resistive, other: _____

Joint: C-spine, T-spine, L-spine, hip, knee, ankle, shoulder, elbow, wrist, other _____

Action	Range+Int		Pain+Int		Ltd+Int		Mvmt+Int	
	(R)	(L)	(R)	(L)	(R)	(L)	(R)	(L)

Directions for charting Range of Motion Results: For each test, fill in the form blanks as follows:
ACTION - Identify the action tested: abd, add, DF, ever, ext, ext rot, flex, int rot, inv, lat flex, PF, pro, SB, and Sup
RANGE - Identify the deviation from normal: ↓ (hypomobility), ↑ (hypermobility)
INTENSITY (INT) - Rate the intensity of each finding. L, M, S; 0–5, 0–10; N, G, F, P (normal, good, fair, poor)
PAIN - Identify if pain is present with movement: √ (present), Ø (absent)
LIMITATIONS (LTD) - Identify the cause of the limitation. For example: Adh, ed, HT, LB, (P), Sp, TP, etc.
MOVEMENT (MVMT) - Identify the quality of the movement. sm, seg, Sp, rig, (smooth, segmented, spastic, rigid)

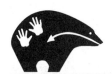

Helena LaLuna, CR
123 Sun Moon and Stars Drive
Capital Hill, WA   98119
TEL   206 555 4446

INSURANCE VERIFICATION

Name _Zamora Hostetter_   Date _4-4-01_

Date of Injury _3-31-01_   Insurance ID# _C98-7654321_

A. Patient Information

Employment
Employer _Howling Moon Cafe_
Phone _555-4444_   Fax _555-3333_
Currenty Employed? ☒Y ☐N
Effective date of benefits _6-24-00_
Expiration date of benefits _6-24-01_
Contact name _Betty_
Date/Time verified _4-4-01   4:00 pm_

Attorney
Name _N/A_
Phone _____ Fax _____
Guarantee of Payment filed? ☐Y ☐N
Medical Lien filed? ☐Y ☐N
    Date _____ Expires _____
    Renewed _____ Expires _____
Copies of patient file requests
    Date requested _____ Date sent _____
    Date requested _____ Date sent _____

Primary Health Care Provider
Name _Manda Rae Yuricich, OC_
Phone _555-3535_   Fax _555-4646_
Attending provider for this injury/illness? ☒Y ☐N
Referring provider for manual therapy services? ☒Y ☐N
Prescription received? ☒Y ☐N
Prescription date _4-1-01_   # of Tx _10_
    Tx duration/frequency _2x wk/5 wks_
    Diagnosis (ICD-10 codes) _724.2, 723.1, 840.9,_
    _728.85, 784.0_
First Renewal date _5-12-01_   # of Tx _3_
    Tx duration/frequency _1x wk-3 wks_
Second Renewal date _____ # of Tx _____
    Tx duration/frequency _____

B. Insurance Information

Workers Compensation Insurance
Contact _Aziz Amaden_
Phone _(360) 555-6655_ Fax _555-5566_
Date/Time verified _4-5-01   9:30 AM_
    Is claim open? ☒Y ☐N
    Date Opened _4-1-01_   Date Closed _____
    Date Reopened _____

Private Health Insurance
Insurer _N/A_
Contact _____
Phone _____ Fax _____
Date/Time verified _____

Personal Injury Insurance
Primary Insurer _N/A_
    Adjuster _____
    Phone _____ Fax _____
    Date/Time verified _____
        PIP policy amount $ _____
        Dates of coverage _____
        PIP available $ _____
        Med Pay policy amount $ _____
        Dates of coverage _____
        Med Pay available $ _____

Secondary Insurer _____
    Adjuster _____
    Phone _____ Fax _____
    Date/Time verified _____
        PIP policy amount $ _____
        Dates of coverage _____
        PIP available $ _____
        Med Pay policy amount $ _____
        Dates of coverage _____
        Med Pay available $ _____

C. Verify Benefits/Authorize Services

Ask the insurance representative the following questions
    regarding the patient's coverage:

1. Is manual therapy a covered benefit? ☒Y ☐N
2. Is the patient eligible for the manual therapy benefit for this
    condition (supply diagnosis/ICD-10 codes)? ☒Y ☐N
3. Am I eligible to provide manual therapy services (supply
    professional license/certification)? ☒Y ☐N

If the answer to any one of these questions is No, bill the patient
    for manual therapy services.
If the answer to all three questions is Yes, continue verification
    on page two, and bill the insurance company for manual therapy
    services.

C. Verify Benefits/Authorize Services, cont.

Record the answers you get to questions 4, 5, and 6 in this table. In the first column list the services you provide. In the second column, record the corresponding CPT code. Complete the table with the answers you get to questions 4, 5, and 6.

4. Which manual therapy services are authorized? (Go through each one listed below.)
5. Are there any restrictions or limitations to each authorized service?
6. What is the maximum allowable reimbursement rate for each authorized service?

Service Item	CPT code	4. Authorized?	5. Restrictions?	6. Max Rate?
1. myofascial	97140	☒Y ☐N	4 units max/tx	28.78
2. Polarity	97139	☐Y ☒N		
3. hot/cold packs	97010	☐Y ☒N	bundled	
4.		☐Y ☐N		
5.		☐Y ☐N		
6.		☐Y ☐N		
7.		☐Y ☐N		
8.		☐Y ☐N		
9.		☐Y ☐N		
10.		☐Y ☐N		

Complete 7-17 as applicable

7. Does a deductible apply? ☐Y ☒N Amount $ _____
   Paid to date $ _____
   Policy year dates _____
8. Does a co-pay apply? ☐Y ☒N Amount $ _____
9. Does a co-insurance apply? ☐Y ☒N Amount % _____
10. Is there a limit on the # of sessions per policy year?
    ☐Y ☒N Total per year 12 per incident
    Number available to date 12
11. Is there a limit on the total $ spent on these services or similar services per policy year? ☐Y ☒N Amount $ _____
    Amount available to date _____
12. Treatment dates authorized 4-1 → 5-1
13. Number of sessions authorized 6
14. Preferred billing method/form:
    ☒HCFA 1500 ☐Electronic ☐Other _____
15. Send with each bill:
    ☒Prescription ☐SOAP notes ☒Progress Reports
    ☐License/Certification ☐Other _____
16. What is the expected turnaround time on claim reimbursement? 30 days
17. Are you able to authorize payment? ☒Y ☐N
    If Yes, authorization # 47329
    If No, can you connect me with someone who is able to authorize payment? ☐Y ☐N
    Name _____
    Phone _____ Fax _____

Send a copy of this form to the insurance representative with a letter confirming the information gathered.
Date sent 4-6-01

Re-Authorization/Verification

Contact Terry Farr
Phone (360) 555-6655 Fax 555-5566
Date/Time verified 4-24-01   10:00 AM
Treatment dates authorized 4-25-01 → 5-25
Number of sessions authorized 6
Is payment authorized? ☒Y ☐N
  Authorization # 47499
Confirmation sent? ☒Y ☐N Date sent 4-24-01
Verify remainder of policy year, if applicable:
1. Deductible paid to date $ _____
2. Total # of sessions to date _____
3. Total $ spent to date $ _____

Re-Authorization/Verification

Contact _____
Phone _____ Fax _____
Date/Time verified _____
Treatment dates authorized _____
Number of sessions authorized _____
Is payment authorized? ☐Y ☐N
  Authorization # _____
Confirmation sent? ☐Y ☐N Date sent _____
Verify remainder of policy year, if applicable:
1. Deductible paid to date $ _____
2. Total # of sessions to date _____
3. Total $ spent to date $ _____

HEALTH INSURANCE CLAIM FORM

PICA | | PICA

CARRIER →

1. MEDICARE	MEDICAID	CHAMPUS	CHAMPVA	GROUP HEALTH PLAN (SSN or ID)	FECA BLK LUNG (SSN)	OTHER	1a. INSURED'S I.D. NUMBER (FOR PROGRAM IN ITEM 1)
(Medicare #)	(Medicaid #)	(Sponsor's SSN)	(VA File #)			☒ (ID)	C98-7654321

2. PATIENT'S NAME (Last Name, First Name, Middle Initial)
Hostetter Zamora

3. PATIENT'S BIRTH DATE
MM 05 DD 22 YY 80   SEX M☐ F☒

4. INSURED'S NAME (Last Name, First Name, Middle Initial)
same

5. PATIENT'S ADDRESS (No., Street)
63 18TH Ave W

6. PATIENT RELATIONSHIP TO INSURED
Self ☒ Spouse ☐ Child ☐ Other ☐

7. INSURED'S ADDRESS (No., Street)

CITY Capitol Hill   STATE WA

8. PATIENT STATUS
Single ☒ Married ☐ Other ☐
Employed ☒ Full-Time Student ☐ Part-Time Student ☐

CITY   STATE

ZIP CODE 98119   TELEPHONE (Include Area Code) (206) 555-1221

ZIP CODE   TELEPHONE (INCLUDE AREA CODE) (   )

9. OTHER INSURED'S NAME (Last Name, First Name, Middle Initial)
same

10. IS PATIENT'S CONDITION RELATED TO:

11. INSURED'S POLICY GROUP OR FECA NUMBER

a. OTHER INSURED'S POLICY OR GROUP NUMBER
555-63-1819

a. EMPLOYMENT? (CURRENT OR PREVIOUS)
☒ YES ☐ NO

a. INSURED'S DATE OF BIRTH
MM DD YY   SEX M☐ F☐

b. OTHER INSURED'S DATE OF BIRTH
MM DD YY   SEX M☐ F☐

b. AUTO ACCIDENT?   PLACE (State)
☐ YES ☒ NO

b. EMPLOYER'S NAME OR SCHOOL NAME
Howling Moon Cafe

c. EMPLOYER'S NAME OR SCHOOL NAME

c. OTHER ACCIDENT?
☐ YES ☒ NO

c. INSURANCE PLAN NAME OR PROGRAM NAME
WA Dept. L & I

d. INSURANCE PLAN NAME OR PROGRAM NAME
Health Co Selections

10d. RESERVED FOR LOCAL USE

d. IS THERE ANOTHER HEALTH BENEFIT PLAN?
☒ YES ☐ NO *If yes*, return to and complete item 9 a-d.

READ BACK OF FORM BEFORE COMPLETING & SIGNING THIS FORM.

12. PATIENT'S OR AUTHORIZED PERSON'S SIGNATURE I authorize the release of any medical or other information necessary to process this claim. I also request payment of government benefits either to myself or to the party who accepts assignment below.
SIGNED Signature on file   DATE 4-4-01

13. INSURED'S OR AUTHORIZED PERSON'S SIGNATURE I authorize payment of medical benefits to the undersigned physician or supplier for services described below.
SIGNED Signature on file

14. DATE OF CURRENT: ILLNESS (First symptom) OR INJURY (Accident) OR PREGNANCY(LMP)
MM 03 DD 31 YY 01

15. IF PATIENT HAS HAD SAME OR SIMILAR ILLNESS. GIVE FIRST DATE MM DD YY

16. DATES PATIENT UNABLE TO WORK IN CURRENT OCCUPATION
FROM MM DD YY   TO MM DD YY

17. NAME OF REFERRING PHYSICIAN OR OTHER SOURCE
Manda Rae Yuricich, DC

17a. I.D. NUMBER OF REFERRING PHYSICIAN

18. HOSPITALIZATION DATES RELATED TO CURRENT SERVICES
FROM MM DD YY   TO MM DD YY

19. RESERVED FOR LOCAL USE

20. OUTSIDE LAB? ☐ YES ☐ NO $ CHARGES

21. DIAGNOSIS OR NATURE OF ILLNESS OR INJURY. (RELATE ITEMS 1,2,3 OR 4 TO ITEM 24E BY LINE)
1. 724.2   3. 840.9
2. 723.1, 784.0   4. 728.85

22. MEDICAID RESUBMISSION CODE   ORIGINAL REF. NO.

23. PRIOR AUTHORIZATION NUMBER

24. A. DATE(S) OF SERVICE From MM DD YY	To MM DD YY	B. Place of Service	C. Type of Service	D. PROCEDURES, SERVICES, OR SUPPLIES (Explain Unusual Circumstances) CPT/HCPCS	MODIFIER	E. DIAGNOSIS CODE	F. $ CHARGES	G. DAYS OR UNITS	H. EPSDT Family Plan	I. EMG	J. COB	K. RESERVED FOR LOCAL USE
4 4 01		3	9	97140		1,2,3,4	25	1				
4 4 01		3	9	97140		1,2,3,4	25	1				
4 4 01		3	9	97140		1,2,3,4	25	1				
4 4 01		3	9	97140		1,2,3,4	25	1				

25. FEDERAL TAX I.D. NUMBER 91-1777771   SSN ☐ EIN ☒

26. PATIENT'S ACCOUNT NO.

27. ACCEPT ASSIGNMENT? (For govt. claims, see back) ☐ YES ☐ NO

28. TOTAL CHARGE $ 100 —

29. AMOUNT PAID $ 0

30. BALANCE DUE $ 100

31. SIGNATURE OF PHYSICIAN OR SUPPLIER INCLUDING DEGREES OR CREDENTIALS (I certify that the statements on the reverse apply to this bill and are made a part thereof.)
SIGNED Helena La Luna, CR   DATE 4-4-01

32. NAME AND ADDRESS OF FACILITY WHERE SERVICES WERE RENDERED (If other than home or office)

33. PHYSICIAN'S, SUPPLIER'S BILLING NAME, ADDRESS, ZIP CODE & PHONE #
Helena La Luna, CR
123 Sun Moon and Stars Dr.
Capitol Hill, WA 98119
PIN# (206) 555-4446 GRP#

PHYSICIAN OR SUPPLIER INFORMATION →
PATIENT AND INSURED INFORMATION →

FORM HCFA-1500 (12-90)
NORTHWEST BUSINESS FORMS (206) 728-8181

PLEASE PRINT OR TYPE

FORM OWCP-1500   FORM RRB-1500   APPROVED OMB-0938-0008
(APPROVED BY AMA COUNCIL ON MEDICAL SERVICE 8/88)

300

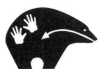

Helena LaLuna, CR
123 Sun Moon and Stars Drive
Capital Hill, WA   98119
TEL   206 555 4446

PAYMENT LOG

Name _Zamora Hostetter_   Date _6-18-01_

Date of Injury _3-31-01_   Insurance ID# _C98-7654321_

Billing Date: _5-18-01_   Total Billed: $ _100-_

Patient Paid: $ _0_   Insurance Paid: $ _0_   Total Paid: $ _0_

If Total Paid does NOT equal Total Billed, complete below for each date of service (from lines 1-6, Section 24 of HCFA 1500)

Line 1, Initial Billing
Treatment Date: _5-18-01_ Bill Date: _5-18-01_
Charges: _100_ Adjustments: _0_ Amount Billed: _100_
Due from patient: _0_ Due from Insurance: _100-_
Patient Paid: _0_   Insurance paid: _0_

Line 1, Rebilling
Rebill Date: _6-18-01_ Rebilled to: _Ins._
Outstanding: _100-_ Interest: _0_ Amount Billed: _100-_
Rebill Date: _____ Rebilled to: _____
Outstanding: _____ Interest: _____ Amount Billed: _____
Rebill Date: _____ Rebilled to: _____
Outstanding: _____ Interest: _____ Amount Billed: _____

Line 2, Initial Billing
Treatment Date: _____ Bill Date: _____
Charges: ____ Adjustments: ____ Amount Billed: _____
Due from patient: _____ Due from Insurance: _____
Patient Paid: _____ Insurance paid: _____

Line 2, Rebilling
Rebill Date: _____ Rebilled to: _____
Outstanding: _____ Interest: _____ Amount Billed: _____
Rebill Date: _____ Rebilled to: _____
Outstanding: _____ Interest: _____ Amount Billed: _____
Rebill Date: _____ Rebilled to: _____
Outstanding: _____ Interest: _____ Amount Billed: _____

Line 3, Initial Billing
Treatment Date: _____ Bill Date: _____
Charges: ____ Adjustments: ____ Amount Billed: _____
Due from patient: _____ Due from Insurance: _____
Patient Paid: _____ Insurance paid: _____

Line 3, Rebilling
Rebill Date: _____ Rebilled to: _____
Outstanding: _____ Interest: _____ Amount Billed: _____
Rebill Date: _____ Rebilled to: _____
Outstanding: _____ Interest: _____ Amount Billed: _____
Rebill Date: _____ Rebilled to: _____
Outstanding: _____ Interest: _____ Amount Billed: _____

Line 4, Initial Billing
Treatment Date: _____ Bill Date: _____
Charges: ____ Adjustments: ____ Amount Billed: _____
Due from patient: _____ Due from Insurance: _____
Patient Paid: _____ Insurance paid: _____

Line 4, Rebilling
Rebill Date: _____ Rebilled to: _____
Outstanding: _____ Interest: _____ Amount Billed: _____
Rebill Date: _____ Rebilled to: _____
Outstanding: _____ Interest: _____ Amount Billed: _____
Rebill Date: _____ Rebilled to: _____
Outstanding: _____ Interest: _____ Amount Billed: _____

Line 5, Initial Billing
Treatment Date: _____ Bill Date: _____
Charges: ____ Adjustments: ____ Amount Billed: _____
Due from patient: _____ Due from Insurance: _____
Patient Paid: _____ Insurance paid: _____

Line 5, Rebilling
Rebill Date: _____ Rebilled to: _____
Outstanding: _____ Interest: _____ Amount Billed: _____
Rebill Date: _____ Rebilled to: _____
Outstanding: _____ Interest: _____ Amount Billed: _____
Rebill Date: _____ Rebilled to: _____
Outstanding: _____ Interest: _____ Amount Billed: _____

Line 6, Initial Billing
Treatment Date: _____ Bill Date: _____
Charges: ____ Adjustments: ____ Amount Billed: _____
Due from patient: _____ Due from Insurance: _____
Patient Paid: _____ Insurance paid: _____

Line 6, Rebilling
Rebill Date: _____ Rebilled to: _____
Outstanding: _____ Interest: _____ Amount Billed: _____
Rebill Date: _____ Rebilled to: _____
Outstanding: _____ Interest: _____ Amount Billed: _____
Rebill Date: _____ Rebilled to: _____
Outstanding: _____ Interest: _____ Amount Billed: _____

Wellness

This flow chart demonstrates which forms are recommended for use with patients involved in workers' compensation cases: who completes the form, how often the form is used, and any additional comments for using the form.

Wellness Care	Who	Frequency	Comments
INTAKE FORMS			
Fees and Policies	Patient	initial visit	update as needed
Health Information	—		
History section of HxTxC	Patient	initial visit	update annually
Injury Information, part 1	—		
Injury Information, part 2	—		
Billing Information	—		
Prescription	HCP (optional)	as needed	a progress report should precede each renewal
PROGRESS SUMMARIES			
Health Report	Patient	bi-annually	patient reports current status
Pain Questionnaires	Patient	as needed	if Health Report indicates
Initial Report W/O Tx	MT	as needed	if referred by HCP but does not receive tx
Initial Report w/ Tx	MT	as needed	if referred by HCP
Progress Report	MT	as needed	if referred by HCP
Narrative Report	—		
TREATMENT NOTES			
Initial SOAP	—		
Subsequent SOAP	—		
Progress SOAP	—		
Discharge SOAP	—		
HxTxC	MT	each visit	
Range of Motion	—		
BILLING FORMS			
Insurance Status–Personal Injury	—		
Guarantee of Payment	—		
Insurance Verification	—		
HCFA 1500 billing form	—		
Payment Log	—		

Naomi Wachtel
567 Sunnydale Dr.
Flat Irons, CO   80302
TEL   303 555 8866

A. Fee Schedules

My Fees For Services Are As Follows:

| Massage Therapy | $72 per hour |
| 97124 | $18 per 15 minute unit |

B. Payment Policies

Payment for services are as follows:
Cash or Check, 10% discount for payment at the time of service ($65).

I will bill your insurance company directly under the following conditions:
Auto Accident: HCP referral only, PIP only

All billing accounts not paid in full within 30 days from date of service will be charged interest. Interest rates are 12% annually and are charged at 1% monthly. Interest is calculated on the principal amount; interest is not compounded.

C. Office Policies

Cancellations

Cancellations must be made 24 hours in advance of the scheduled appointment time. If cancellations are not made within 24 hours, payment in full is required. This charge will be waived if a replacement can be found for your appointment time. Your insurance company will not be charged for your missed appointment; you will be responsible for payment out-of-pocket.

Right of Refusal

I reserve the right to refuse service to anyone. This includes but is not limited to anyone who requests treatment or services that are outside my scope of practice. I will exercise this right if anyone arrives for treatment under the influence of alcohol or recreational drugs; I reserve the right to charge for the session time, whether or not services were rendered, if I so choose.

Patient Agreement

I have read the policies stated above and agree to abide by them.

Signature   _Lin Pak_____   Date _7-27-01_____

Naomi Wachtel
567 Sunnydale Dr.
Flat Irons, CO   80302
TEL   303 555 8866

STANDARD HxTxC Chart

Name Lin Pak   Date 7-27-01

Phone (303) 555-0033x253   Address   IBM 3rd Floor

1. What are your goals for health, and how may I assist you in achieving your goals? Limit
   longterm complications of diabetes through relaxation and stress reduction   .

2. Are you currently experiencing any of the following? If yes, please explain.

pain, tenderness	☒ No ☐ Yes: _____	stiffness	☒ No ☐ Yes: _____
numbness or tingling	☒ No ☐ Yes: _____	swelling	☒ No ☐ Yes: _____
allergies	☒ No ☐ Yes: _____		

3. List all illnesses, injuries, and health concerns you have now or have had in the past 3 years.
   (Examples: arthritis, diabetes, car accident, pregnancy) diabetes, boarderline high
   blood pressure

4. List medications and pain relievers taken today.   insulin

5. I have provided all my known medical information. I acknowledge that manual therapy is not
   a substitute for medical diagnosis and treatment. I give my consent to receive treatment.

   Signature Lin Pak   Date 7-27-01

   Tx: FB Sw Ⓜ, LDT neck, chest, axillary
        45 min.
   C: HW-relaxation ex., V BP pre & post Ⓜ

initials   NW, LMT

306

Naomi Wachtel
567 Sunnydale Dr.
Flat Irons, CO   80302
TEL   303 555 8866

PRESCRIPTION

Patient Name __Lin Pak__   Date __7-15-01__

Date of Injury __∅__   Insurance ID# __∅__

A. Diagnosis

(Include ICD-10 codes that specifically
address Manual Therapy Treatment)

__diabetes s̄ complications__

__↑ BP (boardline) no meds__

Condition is related to
☐ Auto Accident
☐ Work Injury
☐ Illness
☒ Other: __stress__

B. Medically Necessary Treatment: Implement Plan as Prescribed Below

Application (Direct & Indirect)

☐ Head _____
☒ Neck _____
☒ Chest _____
☒ Shoulders _____
☐ Abdomen _____
☒ Back _____
☐ Lowback/Hips _____
☐ Upper extremities _____
☐ Lower extremities _____
☐ All of the above
☒ Other: __As needed__

Treatment Type
☐ Manual Therapy _____
☐ Hydrotherapy _____
☐ Self-Care Education _____
☐ Other _____

Treatment Goals
☐ Decrease Pain
☐ Decrease Inflammation
☐ Decrease Muscle Tension/Spasms
☐ Decrease Compensatory Patterns
☐ Increase Mobility
☐ Increase Strength
☐ Restore Function
☐ Restore Posture
☐ Maintain Associated Structures
☐ All of the Above
☐ Other _____

Duration & Frequency
☐ 1× wk for _____ wks
☐ 2× wk for _____ wks
☐ 3× wk for _____ wks
☒ 2× month for __6__ months
☐ 1× month for _____ months

Specific Instructions:
__No cautions for Tx currently__
__Apply tx as needed__

C. Referring Health Care Provider (HCP)

Contact Information
HCP Name __Tami Chan OMD__
Provider No. _____
Address __675 Arapahoe Dr.__
City __Flat Irons__ State __CO__ Zip __80302__
Phone __(303) 555-0202__
Fax __555-2020__

Reporting
☐ Send Report After Initial Visit
☒ Send Report at End of Prescription
☐ Send Copies of Chart Notes at End of Prescription
☒ Fax Information
☐ Mail Information
☐ Email Information

HCP Signature: __Tami Chan OMD__   Date __7-15-01__

Revised and reprinted with permission, Adler ♦ Giersch, PS

307

DAILY HEALTH REPORT

Patient Name _Lin Pak_   Date _7-27-01_

Date of Injury _Ø_   Insurance ID# _Ø_

A. Draw today's symptoms on the figures.

1. Identify CURRENT symptomatic areas in your body by marking letters on the figures below. Use the letters provided in the key to identify the symptoms you are feeling today.
2. Circle the area around each letter, representing the size and shape of each symptom location.

Key
P = pain or tenderness
S = joint or muscle stiffness
N = numbness or tingling

B. Identify the intensity of your symptoms.

1. Pain Scale: Mark a line on the scale to show the amount of pain you are experiencing today.

   No Pain |—————————————————————————————| Unbearable Pain

2. Activities Scale: Mark a line on the scale to show the limitations you are experiencing today in your daily activities.

   Can Do Anything I Want |—————————————————————————————| Cannot Do Anything

C. Comments

I get stiff in my chest, neck, and between my shoulder blades w/ long work days.

Tx: FB (M)SW & LDT to ↓ stiffness ↑ circ & ↑ relaxation

M SH rot BL, HT chest, neck, midback L → L⁺, L Adh teres BL   NW, LMT

Signature _Lin Pak_   Date _7-27-01_

308

Naomi Wachtel
567 Sunnydale Dr.
Flat Irons, CO   80302
TEL   303 555 8866

Name   _Lin Pak_   Current Meds   _IBM 3rd Floor_

Tx: FB SW Ⓜ LDT
45 min
C: _HW con't_

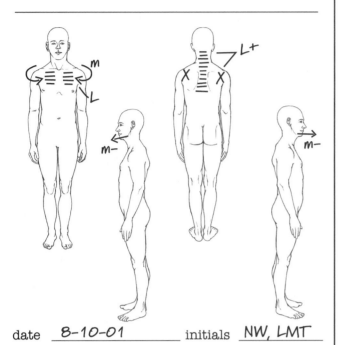

date   _8-10-01_   initials   _NW, LMT_

Tx: FB SW Ⓜ LDT
45 min
C: _HW con't_

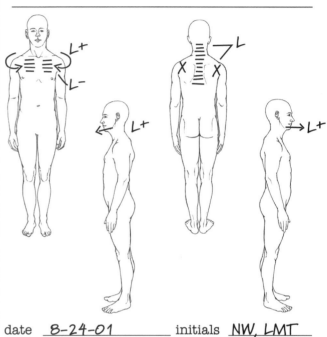

date   _8-24-01_   initials   _NW, LMT_

Tx: FB SW Ⓜ LDT
45 min
C: _pt rpt. BP ↓ post Ⓜ and overall_

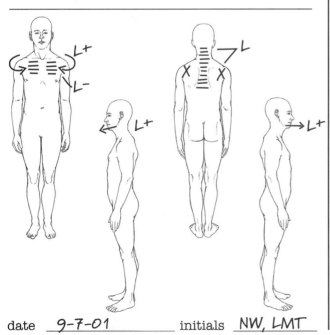

date   _9-7-01_   initials   _NW, LMT_

Tx: FB SW Ⓜ LDT
45 min
C: _flare-up worked overtime all wk_

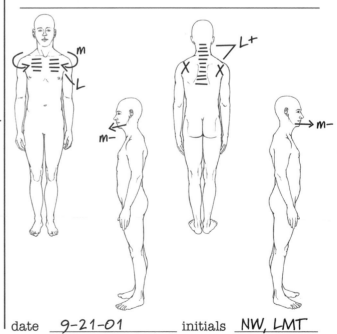

date   _9-21-01_   initials   _NW, LMT_

309

Appendix:
Abbreviations List

312

HANDS HEAL:
COMMUNICATION,
DOCUMENTATION,
AND INSURANCE BILLING
FOR MANUAL THERAPISTS

Symbols

ā, pre	before
@	at
&, +	and
~ , ≈	approximate
c̄, w/	with
Δ	change
↓	down, decrease
=	equals
♀	female
>	greater than
→	leading to, resulting in, through
<	less than
♂	male
–	minus, negative
#	number
Ø	no, none
p̄, post	after
//	parallel
/	per
1°	primary
+	plus, positive
s̄, w/o	without
2°	secondary, due to
x	times, repetitions
↑	up, increase

Symbols for figure drawing:

╳	adhesion
╱	elevation
≡	hypertonicity, tension
⟷	longer than normal
≋	numbness, tingling
℗	pain
↻	rotation
⟩⟨	shorter than normal
≈	spasm
✳	swelling, inflammation
●	tender points
ℂ	trigger point

Anatomy: (Sample list of common landmarks. Follow suit with additional terms by shortening words or using initials.)

abs	abdominals
AC	acromioclavicular
ACL	anterior crutiate ligament
AIIS	anterior inferior iliac spine
ASIS	anterior superior iliac spine
ATFL	anterior talofibular ligament
AW	abdominal wall
BBB	blood brain barrier
BEF	bio-energetic field
bi	biceps
BJM	bones, joints, and muscles
BR	breath
C, C 1-7	cervical, cervical vertebrae
CN 1-8	cervical nerves
CrN 1-12	cranial nerves
CSF	cerebral spinal fluid
ch	chest
Cl	clavicle
CM	carpometacarpal
CNS	central nervous system
coc	coccygeal
Cr	cranium
delt	deltoid
DH	dominant hand
dia	diaphragm
E	energy
elb	elbow
EMF	electromagnetic field
ES	erector spinae muscle group
FE	femur
gastroc	gastrocnemius
GHL	glenohumeral ligament
gluts	gluteal muscle group
GT	greater trochanter
hams	hamstring muscles
he	heart
hd	head
H&N	head and neck
hum	humerous
IC	ileocecal, iliococcygeal, intercarpal, intercostal, intracranial
IF	iliofemoral
IP	iliopsoas
ISF	interstitial fluid
ITB	iliotibial band
IT	ischial tuberosity
IVD	intervertebral disk
IVJC	intervertebral joint complex
J, jt	joint
JV	jugular vein
L, L 1-5	lumbar, lumbar vertebrae
LC	lymph capillaries
LCL	lateral collateral ligament
lats	latissimus dorsi
lev scap	levator scapula
LI	large intestine
LN	lymph node
LV	lymph vessel
mas	masseter
meta	metacarpal, metatarsal
mm	muscles
MN	median nerve
ms	musculoskeletal
nn	nerves
NR	nerve root
NS	nervous system
occ	occiput
OF	occipitofrontal
os	bone
PCx	paracervical
pecs	pectoralis major and minor
M&m	minor
PNS	parasympathetic nervous system
PSIS	posterior sacroiliac spine, posterior superior iliac spine
Q	radiant energy
QL	quadratus lumborum
quads	quadricep muscles
RC	rib cage
rhomb	rhomboids
SB	sternal border
SC	subclavian, sternoclavicular, sternocostal
sc	subcutaneous
SC	sternoclavicular
SCM	sternocleidomastoid
ScM	scalene muscle group
SCV	subclavian vein
SI	sacroiliac, small intestine
sh	shoulder
sol	soleus
ST	soft tissue
st	sternum
T, T 1-12	thoracic, thoracic vertebrae
TC	thoracic cage
TD	thoracic duct
TFA	tibiofemoral angle
TFL	tensor fascia lata
th	throat
tib	tibia, tibialis
tibfib	tibia and fibula
TMJ	temporal mandibular joint
traps	trapezius
	vertebrae
tri	triceps
UN	ulnar nerve
vert	vertebrae
visc	viscera

Descriptive Terms:

Abn	abnormal
aux	auxiliary
avg	average
cons	constant
F	fair
freq	frequent
G	good
G&B	good and bad (days)
grad	gradual
interm	intermittant
L	light, low, mild
Ltd	limited, limitation
M	moderate
max	maximum
min	minimum
N	normal
OK	all right, acceptable
P	poor
QOL	quality of life
QWL	quality of working life
rig	rigid
S	severe
seg	segmented
seld	seldom
sm	smooth
sp	spastic
sym	symmetrical
VGH	very good health
WNL	within normal limits
xs	excessive

Directions and Positions

adj	adjacent, adjoining, adjuctive
ant	anterior
Ⓑ, ⒝	bilateral, both
cd	caudal
ceph	cephalic
D/3	distal third
dist	distal
dp	deep
ext	external
glob	global
inf	inferior
int	internal
inter	between
intra	within
Ⓛ	left
L/3	lower third
lat	lateral
LE	lower extremities
LQ	lower quadrant
M/3	middle third
med	medial
ML	midline
OL	other location
P/3	proximal third
post	posterior
prox	proximal
pr	prone
Ⓡ	right
SL	sidelying
sup	superior, supine
super	superficial
U/3	upper third
UE	upper extremities
unilat	unilateral
univ	universal
UQ	upper quadrant

Movements and Planes of Movement

abd	abduction
act	activities
add	adduction
ADLs	activities of daily living
art	articulate
circ	circumduction
dep	depression
DF	dorsiflexion
ele	elevation
ever	eversion
ext	external
flex	flexion
FM	functional movement
front	frontal
inv	inversion
lat flex	lateral flexion
mob	mobility
mvmt	movement

opp	opposition
PF	plantarflexion
pro	pronation
Ptx	protraction
ROM	range of motion
AROM	active range of motion
AAROM	active assisted range of motion
PROM	passive range of motion
RROM	resistive range of motion
CPROM	complete and pain free range of motion
rot	rotation
Rtx	retraction
sag	sagittal
SB	sidebending
sh	shear
sup	supination
tor	torsion
trans	transverse

Measurements and Medical Record Terminology

A:	assessment
a.c.	before meals
ACI	after care instructions
am	morning
AMAP	as much as possible
a.p.	before dinner
appt	appointment
ASAP	as soon as possible
b.i.d.	twice a day
bpm	beats per minute
cm	centimeter
CNT	could not test
c/o	complains of
COD	condition on discharge
cont	continue
cpm	counts or cycles per minute
CSR	craniosacral rhythm
CSTx	continue same treatment
D	daughter
da	day
D/C	discharged or discontinued
DD	daily
DKA	did not keep appointment
DNT	did not test
DOB	date of birth
DOI	date of injury
dur	duration
ea	each
EOD	every other day
FB	full body

freq	frequency
ft	foot
GD	granddaughter
GF	grandfather
GM	grandmother
gm	gram
GS	grandson
h.d., h.s.	at bedtime
hr	hour
hgt	height
h.v.	this evening
Hx	history
i.c.	between meals
ID	identification
immed	immediately
in	inches
int	intensity
kg	kilogram
kph	kilometers per hour
l	liter
lb	pound
lpm	liter per minute
LTG	long-term goal
M	mother
m.d., m.g.	as directed
meds	medications
mg	milligrams
min	minutes
ml	milliliters
mm	millimeters
mo	month
mph	mile per hour
nv	next visit
O:	objective
ODAT	one day at a time
o.h., q.h.	every hour
o.m., q.m.	every morning
o.n., q.n.	every night
ons	onset
oz	ounce
P:	plan
p.c., p.p.	after meals
pg	page
pls	please
pm	afternoon, evening
POMR	Problem-Oriented Medical Record
ppm	pulses per minute
prn	as needed
PTD	prior to discharge
q2h	every 2 hours
q3h	every 3 hours
q.i.d	four times daily
q.l.	as much as desired
q.o.d	every other day
reps	repetitions
RR	respiratory rate
Rx	drugs, prescription, medication, therapy
S	son
S:	subjective

S/A	same as
SAA	same as above
SATx	same treatment
sched	schedule
sec	seconds
s.i.d., u.i.d	once a day
SOAP	Subjective, Objective, Assessment, Plan
stat	at once
STG	short-term goal
suc	success
t.d.d., t.i.d.	three times a day
t.i.w.	three times a week
TMTC	too many to count
TST	total sleep time
UFN	until further notice
unk	unknown

314

HANDS HEAL:
COMMUNICATION,
DOCUMENTATION,
AND INSURANCE BILLING
FOR MANUAL THERAPISTS

Symptoms and Maladies

Abr	abrasion
Acc	accident
Adh	adhesion
AE	acute exacerbation
AI	accidental injury
AIDS	autoimmune deficiency syndrome
ANI	acute nerve irritation
AOB	alcohol on breath
ASP	abnormal spine posture
atr	atrophy
BA	back ache
CA	cancer
CFS	chronic fatigue syndrome
CHD	coronary heart disease
CHI	closed head injury
CHS	congestive heart failure
CHT	closed head trauma
CP	cerebral palsy
crep	crepitis
CTS	carpal tunnel syndrome
DDD	degenerative disk disease
DJD	degenerative joint disease
Dx	diagnosis
EC	energy cyst
ed	edema
EM	emotional, early memory
FB	foreign body
flac	flaccid
FLR	funny looking rash
Flat	flatulence
Fl up	flare up
FOOSH	fell on outstretched hand
FM, FMS	fibromyalgia
FT	fibrous tissue
HA	headache
HD	heart disease, herniated disk
HI	head injury
HNP	herniated nucleus pulposus
Hnt	hypertension
HOH	hard of hearing
HT	hypertonicity, tension, tight muscles

HTR	hypertrophy
Infl	inflammation
AI	acute inflammation, phase I
SI	subacute inflammation, phase II
CI	chronic inflammation, phase III
JRA	juvenile rheumatoid arthritis
kyph	kyphosis
lax	laxity
LB	loose bodies
LD	learning disability
les	lesion
LJM	limited joint mobility
LOC	loss of consciousness
LOM	loss of movement
lord	lordosis
MAEW	moves all extremities well
MI	myocardial infarction
MPS	myofascial pain syndrome
NRI	nerve root irritation
NSI	no sign of infection, inflammation
OA	osteoarthritis
℗	pain
para	paraplegia
PCS	postconcussive syndrome
PD	perception disorder
PNP	peripheral neuropathy
POM	pain on motion
PTSD	posttraumatic stress disorder
Px	prognosis
RA	rheumatoid arthritis
RSS	repetitive stress syndrome
RTD	repetitive trauma disorder
SCI	spinal cord injury
SD	sleep disturbances
SFLE	stress from life experience
SL	subluxation
SOB	shortness of breath
SOBOE	shortness of breath on exercise
Sp	spasm, spastic
st	stiffness
STS	soft tissue swelling
STI	soft tissue injury
Sw	swelling
Sx	symptoms
TBI	traumatic brain injury

TeP	tender point
TJA	total joint arthrotomy or arthroplasty
THA	total hip arthrotomy or arthroplasty
TKA	total knee arthrotomy or arthroplasty
TJR	total joint replacement
TAR	total ankle replacement
TER	total elbow replacement
THR	total hip replacement
TKR	total knee replacement
TSR	total shoulder replacement
TOS	thoracic outlet syndrome
TP	trigger point
URI	upper respiratory infection
UTI	urinary tract infection
VGH	very good health
VV	vericose vein

Treatments, Modalities, Findings

AAS	active assisted stretching
AC	acupuncture, acupressure
AKS	arthoscopic knee surgery
aroma	aromatherapy
AT	adjunctive therapy
bal	balance
B&B	bowel and bladder function
BM	bowel movement
BJE	bone and joint exam
BP	blood pressure
BRS	breath sounds
BV	steam bath
C&E	consultation and examination
chak	chakra
contra	contraindicated
coord	coordinate
CP	cold packs
CST	craniosacral therapy
DB	deep breathing
DBE	deep breathing exercise
detox	detoxification
DP	direct pressure
DT	deep tissue
eff	effleurage
erg	ergonomics consultation

EW	energy work
Ex	exercise
exam	examination
FS	facilitated stretching
FWB	full weight bearing
Fx	friction
HARPPS	signs of infection: heat, absence of use, redness, pain, pus, swelling
H&C	hot and cold
HEP	home exercise program
HMP	hot moist packs
HP	hot packs
HW	homework
hydro	hydrotherapy
ICES	ice, compression, elevation, support
IDM	indirect method
immob	immobilize
JM	joint mobility
jos	jostling
LAM	laminectomy
LAP	laproscopy
LBPQ	low back pain questionnaire
LDT	lymphatic drainage technique
LT	light touch
Ⓜ	massage
man	manipulation
mer	meridian
MET	muscle energy technique
MFT	muscle function test
MFR	myofascial release
MH	moist heat
MLD	manual lymphatic drainage
MT	manual therapy
NA	not attempted
N/A	not applicable
NMT	neuromuscular therapy
NP	not palpable
NWB	non-weightbearing
OBE	out-of-body experience
obs	observation
O&E	observation and examination
OE	orthopedic examination
os adj	osseous adjustment
OTB	off the body
PA	postural analysis or assessment
palp	palpation
PB	parafin bath, postural balancing
pet	petrissage

PMP	pain management program
PNF	proprioceptive neuromuscular facilitation
PPR	passive positional release
PR	postural re-education
PRE	progressive resistive exercise
prev	prevention
proc	procedure
PT	physical therapy
PU	props utilized
PVD	percussion, vibration, drainage
PWB	partial weight-bearing
R&E	rest and exercise
re-ed	re-education
reflex	reflexology
RR	respiratory rate
re-x	re-examination
ROS	review of symptoms, review of systems
RR	respiratory rate
RT	recreational therapy
RTW	return to work
SA	skeletal alignment
SAE	specific action exercise
SC	self-care
SDTx	sleeps during treatment
SE	somatic education
SER	somato-emotional release
SET	subtle energy techniques
SLR	straight leg raise
S&S	stretching and strengthening
str	stretching
SU	supports utilized
TENS	transcutaneous electrical nerve stimulation
Tx	treatment
tx	traction
Ptx	pelvic traction
Ltx	lumbar traction
Ttx	thoracic traction
Ctx	cervical traction
VAPS	visual analog pain scale
VS	vascular flush
WB	weight bearing
XFF	cross fiber friction

APPENDIX:
Contact Information– Offices of Insurance Commissioners

Alabama Department of Insurance
Consumer Services Division
201 Monroe St Ste 1700
P.O. Box 303351
Montgomery, AL 36130-3351
(334) 269-3550
www.aldi.org/

Alaska Division of Insurance
Anchorage Office
3601 C Street, Suite 1324,
Anchorage, AK 99503-5948
(907) 269-7900
(907) 269-7910 Fax
www.dced.state.ak.us/insurance/

Arizona Department of Insurance
Phoenix Office
2910 N 44th St. Ste. 210
Phoenix, AZ 85018
(602) 912-8444
(800) 325-2548 (In-State only)
www.state.az.us/id/

Arkansas Insurance Department
Consumer Services Division
Third and Cross Streets
Little Rock, AR 72201
(501) 371-2640
(501) 371-2749 Fax
(800) 852-5494 (In-State only)
www.state.ar.us/insurance/file_a_
    complaint.html

California Department of Insurance
Consumer Communications Bureau
300 South Spring Street, South Tower
Los Angeles, CA 90013
(213) 897-8921
(800) 927-HELP (4357) (In-State only)
(800) 482-4833 TDD
www.insurance.ca.gov/docs/index.html

Colorado Division of Insurance
1560 Broadway, Suite 850
Denver, CO 80202
(303) 894-7499
(303) 894-7455 Fax
(800) 930-3745 (In-State only)
(303) 894-7880 TDD
www.dora.state.co.us/insurance/

Connecticut Insurance Department
P.O. Box 816
Hartford, CT 06142-0816
(860) 297-3800
(860) 566-7410 Fax
(800) 203-3447 (In-State only)
www.state.ct.us/cid/

Delaware Insurance Department
841 Silver Lake Boulevard
Dover, DE 19904
(302) 739-4251
(302) 739-4251 Fax
(800) 282-8611 (In-State only)
www.state.de.us/inscom/index/html

318

HANDS HEAL:
COMMUNICATION,
DOCUMENTATION,
AND INSURANCE BILLING
FOR MANUAL THERAPISTS

District of Columbia Department of Insurance
810 First Street, NE, Suite 701
Washington, DC 20002
(202) 727-8000
www.state.de.us/inscom/index.html

Florida Department of Insurance
200 East Gaines Street
Tallahassee, FL 32399-0300
(850) 413-3100
(850) 488-2349 Fax
1-800-342-2762 (In-State only)
www.doi.state.fl.us/

Georgia Insurance and Fire Commissioner
Two Martin Luther King, Jr. Drive
West Tower, Suite 704
Atlanta, GA 30334
(404) 656-2070
(404) 651-8719 Fax
(800) 656-2298 (In-State only)
www.inscomm.state.ga.us/

Hawaii Insurance Division
Investigation Branch
250 South King Street, 5th Floor
Honolulu, Hawaii 96813
(808) 586-2790
www.state.hi.us/dcca/ins/

Idaho Department of Insurance
700 West State St., 3rd Floor
P. O. Box 83720
Boise, ID 83720-0043
(208) 334-4250
(208) 334-4398 Fax
(800) 721-3272 (In-State only)
www.doi.state.id.us/

Illinois Department of Insurance
320 West Washington Street
Springfield, IL 62767-0001
(217) 782-4515
(217) 782-5020 Fax
(217) 524-4872 TDD
100 West Randolph Suite 15-100
Chicago, IL 60601
(312) 814-2427
(312) 814-5435 Fax
(312) 814-2603 TDD
www.state.il.us/ins/default.htm

Indiana Department of Insurance
311 W. Washington Street, Suite 300
Indianapolis, IN 46204-2787
(317) 232-2385
(317) 232-5251 Fax
http://www.state.in.us/idoi

Iowa Insurance Division
330 Maple St.
Des Moines, IA 50319-0065
(515) 281-5705
(515) 281-3059 Fax
(877) 955-1212 (In-State only)
www.iid.state.ia.us/

Kansas Insurance Department
420 SW 9th St
Topeka, KS 66612
(785) 296-3071
(785) 296-2283 Fax
(800) 432-2484 (In-State only)
www.ksinsurance.org/

Kentucky Department of Insurance
215 West Main Street
Frankfort, KY 40601
(502) 564-3630
(502) 564-1453 Fax
(800) 595-6053 (In-State only)
(800) 462-2081 TDD
www.doi.state.ky.us/

Louisiana Department of Insurance
950 N 5th St.
P.O. Box 94214
Baton Rouge, LA 70804-9214
(225) 342-5900
(225) 342-3078 Fax
(800) 259-5300 (In-State only)
www.ldi.la.gov/

Maine Bureau of Insurance
#34 State House Station
Augusta, ME 04333-0034
(207) 624-8475
(207) 624-8599 Fax
(800) 300-5000 (In-State only)
www.state.me.us/pfr/ins/inshome2.htm

Maryland Insurance Administration
525 St. Paul Place
Baltimore, MD 21202-2272
(410) 468-2000
(410) 468-2020 Fax
(800) 492-6116 (In-State only)
(800) 735-2258 TTY
www.mdinsurance.state.md.us/

Massachusetts Division of Insurance
One South Station, 5th Floor
Boston, MA 02110-2208
(617) 521-7777
(617) 521-7575 Fax
(617) 521-7490 TTD/TDD
www.state.ma.us/doi/

Michigan Division of Insurance
Consumer Services
P.O. Box 30220
Lansing, MI 48909-7720
(517) 241-3991
(517) 335-4978 Fax
(877) 999-6442 (In-State only)
www.cis.state.mi.us/ins/

Minnesota Department of Commerce
85 7th Place East, Suite 500
St. Paul, MN 55101
(651) 296-2488
(651) 296-4328 Fax
(800) 657-3602 (In-State only)
www.commerce.state.mn.us/

Mississippi Insurance Department
Consumer Services Division
P.O. Box 79
Jackson, MS 39205
(601) 359 2453
(601) 359-2474 Fax
(800) 562 2957 (In-State only)
www.doi.state.ms.us/

Missouri Department of Insurance
301 West High Street
P.O. Box 690
Jefferson City, MO 65102
(573) 751-4126
(573) 526-4898 Fax
(800) 726-7390 (In-State only)
(573) 526-4536 TDD
www.insurance.state.mo.us/

Montana State Auditor's Office
P.O. Box 4009
Helena, MT 59604-4009
(406) 444-2040
(800) 332-6148 (In-State only)
www.state.mt.us/sao/

Nebraska Department of Insurance
Terminal Building
941 "O" Street, Suite 400
Lincoln, NE 68508-3639
(402) 471-2201
(800) 833-7352 TDD
www.nol.org/home/NDOI/

Nevada Insurance Division
788 Fairview Drive, Suite 300
Carson City, NV 89701-5491
(775) 687-4270
(775) 687-3937 Fax
2501 East Sahara Avenue, Suite 302
Las Vegas, NV 89158
(702) 486-4009
(702) 486-4007 Fax
doi.state.nv.us/

New Hampshire Insurance Department
56 Old Suncook Rd.
Concord, NH 03301-7317
(603) 271-2261
(603) 271-1406 Fax
(800) 852-3416 (In-State only)
www.state.nh.us/insurance/

**New Jersey Department of Banking and
    Insurance**
20 West State Street
Trenton, NJ 08625
(609) 292-5316
(609) 292-2431 Fax
(800) 446-7467 (In-State only)
states.naic.org/nj/NJHOMEPG.HTML

New Mexico Department of Insurance
P. O. Drawer 1269
Santa Fe, NM 87504-1269
(505) 827-4601
(505) 827-4734 Fax
(800) 947-4722 (In-State only)
www.nmprc.state.nm.us/inshm.htm

New York State Insurance Department
25 Beaver Street
New York, NY 10004
(212) 480-6400
(800) 342-3736 (In-State only)
(800) 220-9250 TDD
www.ins.state.ny.us/

320

HANDS HEAL:
COMMUNICATION,
DOCUMENTATION,
AND INSURANCE BILLING
FOR MANUAL THERAPISTS

North Carolina Department of Insurance
P.O. Box 100105
Columbia, SC 29202-3105
(803) 737-6160
(803) 737-6205 Fax
(800) 768-3467 (In-State only)
www.ncdoi.com/ncdoi/

North Dakota Department of Insurance
600 E Boulevard, Dept. 401
Bismarck, ND 58505-0320
(701) 328-2440
(701) 328-4880 Fax
www.state.nd.us/ndins/

Ohio Department of Insurance
2100 Stella Court
Columbus, OH 43215-1067
(614) 644-2658
(614) 644-3743 Fax
(800) 686-1526 (In-State only)
www.ohioinsurance.gov/

Oklahoma Insurance Department
P.O. Box 53408
Oklahoma City, OK 73152-3408
(405) 521-2828
(405) 521-6652
(800) 522-0071 (In-State only)
www.oid.state.ok.us/

Oregon Insurance Division
350 Winter St. NE Room 440
Salem, OR 97301-3883
(503) 947-7980
(503) 378-4351 Fax
(888) 877-4894 (In-State only)
(503) 947-7280 TTY
www.cbs.state.or.us/external/ins/index.html

Pennsylvania Insurance Department
1326 Strawberry Square
Harrisburg, PA 17120
(877) 881-6388 (In-State only)
(717) 787-8585 Fax
(717) 783-3898 TTY/TDD
www.insurance.state.pa.us/

**Rhode Island Department of Business
  Regulation**
233 Richmond Street
Providence, RI 02903
(401) 222-2246
(401) 222-6098 Fax
www.dbr.state.ri.us/

South Carolina Department of Insurance
1612 Marion Street
Columbia, SC 29201
P.O. Box 100105
Columbia, SC 29202-3105
(803) 737-6160
(803) 737-6229 Fax
(800) 768-3467 (In-State only)
www.state.sc.us:80/doi/

South Dakota Division of Insurance
118 W Capitol
Pierre, SD 57501
(605) 773-3563
(605) 773-5369 Fax
www.state.sd.us/dcr/insurance/

Tennessee Division of Insurance
500 James Robertson Parkway, 4th Floor
Nashville, TN 37243-0574
(615) 741-2218
(800) 342-4029 (In-State only)
www.state.tn.us/commerce/

Texas Department of Insurance
333 Guadalupe
Austin, TX 78701
P.O. Box 149104
Austin, TX 78714-9104
(512) 463-6169
(512) 475-1771 Fax
(800) 578-4677 (In-State only)
www.tdi.state.tx.us/

Utah Insurance Department
State Office Bldg. Room 3110
Salt Lake City, UT 84114-6901
(801) 538-3805
(801) 538-3829 Fax
(800) 439-3805 (In-State only)
(801) 538-3826 TDD
www.insurance.state.ut.us/

**Vermont Department of Insurance
  (BISHCA)**
89 Main Street Drawer 20
Montpelier, VT 05620-3101
(802) 828-2900
(800) 631-7788 (In-State only)
www.bishca.state.vt.us/

Virginia State Bureau of Insurance
P.O. Box 1157
Richmond, VA 23218
(804) 371-9741
(800) 552-7945 (In-State only)
(804) 371-9206 TDD
www.state.va.us/scc/division/boi/index.htm

Washington State Insurance Commissioner
Insurance Bldg. Capitol Campus
14th & Water
P.O. Box 40255
Olympia, WA 98504-0255
(360) 753-7301
(360) 586-3535 Fax
(800) 562-6900 (In-State only)
www.insurance.wa.gov/

West Virginia Office of the Insurance Commissioner
Consumer Services
1124 Smith Street
P.O. Box 50540
Charleston, WV 25305-0540
(304) 558-3386
(304) 558-4967 Fax
(800) 642-9004 (In-State only)
www.state.wv.us/insurance/

Wisconsin Office of the Commissioner of Insurance
121 East Wilson Street
Madison, WI 53702
(608) 266-3585
(608) 266-9935, Fax
(800) 236-8517 (In-State only)
(800) 947-3529 TDD (ask for 608-266-3586)
badger.state.wi.us/agencies/oci/oci_home.htm

Wyoming Insurance Department
Herschler Bldg. 3rd Floor East
122 West 25th Street
Cheyenne, WY 82002
(307) 777-7401
(307) 777-5895 Fax
(800) 438-5768 (In-State only)
insurance.state.wy.us/

American Samoa Insurance Commissioner
Executive Office
American Samoa Government
Pago Pago, American Samoa 96799
011 (684) 633-4116
www.samoanet.com/asg/

APPENDIX:
Contact Information–
Workers' Compensation

For more information, please contact the office below and request the phone number of the specific department you are seeking, for example, provider information, claims authorization, or billing.

ALABAMA
James Barnhart, Commissioner
Department of Labor
P.O. Box 303500
Montgomery, AL 36130
(334) 242-3460
(334) 240-3417 Fax
www.dir.state.al.us

ALASKA
Ed Flanagan, Commissioner
Department of Labor
P.O. Box 21149
Juneau, AK 99802-1149
(907) 465-2700
(907) 465-2784 Fax
www.labor.state.ak.us

ARKANSAS
James Salkeld, Director
Department of Labor
10421 West Markham, #100
Little Rock, AR 72205
(501) 682-4500
(501) 682-4508 Fax
www.state.ar.us/labor

CALIFORNIA
Stephen J. Smith, Director
Department of Industrial Relations
455 Golden Gate Avenue, 10th Floor
San Francisco, CA 94102
415/703-5050 FAX 415/703-5059
www.dir.ca.gov

COLORADO
Vickie L. Armstrong, Executive Director
Department of Labor and Employment
Tower 2, Suite 400
1515 Arapahoe Street
Denver, CO 80202-2117
(303) 620-4701
(303) 620-4714 Fax
http://cdle.state.co.us

CONNECTICUT
Commissioner
Department of Labor
200 Folly Brook Blvd.
Wethersfield, CT 06109-1114
(860) 263-6505
(860) 263-6529 Fax
www.ctdol.state.ct.us

DELAWARE
Harold E. Stafford, Secretary
Department of Labor
4425 North Market Street
Wilmington, DE 19802
(302) 761-8000
(302) 761-6621 Fax
www.delawareworks.com

324

HANDS HEAL:
COMMUNICATION,
DOCUMENTATION,
AND INSURANCE BILLING
FOR MANUAL THERAPISTS

DISTRICT OF COLUMBIA
Gregg Irish, Director
Department of Employment Services
Employment Security Building
500 C Street, NW, Suite 600
Washington, DC 20001
(202) 724-7100
(202) 724-5683 Fax
http://does.ci.washington.dc.us

FLORIDA
Mary B. Hooks, Secretary
Dept. of Labor and Employment Security
2012 Capitol Circle, SE
Hartman Building, Suite 303
Tallahassee, FL 32399-2152
(850) 922-7021
(850) 488-8930 Fax
www.state.fl.us/dles/

GEORGIA
Michael Thurmond, Commissioner
Department of Labor
Sussex Place, Room 600
148 International Blvd. NE
Atlanta, GA 30303
(404) 656-3011
(404) 656-2683 Fax
www.dol.state.ga.us/

HAWAII
Gilbert Coloma-Agaran Director
Dept. of Labor & Industrial Relations
830 Punchbowl Street, Room 321
Honolulu, HI 96813
(808) 586-8844
(808) 586-9099 Fax
www.dlir.state.hi.us

IDAHO
Roger Madsen, Director
Department of Labor
317 W. Main Street
Boise, ID 83735-0001
(208) 334-6110
(208) 334-6430 Fax
www.labor.state.id.us/

ILLINOIS
Robert Healey, Director
Illinois Industrial Commission
100 W. Randolph St. Ste. 8-201
Chicago, IL 60601-3275
(312) 814-6611
www.state.il.us/agency/iic

INDIANA
John Griffin, Commissioner
Department of Labor
402 West Washington Street, Room W195
Indianapolis, IN 46204-2739
(317) 232-2378
(317) 233-5381 Fax
www.state.in.us/labor or
    www.teenworker.org

IOWA
Byron Orton, Labor Commissioner
Division of Labor Services
1000 East Grand Avenue
Des Moines, IA 50319
(515) 281-3447
(515) 281-4698 Fax
www.state.ia.us/iwd/

KANSAS
Richard Beyer, Secretary
Department of Human Resources
401 S.W. Topeka Blvd.
Topeka, KS 66603
(785) 296-7474
(785) 368-6294 Fax
www.hr.state.ks.us/

KENTUCKY
Joe Norsworthy, Secretary
Labor Cabinet
1047 US Highway 127 South, Suite 4
Frankfort, KY 40601
(502) 564-3070
(502) 564-5387 Fax
www.state.ky.us/agencies/labor/labrhome/
    html

LOUISIANA
Garey J. Forster, Secretary
Department of Labor
P.O. Box 94094
Baton Rouge, LA 70804-9094
(225) 342-3011
(225) 342-3778 Fax
www.ldol.state.la.us/

MAINE
Valerie Landry, Commissioner
Department of Labor
20 Union Street, P.O. Box 309
Augusta, ME 04332-0309
(207) 287-3788
(207) 287-5292 Fax
www.workerscompensation.com/maine/

MARYLAND
John P. O'Connor, Secretary
Department of Labor, Licensing, and
    Regulation
500 N Calvert St., Room 401
Baltimore, MD 21202
(410) 230-6020
(410) 333-0853 Fax
www.dllr.state.md.us

MASSACHUSETTS
Angelo Buonopane, Director
Department of Labor & Workforce
    Development
1 Ashburton Place, Rm. 2112
Boston, MA 02108
(617) 727-6573
(617) 727-1090 Fax
www.detma.org/index.htm or
    www.state.ma.us/

MICHIGAN
Kathleen Wilbur, Director
Department of Consumer and Industry
    Services
525 West Ottawa, P.O. Box 30004
Lansing, MI 48909
(517) 373-7230
(517) 373-2129 Fax
www.cis.state.mi.us/bsr/divisions/wh/
    home.htm

MINNESOTA
Gretchen Maglich, Commissioner
Department of Labor and Industry
443 Lafayette Road, N.
St. Paul, MN 55155
(651) 296-2342
(651) 282-5405 Fax
www.doli.state.mn.us/

MISSOURI
Catherine B. Leapheart, Director
Department of Labor and Industrial
    Relations
P.O. Box 504
Jefferson City, MO 65102
(573) 751-9691
(573) 751-4135 Fax
www.dolir.state.mo.us

MONTANA
Patricia Haffey, Commissioner
Department of Labor and Industry
1327 Lockey, P.O. Box 1728
Helena, MT 59624
(406) 444-9091
(406) 444-1394 Fax
http://dli.state.mt.us/

NEBRASKA
Fernando "Butch" Lecuona,
    Commissioner
Department of Labor
550 South 16th Street, Box 94600
Lincoln, NE 68509-4600
(402) 471-9792
(402) 471-2318 Fax
www.dol.state.ne.us

NEVADA
Terry Johnson, Labor Commissioner
555 East Washington Ave., Suite 4100
Las Vegas, NV 89101
(702) 486-2650
(702) 486-2660 Fax
www.state.nv.us/labor

NEW HAMPSHIRE
James D. Casey
Commissioner of Labor
95 Pleasant Street
Concord, NH 03301-3838
(603) 271-3171
(603) 271-6852 Fax
www.state.nh.us/dol

NEW JERSEY
Mark Boyd, Commissioner
NJ Department of Labor
John Fitch Plaza
PO Box 110, 13th Floor, Suite D
Trenton, NJ 08625-0110
(609) 292-2323
(609) 633-9271 Fax
www.state.jn.us/labor

326

HANDS HEAL:
COMMUNICATION,
DOCUMENTATION,
AND INSURANCE BILLING
FOR MANUAL THERAPISTS

NEW MEXICO
Clinton D. Harden, Jr. Secretary
Department of Labor
401 Broadway, NE, P.O. Box 1928
Albuquerque, NM 87103-1928
(505) 841-8406
(505) 841-8491 Fax
http://www3.state.nm.us/dol

NEW YORK
James Dillon, Acting Commissioner
NY State Department of Labor
State Office Campus, Building 12
Albany, NY 12240
(518) 457-2741
(518) 487-6908 Fax
www.labor.state.ny.us

NORTH CAROLINA
Cherrie Berry, Commissioner
Department of Labor
4 West Edenton Street
Raleigh, NC 27601-1092
(919) 733-0360
(919) 733-6197 Fax
www.dol.state.nc.us

NORTH DAKOTA
Mark Bachmeier, Commissioner
Department of Labor
State Capitol, 13th Floor
Bismarck, ND 58505
(701) 328-2660
(701) 328-2031 Fax
www.state.nd.us/labor

OHIO
Gordon Gatien, Superintendant
Division of Labor & Worker Safety
50 West Broad Street, 28th floor
Columbus, Ohio 43216
(614) 644-2239
(614) 728-8639 Fax
www.state.oh.us.objfs/

OKLAHOMA
Brenda Reneau, Commissioner
Department of Labor
4001 North Lincoln Boulevard
Oklahoma City, OK 73105
(405) 528-1500
(405) 528-5751 Fax
www.state.ok.us/~okdol

OREGON
Jack Roberts, Commissioner
Bureau of Labor and Industries
800 NE Oregon Street, #32, Suite 1045
Portland, OR 97232
(503) 731-4070
(503) 731-4103 Fax
www.boli.state.or.us

PENNSYLVANIA
Johnny Butler, Secretary
Department of Labor and Industry
1700 Labor and Industry Building
7th and Forster Streets
Harrisburg, PA 17121
(717) 787-3756
(717) 787-8826 Fax
www.li.state.pa.us

PUERTO RICO
Aura L. Gonzalez Rios, Secretary
Department of Labor and Human
   Resources
505 Munoz Rivera Avenue
GPO Box 3088
Hato Rey, PR 00918
(787) 754-2119
(787) 753-9550 Fax

RHODE ISLAND
Dr. Lee Arnold, Director
Department of Labor & Training
610 Manton Avenue
Providence, RI 02909
(401) 462-8870
(401) 462-8872 Fax
www.det.state.ri.us

SOUTH CAROLINA
Rita M. McKinney, Director
Department of Labor, Licensing &
   Regulation
110 Centerview Drive
Columbia, SC 29211-1329
(803) 896-4300
(803) 896-4393 Fax
www.llr.state.sc.us

SOUTH DAKOTA
Craig Johnson, Secretary
Department of Labor
700 Governors Drive
Pierre, SD 57501-2291
(605) 773-3101
(605) 773-4211 Fax
www.state.sd.us/dol/dol.html

TENNESSEE
Michael E. Magill, Commissioner
Department of Labor
710 James Robertson Parkway, 8th Floor
Nashville, TN 37243-0655
(615) 741-6642
(615) 741-5078 Fax
www.state.tn.us

TEXAS
Cassie Carlson Reed, Executive Director
Texas Workforce Commission
101 East 15th Street, Room 618
Austin, Texas 78778
(512) 463-0735
(512) 475-2321 Fax
www.twc.state.tx.us

UTAH
R. Lee Ellertson, Commissioner
Labor Commission, State of Utah
160 East 300 South, 3rd Floor
P.O. Box 146600
Salt Lake City, UT 84114-6600
(801) 530-6880
(801) 530-6390 Fax
www.labor.state.ut.us

VERMONT
Tasha Wallis, Commissioner
Department of Labor and Industry
National Life Building
Montpelier, VT 05620-3401
(802) 828-2288
(802) 828-0408 Fax
www.state.vt.us/labind

VIRGIN ISLANDS
John Sheen, Acting Commissioner
Department of Labor
2203 Church St.
Christiansted, St. Croix
US Virgin Islands 00820-4612
(340) 773-1994
(340) 773-0094 Fax
www.vidol.org

WASHINGTON
Gary Moore, Director
Department of Labor & Industries
PO Box 44001
Olympia, WA 98504-4001
(360) 902-4213
(360) 902-4202 Fax
www.wa.go/lni

WEST VIRGINIA
Stephen Allred, Commissioner
Division of Labor
Bureau of Commerce
State Capitol Complex, Building 3, Room
  319
Charleston, WV 25305
(304) 558-7890
(304) 558-3797 Fax
www.state.wv.us/labor

WISCONSIN
Jennifer Reinert, Secretary
Department of Workforce Development
201 East Washington Avenue
P.O. Box 7946
Madison, WI 53707
(608) 267-9692
(608) 266-1784 Fax
www.dwd.state.wi.us

WYOMING
Beth Nelson, Director
Department of Employment
122 W. 25th Street
Cheyenne, WY 82002
(307) 777-7672
(307) 777-5805 Fax
http://wydoe.state.wy.us/labstd/

US DEPARTMENT OF LABOR
Office of the Secretary
200 Constitution Avenue, NW
Washington, DC 20210
(202) 219-8271
(202) 219-8822 Fax

SECRETARIAT
The Council of State Governments
Dave Scott, Policy Analyst
444 North Capitol Street, NW, Suite 401
Washington, DC 20001
(202) 624-5460
(202) 624-5452 Fax
email: dscott@csg.org

Index

Page numbers in *italics* indicate figures. *Blank Forms* are designated as such.

329